ROCKY MOUNTAIN MEDICINE

ROCKY MOUNTAIN MEDICINE

*Doctors, Drugs, and Disease
in Early Colorado*

Robert H. Shikes, M.D.

Johnson Books: Boulder

ISBN 1-55566-001-0

LCCCN 86-82974

Printed in the United States of America by
Johnson Publishing Company
1880 South 57th Court
Boulder, Colorado 80301

To
PATRICIA,
our children,
JONATHAN AND SARAH
and their grandparents,
JACK AND THELMA SHIKES
MEYER AND EDNA GORDON

CONTENTS

PREFACE

Colorado is truly the watershed of the Rocky Mountain West. It is the source of great rivers which ultimately flow into both oceans—the Rio Grande, the Platte, the Arkansas, and the Colorado. Its mountainous core provides a majestic centerpiece for the high plains of the east, the pueblos and piñon country of the south, the great basin and canyons of the west, and the big sky country of the north. Colorado is a crucible of Western frontier history—explorers and mountain men, Indians and cavalry, cowboys and miners, railroadmen and outlaws, homesteaders and ranchers—as well as ethnic minorities, urban problems, smokestack industry, and labor strikes.

Early Colorado is also a watershed of western medical history, of health and disease, doctors and patients. Beginning with the gold rush of 1858-1859 and ending in the 1920s, the first seven decades of Colorado's history mirrored the enormous changes that occurred in American medicine during that era. This transitional phase marked the end of nearly two thousand years of medical dogma, much of it incorrect, and witnessed the gradual acceptance of scientific medicine. It saw enormous changes in medical care, technology, and education, as well as in the social, ethical, and economic aspects of medical practice. This era marked the demise of bloodletting and purging, and the introduction of antisepsis and the appendectomy, X-rays and the biopsy, pure drinking water and sanitation. It saw the beginning-of-the-end for such dreaded diseases as smallpox, childbirth fever, and diphtheria and the emergence of cardiovascular disease, lung cancer, and narcotics addiction. It saw the rise of good medical schools, hospitals, and scientific research, medical licensure, public health measures, and pure food and drug laws. It also saw increases in the cost of medical care and concerns over indigent care, malpractice and medical marketing, corporate and state medicine, physician glut and "alternative" medicine. It was an era of increasing pride in medicine's technological advances and increasing concern over the profession's image.

It is within the context of this medical transition that this book is presented; Colorado provides the setting. And the setting is as varied as the history and geography of the state. Thus, we will consider such diverse topics as the medical aspects of the battle between Indians and soldiers at Beecher Island, an outbreak of typhoid in Leadville, an immigrant consumptive's battle for survival in Colorado Springs, the shenanigans of Schlatter "The Healer," "Doctor" Gun Wa, and other quacks in Denver, a coal miners' strike in Ludlow, a cowboy's appendectomy in Saguache, and a vigilante lynching in Golden. There are features of health and disease in early Colorado which, though by no means unique, deserve special consideration: medicine in the early gold and silver camps and the later coal camps, the huge influx of tuberculous patients and the sanitaria, the mysterious "mountain fever," the alleged effects of high altitude, and the supposed healthful effects of Colorado's climate. Many of Colorado's early doctors are worthy of special consideration as well, the frontier having attracted some of the best and some of the worst physicians to the state.

In researching Colorado's early medical history, I have surveyed the standard references on the West and Colorado, as well as American, western and Colorado medicine. I have utilized such periodicals as *Colorado Magazine* and *The Trail*, various early newspapers, and the numerous early medical journals which, fortunately for the student of the state's medical history, were published in Colorado's early days. I obtained valuable information not only from such obvious sources as the annual reports of the State Board of Health but from the reports of the Bureau of Mines and of the Adjutant General. I have used quite a few of the nearly six thousand publications in my own collection of western Americana and Coloradoana as well as card files, clippings, books, and other materials in institutional collections. The huge amount of information which resulted has been condensed into what I hope is a reasonable presentation, and I apologize for the omission of a number of names, places, items, and events that could not be included. My own specialty for example, pathology, is hardly mentioned in the book.

My special thanks to Charles Bandy and the staff of the University of Colorado Health Sciences Center's Denison Memorial Library. In addition, I want to thank the Denver Medical Library, the Colorado Medical Society, the Colorado State Historical Society, the Colorado State Archives, the Western History Department of the Denver Public Library, the Western Collections of the Norlin Library of the University of Colorado at Boulder, the Archives of the Penrose Library of the University of Denver, the Aspen Historical Museum, and the Ouray County Historical Museum. I also want to thank the following individuals who helped in many different ways: Dr. Michael Arnall, Ed and Nancy Bathke, Alan Culpin, Mary De Mund, Dr. James Delaney, Darlene Edgerton, Scotty Ellis, Steve Fisher, Dr. Robert Gordon, Marjorie Hornbein, Paul Mahoney, Dr. Tom Noel, Dr. Peter Olch, John Robinson, Dr. Frank Rogers, Jonathan Shikes, Patricia Shikes, Sarah Shikes, Steven Shikes, Dr. Henry Toll, Bob Topp, and many friends in the Denver Westerners, the Colorado Corral of the Westerners, and the Ghost Town Club of Colorado. I am grateful to the late Caroline Bancroft, Don Bloch, Dr. Nolie Mumey, and Fred Rosenstock.

Finally, a special acknowledgement, for his support and encouragement, to the late Dr. Joseph W. St. Geme, Jr. In his brief tenure as dean of the University of Colorado School of Medicine, he taught us so much.

ROBERT H. SHIKES, M.D.
University of Colorado
School of Medicine
Denver, Colorado
November 1986

1 NINETEENTH CENTURY MEDICINE

If the whole materia medica, as now used, could be sunk to the bottom of the sea, it would be all the better for mankind, and all the worse for the fishes.

Oliver Wendell Holmes, 1860[1]

AT THE BEGINNING OF THE nineteenth century, the Rocky Mountain West was little changed from its appearance thousands of years ago. A millenium had seen the cultural zenith and then the disappearance of the Anasazi, the introduction of the horse to Indian culture, and some tentative inroads by European explorers. Within a century, the area would be explored, conquered, settled, and assimilated into the United States. The early part of the century would see exploration by Anglo-Americans, the culmination of the fur trade, a war with Mexico and the annexation of new lands, and, finally, the great overland migrations by gold seekers and settlers. The Civil War, which barely touched the area, was followed by the unifying influences of the telegraph, telephone, and railroads, the subjugation of the Indians and their sequestration on reservations, the development of mining, ranching, and farming, and the establishment of homesteads, settlements and cities. By the 1890s, the western frontier had been officially designated as "closed."

The same one hundred year span saw profound changes in American medicine. In the early nineteenth century, medicine was little changed from that of the seventeenth century, the Renaissance and Medieval eras, or for that matter, even Greek and Roman times. True, Harvey had described the circulation of the blood, Sydenham had made clinical description a virtue, and some useful drugs, instruments, and procedures had been introduced. Essentially, however, mankind's major afflictions remained the same, and the physician's inablility to prevent and treat those afflictions continued unchanged—i.e. he was generally ineffectual. Premature birth was frequently lethal in the newborn, as were infectious diarrhea in the infant, diphtheria in the child, appendicitis in the adolescent, and pneumonia in the adult.

Early in the century, the realms of human biology and disease were as uncharted as the mountains, deserts, and canyons of the American West. For most physicians, the pathogenetic concept of disease was still based on the four elements of the ancient Greeks—earth, air, fire, and water. Corresponding to the elements were the body's four humours—blood, phlegm, and black and yellow bile. Medical dogma ascribed virtually all human disease to imbalances among these four humours. The role of the physician was to determine the nature of these imbalances and to correct them, usually by purging noxious elements from the patient. His main therapeutic tools included bleeding, cupping, and the use of various purging medicines, often in combination.

Bleeding, or phlebotomy, involved the incision of a vein, usually in the forearm, and draining the patient of one or more pints of blood. In general, the sicker the patient, the greater the volume of blood removed. The technique was so common that the lancet became the sym-

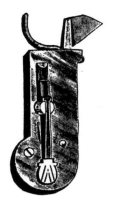

1.1 Bleeding was so much a part of standard medical practice that the lancet became a symbol of the physician.

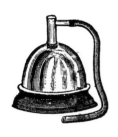

1.2 Cupping was another widely used method of relieving the patient of noxious humours.

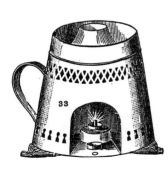

1.3 Mercury, often in the form of calomel, was widely used in the first half of the nineteenth century. It was administered in a variety of ways, including as a vapor.

bol of the physician, an unfortunate association, but preferable to another popular means of bleeding, the leech. Cupping, or blistering, was another means by which the body could be relieved of its bad humours. Superficial incisions were made in the skin and heated glass cups were applied. As the cup cooled, the resultant vacuum drew out noxious vapors and blisters were raised. Still another approach was the sweating out of disease, a timeless and nearly universal technique of eliminating toxins. In addition to variations on European "Turkish" baths and Native American sweat lodges, physicians prescribed such diaphoretic agents as Virginia snake-root, Dover's powders, and sweet spirit of nitre.

The induction of vomiting was a more direct method of purging, and such vomitives as ipecac, lobelia inflata, and tartar emetic were widely used. The most widely used, and probably the most noxious purgatives, however, were the cathartics, those agents whose effect was to "increase the natural expulsive action of the bowels."[2] Of these, the favorite was calomel—bichloride of mercury. Not far behind was jalap, a derivative of the Mexican plant, *Convolvulus jalapa*. The effect of these agents was dramatic, even explosive, and one or both were used to treat almost every disease imaginable. Clysters, or enemas, were also used, a typical prescription beginning with "To a pint of thin broth or gruel, add two table spoonfuls of sugar or molasses . . . [to which may be added] hog's lard . . . ."[3]

This therapeutic regimen has been referred to as "heroic" medicine—the hero, presumably, being the patient. Such heroic medicine accelerated the demise of many of our forefathers, including some national heroes. Today one has difficulty picturing a patient being bled and purged to death by his physician, but George Washington was blistered, administered calomel and tartar emetic, and relieved of as much as two gallons of blood before he died.[4] Many of these same procedures were still being used well into the second half of the nineteenth century.

A few specific medications such as quinine (for "fever"), colchicine (for gout), and digitalis (for "dropsy") were used, but such later standbys as antibiotics, insulin, diuretics, and antihypertensives were not even dreamt of. Oxygen, intravenous solutions, and blood transfusion were unavailable, as were hypodermic needles, X-rays, and most laboratory tests. Anaesthesia was introduced in the 1840s, but surgeons and obstetricians did not bother to wash their hands

and still operated in their street clothes. The Civil War trained a whole generation of surgeons in the art of the two minute amputation and setting broken bones, but for years after the war, they continued to avoid entering the abdominal, thoracic and cranial cavities. Appendicitis, untreated, had a high mortality until surgeons finally "discovered" the appendectomy in the 1880s. Most deliveries and operations were done in the patient's home, and hospitals were regarded as places for the poor and the dying until the second half of the nineteenth century. Mental illness was looked on as an expression of God's wrath, and as the century progressed, the "insane" were simply transferred from the streets and prisons to vast asylums, there to be forgotten.

During the nineteenth century, the average American's life expectancy improved from about forty to fifty years. High mortality rates were due, to a large extent, to the prevalence of such infectious diseases as yellow fever, malaria, cholera, and later in the Rocky Mountain West, tuberculosis, smallpox, typhoid, pneumonia, and influenza. Childhood mortality was especially high, and among children, the major killers were cholera infantum (infectious diarrhea of infancy), diphtheria, scarlet fever, whooping cough, and measles. One by one, in the latter part of the century, the bacterial agents which caused some of these diseases were identified. Gradually, as the germ theory of infectious disease was accepted, the use of antiseptic solutions was expanded to include such aseptic techniques as the sterilization of surgical instruments and the wearing of surgical gloves, gowns, and masks. The simple expedient of obstetric cleanliness saw a marked reduction in the deadly killer of post-partum women, "childbirth," or puerperal, fever. In addition, and prior to antibiotics, the only effective means of dealing with infectious diseases, public health measures were introduced. Slowly and not without opposition, sanitary measures, water purification and proper sewage disposal, vaccination, isolation and quarantine, and other measures, were accepted, legislated, and implemented.

On the other hand, many of today's major causes of morbidity and mortality were of little concern to nineteenth century physicians. Some diseases were simply unrecognized as yet, while others, common today, were infrequent or even rare in those days. A typical medical textbook of the mid-century, Watson's *Lectures on the Principles and Practice of Physic*,[6] paid little attention to today's major cause of adult mortality, atherosclerosis. In fact, the nature of myocardial

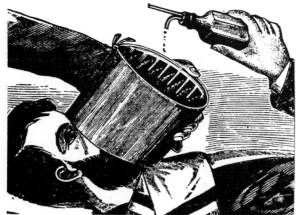

infarction and its relationship to coronary artery disease were not discovered until decades later. Only ten pages of the thousand page book were devoted to cancer and, in the pre-cigarette era, lung cancer was so rare that it was not even mentioned. Cirrhosis, emphysema, diabetes, peptic ulcer, and gallstones were given only modest attention.

In the first half of the nineteenth century, most American physicians had either attended a two-year medical school or had earned their M.D. by apprenticing with a physician in practice. After the Civil War, the number of medical schools began to increase, but there were still no uniform standards or requirements for admission or graduation. Many schools were proprietary, or profit making, institutions organized by a few interested physicians, and even the university-affiliated schools relied on part-time faculty. Upon "graduation," the student was awarded a certificate, the equivalent of a license to practice medicine. In the absence of any real licensing authority, virtually anyone could practice medicine—with or without a degree. With regular medicine unable to offer much more than a variety of useless, and frequently harmful, purging procedures and medicines, many Americans either medicated themselves and their families—using innumerable home remedies, patent medicines and health manuals—or turned to a growing number of "irregulars"—homeopaths, osteopaths, chiropractors, herb doctors and faith healers, and quacks and charlatans of all types. There were almost no minority or women physicians.

The second half of the nineteenth century saw regular medicine begin to, and eventually, totally discard the theories and therapeutics of the past and to replace them with pragmatic and increasingly scientific approaches and methods. Continued progress resulted in increasing specialization and major changes in the nature, as well as the quality, of medical practice. The expanded roles of medical societies led to the adoption of uniform standards of practice, reforms in medical education, and the establishment of state licensing boards with relatively stringent requirements. By the end of the century, remarkable advances were being made in the understanding of fundamental pathogenetic processes and in applying such knowledge to the diagnosis and treatment of disease. As the standards of practice were raised and as he began to achieve increasing therapeutic success, the physician began to enjoy an improvement in professional, economic, and social status. By 1900, the profession had not only survived, it had reestablished its credibility. The physician had become an important, valued, and respected member of the community. The second half of the nineteenth century had laid the foundations for the remarkable progress which was to come in the twentieth century.

1.4 There were some notable medical advances in the first half of the century. The introduction of general anaesthesia in the 1840s was a boon to patient and surgeon.

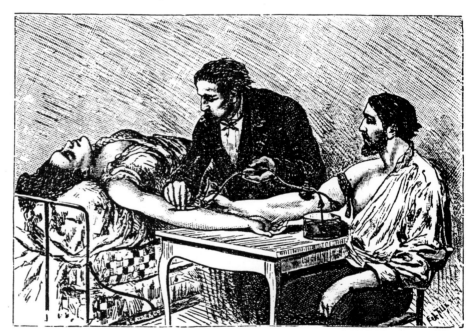

1.5 Such latter-day standbys as blood transfusion were not available until later in the century, and then only in primitive fashion.

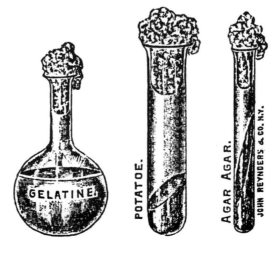

1.6 The second half of the century saw the identification of the bacterial agents of such diseases as diphtheria, cholera, and tuberculosis.

2 EARLY WEST

Dr. Robinson will accompany you [Lt. Pike] . . . He will be furnished medicines and . . . he is bound to attend to your sick.

General James Wilkinson, 1806[1]

2.1 Dr. John Robinson.

IN 1806, THE SAME YEAR THAT Lewis and Clark returned from their overland journey to the Pacific Northwest, Lieutenant Zebulon Pike set out on the first American expedition to Colorado. Pike's party included a doctor, Dr. John H. Robinson, Colorado's first American physician.[2] Robinson, a Virginian, had come to St. Louis in 1805 and married the sister-in-law of that city's first physician, Dr. Antoine Saugrain.[3] While working at a nearby military camp, the doctor was recruited by General James P. Wilkinson to accompany Pike's expedition. As is indicated throughout Pike's journal, he and Robinson became good friends and Pike clearly relied upon the doctor as a companion and "right hand man." Those who believe that the Pike expedition was part of a Burr-Wilkinson conspiracy against the federal government and part of a plan to create an independent nation out of the western United States and Mexico have suggested that both Pike and Robinson served as as spies for Wilkinson. There is no real evidence for this, however.

At any rate, the expedition left its base on the Missouri River in July 1806, trekked across Kansas, and followed the Arkansas River into Colorado. They reached the Rocky Mountains, and Pike and Robinson made an unsuccessful attempt to climb the great peak that, years later, would be named for Pike. They soon found themselves wandering around the mountains. Dressed in mid-winter in lightweight uniforms, they nearly froze and starved to death. At this time, Dr. Robinson suddenly left the expedition on a mysterious business trip to Santa Fe. Three months later, still wandering around Colorado, Pike and his party were arrested by Spanish troops for trespassing on what was then Mexican territory. Robinson, who had already been arrested, and Pike found themselves reunited in a Mexican jail. Ultimately they were released and escorted back to American territory.

Pike subsequently praised Dr. Robinson's contributions to the expedition:

> I have received important services [from Dr. Robinson], as my companion in dangers and hardships, counsellor in difficulties and to whose chymical, botanical and mineralogical knowledge the expedition was greatly indebted: in short, sir, he is a young gentleman of talents, honor and perseverance . . .[4]

There must have been a number of medical "events" on the Pike expedition. Unfortunately, Pike doesn't mention any and Dr. Robinson kept no records. About the only comment of medical interest is Pike's observation that Robinson had offered his medical services to the local Mexican hospital during their incarceration. Much to their chagrin, the offer was rejected, allegedly because of the local Spanish doctor's jealousy.[5] For more than a decade after his return to the States, Dr. Robinson engaged in a series of mysterious and ineffectual "revolutionary" schemes involving Mexico. A map he drew of the Mexican, Louisiana, and Missouri territories, is said to be notable for its inaccuracies. He died in Mississippi in 1819 at the age of thirty-seven.

In the spring of 1820 an exploring party under Major Stephen H. Long, Chief Topographic Engineer of the U.S. Army, left its encampment on the Missouri River near present-day Omaha. During the next year they followed the South Platte to its headwaters in Colorado, headed south along the Front Range, and returned via the Canadian River (which they mistook for the Red River) to the East. The group was accompanied by a physician who was also a geologist and botanist, Dr. Edwin James. At the age of fourteen, James had published the first botanic survey of his home state, Vermont.[6] Now twenty-two, having studied under Professors John Torrey and Amos Eaton, James was a bona fide scientist. His medical degree was equally authentic though less distinguished, having been awarded on the basis of study with his physician-brother rather than at a medical school. In addition to his other responsibilities on the expedition, James served as its chronicler. When the expedition was completed, the doctor wrote its official report, the classic *Account of an Expedition from Pittsburg to the Rocky Mountains*.[7] The *Account* provided a valuable compendium of geological, botanical, ethnological and other data.

James had plenty to do medically. Soon after the expedition entered what is now Colorado, for example, two men became quite ill shortly after drinking water from the South Platte. Dr.

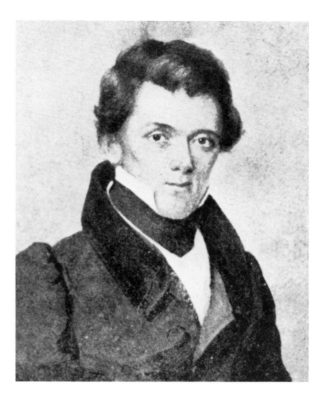

2.2 Dr. Edwin James

James treated them with various medicines and whiskey and they recovered. That night, however, a number of men came down with an illness characterized by headache, chest pain, and vomiting. One of the party later wrote:

> They had all eaten of wild currants . . . We attribute the sickness to that cause. A dose of calomel and jalap . . . soon gave relief. We eat no more currants.[8]

Dr. James, himself, wrote of the incident:

> It is not to be supposed that this illness was caused by any very active deleterious quality in the fruit, but that the stomach, by long disuse, had . . . lost the power of digesting fruits. Several continued unwell during the night.[9]

The doctor attempted to improve the men's general health by bleeding them.[10] The phlebotomy may have made them feel better, but it could not have made it any easier when they attempted to climb the the 14,000 foot peak which Long named for Dr. James. This was the same mountain which Pike and Robinson had failed to climb and which Fremont later renamed Pike's Peak.

When the expedition was completed, James continued as an army surgeon and served at a number of forts in the mid-West.[11] During his tour at Fort Brady in Michigan, the scholarly doctor learned to speak Ojibway and translated the New Testament and other books into that language. He also wrote one of the classic narratives of Indian captivity, that of John Tanner.

In 1833 James moved to Iowa where he practiced medicine, farmed, and wrote on a variety of topics, including agriculture and western history. He was an active abolitionist and his house was a station on the Underground Railway. James died in 1861.

In the late fall of 1848, thirty-three men under Colonel John C. Fremont, guided by the old mountain man, Bill Williams, set out for Colorado's San Juan Mountains.[12] The party included the Kern brothers of Philadelphia—artists Richard and Edward and the expedition's physician, Dr. Benjamin Kern. Within a short time the San Juan's huge annual snowfall had begun and the party soon found itself lost and trapped in the drifts. On December 16, Dr. Kern wrote in his diary:

> Many had their noses, etc. frozen and some became stupid from the cold . . . My eyelids stuck together from cold and for a time I saw nothing but red . . .[13]

Dr. Kern saw nothing but red when it came to Colonel Fremont as well, and the feeling was mutual. The Kern brothers blamed Fremont for getting them into the mess. Dr. Kern himself spent the day after Christmas " . . . sick . . . with severe vomiting."[13] He wrote of

> days of horror, desolation, despair . . . almost continued heavy winds, intense cold and snow storms . . . blankets, coats and one's hair frozen indiscriminately together . . . , the packing of saddles, manes and mule tails eagerly devoured by the starving animals.[13]

There was little that any physician could do to alleviate the situation. Soon men as well as mules began to starve and freeze to death. After nearly two months of such misery, the party emerged from the San Juans, but not before ten men had died. The following month, after recuperating in Taos, Dr. Kern and Bill Williams returned to the mountains to try to recover the expedition's abandoned possessions. They never returned. According to the army surgeon stationed in Taos, they were killed by a band of Utes. Others blamed it on "Mexicans."[14] Dr. Kern was thirty years old.

In 1853 the U.S. government sent several expeditions across the West to explore possible routes for the proposed transcontinental railway. The expedition that crossed Colorado was led by Captain John Gunnison and was accompanied by "surgeon and geologist" Dr. Jacob Schiel. The doctor was a well-trained physical scientist, and Gunnison, who had been quite ill on a previous expedition, was probably delighted to have someone who could serve as a physician as well.[15] Schiel outfitted himself with medicines in St. Louis and attended to the inevitable medical problems of the journey. When, for example, the expedition's astronomer suffered the torments of poison ivy, Schiel applied "a thin dilution of acid sublimate" to his rash and, "to complete the cure," had him drink a mild purgative and lemonade.[16] There was little Schiel could do for Gunnison, however, when the Captain and a detachment of men were massacred by Indians.

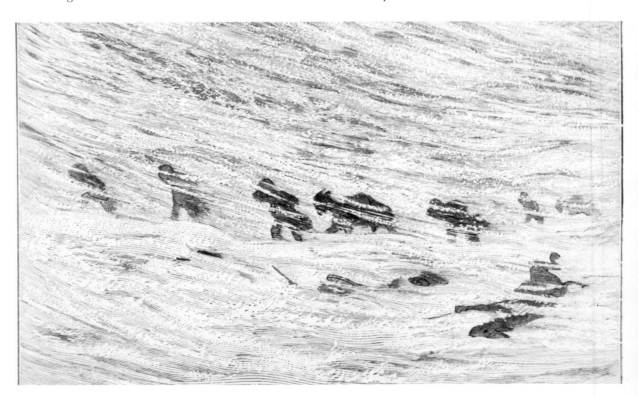

2.3 An early illustration depicts the Fremont Expedition trapped by a blizzard in Colorado's San Juan mountains. Dr. Kern could do little under these conditions.

Apparently, Gunnison never knew that Schiel was not really a physician. Although the doctor's official report was signed "M.D.," it turns out that he had never received any medical training, and the title of "doctor" referred to his Ph.D. in geology. Schiel later returned to Germany, published a descriptive journal of the expedition, and became a distinguished professor and author of works in geology, chemistry, and philosophy.

A number of other physician-explorers and scientists have been associated with early Colorado. These include Dr. Benjamin Fellowes, who accompanied Colonel Dodge's dragoons on their expedition into eastern Colorado in 1835 and, although he did not use his M.D. professionally, the famed government explorer, Ferdinand V. Hayden.

Mountain Men

I have not known at any time a single instance of bilious fever among [the mountain men] or any other disease prevalent in the settled parts of our country, except a few instances . . . of slight fevers produced by colds or rheumatic affections.

General William Ashley,[17]
Head of the American Fur Company, 1820s

The fur trade had existed for more than a century, when, stimulated by fashion's demand for beaver hats, it reached a frenetic peak between 1820 and 1840. For two decades, trappers headed out from St. Louis and Taos-Santa Fe to range over virtually the entire West, including Colorado. Hired by such outfits as the Rocky Mountain Fur Company and the American Fur Company, or on their own as "free" trappers, they scoured the waterways of the West searching for enough beaver to satisfy the sartorial needs of urban American and European gentlemen. More importantly, the mountain men, as they came to be known, provided much valuable information on the new territories.

In all, there were never more than a few thousand mountain men, of whom several hundred have been identified by name. Nevertheless, they were a remarkable group of men who, rightfully, have become part of the nation's heroic lore. Usually in·small groups, they made their way for hundreds, sometimes thousands of miles, through uncharted, rugged, and often hostile territory—away from any semblance of civilization for months or years. Their annual rendezvous, usually at previously chosen sites in the Teton country, were vivid panoramas of early western Americana. These gatherings drew trappers, travelers, and Indians together from all over the West for an annual extravaganza of buying and selling, bartering and trading, and drinking, gambling, womanizing, and story-telling. Some of their stories are of medical interest.

The mountain men seem to have been a remarkably healthy lot. Presumably, sickly men were smart enough not to come in the first place, or if they did, they weren't around long enough to have their presence recorded. The high mortality rates of the East and the South were due to infectious diseases, most of them spread by human contact and maintained by populations which were increasing in size and density. Diseases such as typhoid, yellow fever, cholera, smallpox, and diphtheria depended upon such populations for their survival. The mountain men were few in number and spread over vast distances. As a result, they were little bothered by most of the contagious diseases. In addition, the climate and altitude of the beaver country were considered to be good for one's health. George Ruxton, a young Englishman who lived with the mountain men, wrote of the "wonderfully restorative effects" of the Rocky Mountains and of friends whose health had been renewed by their "reinvigorating climate."[19] Another visitor told of "old mountaineers who have traded among the Indians here [in Colorado] for many years [who] assert that they have never known a man to die in this region from any disease contracted here."[19]

On the other hand, the mountain men did face many medical challenges—heat and cold, exposure and altitude, starvation and dehydration, grizzlies and rattlesnakes, drownings and accidents, a misfired rifle, an Indian's arrow, a former friend's Green River knife. The chronicles of the mountain men are replete with memories of such "macho" medical concerns; more common and more mundane problems such as diarrhea were recalled with much less frequency.

Under the best of circumstances, the mountain man's diet might be regarded as "nutritionally unbalanced;" under the worst of circumstances he faced starvation. He expected to live off the land and he carried as little food with him as possible—perhaps a little flour for biscuits, some salt, and a little beef jerky for emergencies. Fortunately, he had learned many Indian ways and could tell edible berries, plants and roots from those which were not. The mountain men must have had at least a modicum of fruits and vegetables since scurvy does not seem to have been a problem. Whenever he had the choice, however, the mountain man's diet consisted of fresh meat. Fur trade entrepreneur General William Ashley commented that "nothing more is necessary for the support of men in the wilderness than a plentiful supply of good fresh meat. It is all that our mountaineers ever require or even seem to wish."[20]

Mountain man Rufus Sage and his fellows were in Colorado on their way to Bent's Fort when they ran out of food, could find no game, and " . . . began to talk seriously of the imminent danger of starving to death."[21] Finally, they found a few pieces of buffalo hide which had apparently been rejected by the wolves as too tough. They boiled the hide for several hours, but the result was "of so glutinous a nature [as to] cement [one's] teeth." Someone next suggested roasting some of the ubiquitous cactus. The taste was acceptable, and a number of the group were "induced to partake quite heartily." Unfortunately,

> the inherent properties of the cacti began to have their effect . . . a weakness in the joints, succeeded by a severe trembling and desire to vomit, accompanied by an almost insufferable pain in the stomach and bowels. [Some] were in such extreme pain they rolled upon the ground for agony, with countenances writhing in every imaginable shape . . .[21]

This was too much! The starving mountain men finally sacrificed and feasted on one of their treasured mules.

Hunger was bad enough, but according to Sage, thirst was even worse.[21] On one occasion, instead of following the Colorado branch of the Santa Fe Trail, Sage and his party chose the virtually dry Cimarron cutoff. They made a bad choice. After the "indescribable torments of burning thirst . . . had rendered us almost frantic with agony," the literary Sage recalled the exhilaration which he and his comrades felt when they finally discovered water:

> What tongue can tell the sweetness of the draught that first greeted our parched lips . . . What mind can conceive the inestimable value of water, until destitution unfolds its real merits . . . Thirst, withering thirst, can never be forgotten while it continues . . . it will burn as if to scorch the vitals and dry up the heart's blood.[21]

The winter's cold was even more dangerous than the summer's heat. Crossing Colorado's Sangre de Cristo range one winter, Ruxton experienced "cold . . . more intense than I ever remember."[22] Entertained all evening by howling wolves, the next morning he awoke to find his blanket as stiff as a board and "suffered extremely." He was surprised that he survived—"I really thought I should have frozen bodily." Winter on the plains could be just as cruel. Caught in a blizzard north of present-day Pueblo, Ruxton nearly froze to death and spent "two days in nursing my frozen fingers and feet."[22] Frostbite was common. Rufus Sage recalled that when he and his fellows were caught in a Colorado blizzard, "the feet of one poor fellow were so badly frozen, it was three months before he entirely recovered. Another lost a portion of one of his ears."[23]

Indian attacks presented another source of danger, and arrow and bullet wounds were a common medical problem. Kit Carson, a mountain man in his early days, encountered a hostile Indian's bullet one day:

> The ball grazed my neck and passed through my shoulder . . . I passed a miserable night from the pain of the wound [it having bled freely], which was frozen.[24]

In a few days, Carson and his companions set out on their spring hunt. There is no further mention of his wound—typical of the mountain man's nonchalant attitude to such inconveniences. Physical trauma was not always the result of accidents or Indian attacks. The frenzied activities of rendezvous, for example, often saw a trapper's fists, knife, or gun turned against his fellow. Such was the case at Fort Lancaster (now Fort Lupton, Colorado) in 1844 when "an old mountaineer" died as the result of a "pistol wound received at a drunken frolic on the Fourth of July." With clinical precision, Rufus Sage described the man's injury:

> The ball entered the back about two inches below the head, severely fracturing the vertebrae and nearly severing the spinal marrow . . . His body below the wound was entirely devoid of feeling or use. He lived one week . . . but meanwhile suffered more than the agonies of death.[25]

Biting insects were one of the banes of the trapper's life. Warren Ferris recalled mosquitos "which . . . kept sucking at the vital currents in our veins in spite of every precaution."[26] Such annoyances yielded to abject fear, however, when rumors of a "mad wolf" and hydrophobia (i.e. rabies) circulated among the trappers. In 1833, after a season of trapping, and "returning, richly laded with spoils," J.S. Robb and three companions were camped somewhere in what appears to have been northwestern Colorado or southwestern Wyoming. Suddenly, the peace of the camp was broken by a wolf which attacked and bit all of them. They killed the animal and, the next day, resumed their trek. Unfortunately, however, though they had successfully avoided the savage foe, a hidden one was at work in our midst more terrible than the painted warriors . . . , more appalling in its promised fatality than the torturing knife of the ruthless red man. *Hydrophobia*, in all its horrid panoply of terrors, looked out from the eyes that surrounded me.[27]

Robb went on to describe his friends' bizzare behavior, "violent paroxysms" and grimacing mouths covered with "blood and foam." Two were soon dead and the other committed suicide, leaving Robb "alone—far in the wilderness—a dreadful apprehension of the poison being in my veins ever present to my thoughts." Robb survived the episode, however, later ascribing his good fortune to the "free use of liquor and salt." The tale is interesting, but possibly apocryphal.

The sick or injured mountain man might be, literally, a thousand miles by trail away from the comforts of a bed and the ministrations of a doctor. Some carried a few items of medical use in their packs, such as a lancet or a pocket knife for phlebotomy or for performing some minor surgical task.[28] The experienced trapper might even carry a few medications—anti-fever pills (quinine), calomel or jalap for intestinal problems, or tartar emetic to induce vomiting. Whiskey was a popular medicine and was often used as an anaesthetic of sorts. The inventories of the fur trading posts included medicines, and such standard items as Essence of Peppermint and Turlington's Balsam of Life were especially popular. The latter was recommended as " a specific remedy for the stone, gravel, cholick, vomiting and spitting of blood and other inward weaknesses and decays."[29]

Many other mountain man remedies and treatments were adopted from the Indians—all sorts of animal and, especially, plant materials— used to prepare various teas, decoctions, ointments, poultices, linaments, and the like. Beaver oil and castoreum, for example, were commonly rubbed into wounds. Rufus Sage extolled the medicinal benefits of cherry bark tea,

> a drink quite common among mountaineers and Indians in the Spring season. It is used for purifying the blood and reducing it to suitable consistency for the temperatures of summer . . . I recommend it as the most innocent and effective medicine . . .[30]

Pehaps less "innocent" was the "bitters [which was] very common among mountaineers." Bitters consisted of "one gill of buffalo gall" in a pint of water. Sage recommended the virtues of mountain man bitters with enthusiasm:

> Upon the whole system its effects are beneficial.

As a stimulant it braces the nerves . . . It also tends to restore an impaired appetite and invigorate the digestive powers . . . [and] to make sound an irritated and ulcerated stomach . . . striking an effective blow at that most prolific source of so large a majority of the diseases common to civilized life.[30]

Without access to professional help, the mountain men had to rely on each other for medical treatment. Kit Carson's biographer, Dr. De Witt Peters, commented on the "careful and sympathizing care which the mountaineers . . . ever exhibit towards each other in distress."[31] Such was the case when one of the most famous of the mountain men, Jedediah Smith, had much of his scalp and an ear removed by a grizzly bear. The wounds, which were apparently extensive, were repaired by one of Smith's comrades using a needle and thread. In another incident, Dick Wootten and a party of trappers were long gone from Bent's Fort when one of the group, in a free-for-all with some Indians, broke both of his legs. Wootten recalled:

> There were no surgeons within five hundred miles . . . so we had to set the broken bones ourselves. Then we made a litter out of poles which we placed on two pack animals, and in this way we carried him from place to place for nearly two months.[32]

Perhaps the most controversial medical event in mountain man history involved Tom Smith. In 1827 Smith was with a party of trappers in North Park, Colorado, when he sustained a severe leg injury—possibly having been shot by an Indian's arrow or bullet. The bone was shattered and an amputation was clearly necessary. There are several different accounts of the events that followed.[33] In later years, Tom himself claimed that he had become impatient with his fellows' hesitancy, fortified himself with Taos lightning, fashioned a tourniquet, made a rude saw from a knife, and amputated his own leg. Other stories have Tom beginning the procedure himself, with a companion finishing the amputation. According to another story, it was Milton Sublette who

> took the sharp knife and cut down to the bones just below the knee. He stood that pretty well for the leg was numb from the tight band [of green deer's hide . . . above the knee]. Then [someone] pulled down the bottom flesh and [Milt] took the sawknife and sawed off both bones. *That* was a teaser, but it was nothing to what was comin', for as soon as the leg dropped, [someone] handed [Milt] the red hot gun barrel and he rubbed it over the stump till it fizzled and smoked worse nor a venison steak![34]

Known thereafter as "Pegleg," Smith was taken

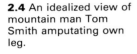

2.4 An idealized view of mountain man Tom Smith amputating own leg.

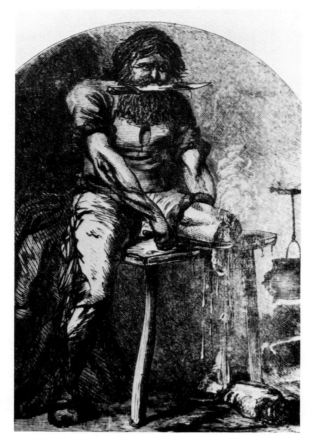

2.5 Mountain man Dick Wootten about the time he was Dr. Beshoar's patient.

and sewing up the lacerations.[36] Another old time trapper, Jim Baker, was a patient of Colorado's Dr. J.N. Hall. Hall commented on Baker's pigmented facial scars. Such scars, seen especially around the right eye and upper cheek, were characteristic of powderburns in old-timers who used to fire their rifles while seated on a galloping horse.[37]

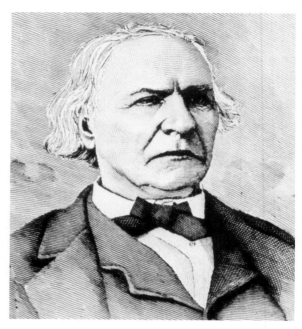

to a Ute village, where the women chewed herbs and roots into a poultice, dressed his wound, and nursed him back to health. Regardless of the details, there is no question that this was major surgery and, apparently, the first recorded instance of such surgery in Colorado.

Eventually, as men's fashions changed, the demand for beaver pelts declined, and the mountain men drifted off to other locales and other pursuits. Some, like Kit Carson, continued to participate in the history of the West, as scouts, Indian fighters, and settlers, while others passed into obscurity. Pegleg Smith became an established western "character," earning many a complimentary whiskey by showing off his wooden leg and telling progressively more dramatic tales of his amputation. Milton Sublette, credited by some with having been Smith's surgeon, had his own leg amputated some years later—the result of chronic osteomyelitis from an old arrow wound.[35] "Uncle Dick" Wootten became a buffalo hunter, scout, and pioneer settler in southern Colorado. In his later years, Wootten fondly remembered the wild days of the rendevous. Apparently, this was the case in 1869 when, in a bar in Trinidad, Colorado, the old trapper decided to demonstrate his toughness—by chomping down on a whiskey glass. Dr. Michael Beshoar spent a considerable amount of time picking glass out of Wootten's mouth

One of the most poignant medical events of the old West was the death of Kit Carson in 1868 at Fort Lyon, Colorado.[38] Way back in 1826, as a boy of seventeen, Carson was said to have amputated the shattered arm of a fellow traveler on the Santa Fe trail.[39] During the next four decades, Carson participated in much of the early West's history—the fur trade, several Fremont expeditions, Bent's Fort, the Mexican War and Californian independence, Indian Wars, and more.[40] Carson had been having chest pains while serving as commanding officer at Fort Garland, Colorado, in 1867. The pains had become so severe and incapacitating that the old scout had to travel in a wagon. Nevertheless, Carson consented to accompany a delegation of Utes to Washington, D.C. While in the East, he consulted a number of physicians, all of whom agreed that nothing could be done for his medical problem. General Fremont's wife was distressed by Carson's appearance, and one doctor commented that although he might survive the trip back to Colorado, the old scout might die at any moment. Carson's problem was, indeed, a serious one—he had an aneurysm of his thoracic aorta.[41] The aneurysm was enlarging and impinging upon the trachea and bronchi, making him perpetually short of breath and causing him increasing pain.

Carson resigned from the army and moved to Boggsville, Colorado, where he met the assistant surgeon at nearby Fort Lyon, Dr. H.R. Tilton.[42] Tilton was an amateur trapper and he and the old mountain man became good friends. As Carson became increasingly ill, Tilton made more and more visits to his home. When, after the birth of their seventh child, Carson's wife died, the doctor pursuaded him to move in with him at the fort. Carson did so and promptly made his will. Years later, Dr. Tilton described Carson's last days.

> The aneurysm . . . had progressed rapidly . . . pressing on the pneumo-gastric nerves and trachea [and] caused frequent spasms of the bronchial tubes.
> I explained to him the probable mode of termination of his disease, that he might die from suffocation or, more probably, the aneurysm would burst and cause death by hemorrhage. He expressed a decided preference for the latter mode.[43]

Tilton eased the old man's pain with chloroform. One evening, he coughed up blood. The next afternoon, Carson suddenly cried out, " Doctor, compadre, adios." With that, a gush of blood poured from his mouth and he died. Although an autopsy was not done, the aneurysm had apparently ruptured into the trachea or a bronchus.

The doctor had read Peter's biography of Carson during the mountain man's last days. He later commented, "It was wonderful to read of the stirring scenes, thrilling deeds, and narrow escapes, and then look at the quiet, modest, retiring, but dignified little man who had done so much."[44]

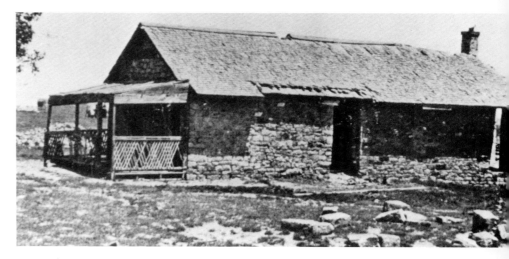

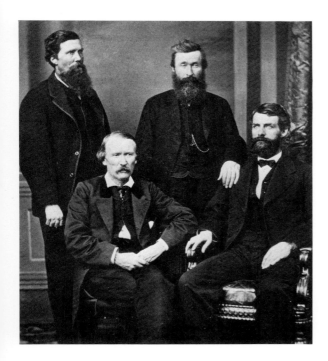

Bent's Fort

Bent's Fort . . . is the finest and largest fort which we have seen on this journey. The outer wall is built of imperfectly burnt brick; on two sides arise two little towers with loop holes . . . The fort is about one hundred and fifty miles from Taos in Mexico.

F.A. Wislizenus, M.D., 1839[45]

In 1833 Colonel William Bent and his brothers completed their fortified adobe trading post on the Santa Fe Trail, along the Arkansas River near present-day La Junta, Colorado. The Bents, successful fur traders and merchants, had picked an ideal site, the intersection between the Santa Fe Trail and the North-South trail between Santa Fe—Taos in the South and the Oregon Trail and, later, Fort Laramie in the North. Over the years nearly every famous visitor to the early West stopped at Bent's fort. As well as acting as a trading post, it provided every available facility to the traveler; it was a combined rest stop, information center, and sanctuary. And it was the only source of medical care in a vast area.

Although for most of its existence there was no bona fide physician at the fort, the Colonel served as doctor to many trappers, travelers, and Indians. According to George Bird Grinnell, Bent

> possessed an ample medicine chest which he replenished on his trips to Westport and St. Louis. He had a number of medical books, and no doubt these, and such practical experience as came to him with the years, made him reasonably skillful in the rough medicine and surgery that he practiced. [Away from the fort] he carried a small medicine chest.[46]

In 1829, while the fort was under construction, there was an outbreak of smallpox among the "Mexican" workers. Bent, Kit Carson, and others soon fell victim. The major medical effort

2.7 Surgeon Tilton's residence at Fort Lyon. Kit Carson spent his last days here under the doctor's care.

2.6 This photo of Kit Carson (seated, left) was taken shortly before his death from a ruptured aortic aneurysm.

was preventive—keeping the Indians, who were highly susceptible to the pox, away from the fort. Years later, Bent himself was the patient of a Cheyenne "doctor." According to a witness, Bent's friend William Boggs, the Colonel had developed a

> putrid sore throat [which] had become so bad that he had ceased to swallow food and . . . his wife fed him with broth by taking a mouthful and squirting it through a quill which she forced down his throat.[47]

Knowing that he would soon die if something were not done, Bent called for an Indian doctor named "Lawyer," a plain looking man "without show or ornamentation." The Indian examined Bent's throat by using a spoon handle as a tongue depressor, "just as any doctor would do," shook his head and left. He soon returned with a handful of small sandburs with barbs "as sharp as fish hooks," used an awl to run strands

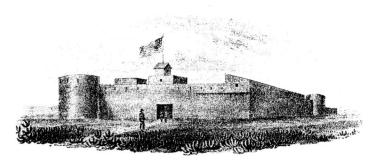

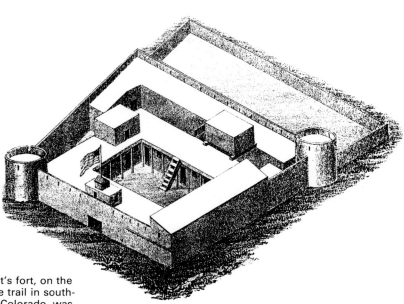

2.8 Bent's fort, on the Santa Fe trail in southeastern Colorado, was the site of many medical "happenings" prior to 1850.

of sinew through the sandburs, rubbed marrow grease around them, and attached them to a stick. Then he pushed the burrs down Bent's throat

> the length of the stick, and drew it out . . . and repeated it, . . . drawing out all the dry and corrupt matter each time, and opened the passage so that

Bent could swallow soup. In a day or two he was well enough to eat food . . . But for this simple remedy Bent would have died. No one but an Indian would ever have thought of resorting to such a remedy.[47]

Bent's Fort was the home of Colorado's first resident physician, Dr. Edward L. Hempstead. Hempstead was a member of a prominent St. Louis family, connected by marriage and business to the famous fur trader and entrepreneur, Manuel Lisa. Although little is known about the doctor, it has been said that he spent several years at the fort.[48] Several visitors commented on his presence there in 1846 and 1847. Garrard described him as "affable," possibly shy (" . . . [he] did not join the festive throng [at a dance]") and scholarly (" . . . his well stocked library afforded recreation and pastime during the dull intervals of the day").[49] Another visitor-chronicler, Lieutenant Abert, was presented with mineral and botanic specimens by the doctor for his scientific collection.[50]

There was much medical activity at the fort during the years 1846 - 1847. In June 1846, one famous patient, young Susan Magoffin, arrived. The eighteen-year-old wife of a prominent St. Louis businessman, Susan was accompanying her husband and a wagon train of merchandise to Santa Fe. Although she had brought a maid and whatever other comforts that could be taken on the trail, it was not easy for the genteel, eastern bred young woman, especially as she was pregnant. As they approached the fort, Susan became ill, and Mr. Magoffin pursuaded a physician, Dr. Philippe Masure, to join them from another wagon train. Masure, a Belgian, was described by Susan as a "polite . . . delicate . . . and excellent physician, especially in female cases . . . I have great confidence in his knowledge and capacity for relieving me."[51] She added: " The idea of being sick on the plains is not at all pleasant to me; it is rather terrifying".

The party arrived at Bent's Fort where Susan was provided with a room. Dr. Masure remained with her and attempted to prevent the threatened abortion. His advice, Susan noted, was easier to take than his medicine. On her nineteenth birthday she wrote in her diary: "I am sick! Strange sensations in my head, my back, and hips . . . I am obliged to lie down most of the time . . ."[51]

On the following day:

> My pains commenced and continued until midnight when, after much agony . . . , which was relieved a little at times by medicine given by Dr. Masure, all was over. I sunk off into a kind of lethargy in [my husband's] arms.[51]

Susan could not help but contrast her situation with that of an Indian woman in the room below her.

> She gave birth to a fine healthy baby, about the same time, and in half an hour after she went to the [Arkansas] River and bathed herself . . . Some gentlemen here [have seen] them immediately after the birth of a child go to the water and break the ice to bathe themselves! It is truly astonishing to see what customs will do. No doubt many ladies in civilized life are ruined by too careful treatments during child-birth, for this custom of the heathen is not known to be disadvantageous, but is considered a "heathenish" custom.[51]

Susan Magoffin continued on with her husband to Santa Fe, and then to Mexico, where she contracted yellow fever. In three subsequent pregnancies, one child survived. Shortly after the birth of this child, in 1855, Susan died at the age of twenty-eight.

Shortly before the Magoffins left Missouri for Santa Fe, President Polk declared war on Mexico. In June and early July 1846, Colonel Stephen Kearny raised an army of 1,700 men, mostly volunteers. They soon left Missouri and headed down the Santa Fe trail. From the beginning, illness, especially dysentery, plagued the Army of the West and continued to do so throughout its sojourn in the Southwest and Mexico, accounting for more deaths than did war wounds. One victim who survived was William Gilpin, later the first territorial governor of Colorado.[52] Another was young Lieutenant James Abert, who wrote:

> On the 22 of July I was taken ill, to such a degree that it was necessary to carry me in a wagon . . . until we arrived at Bent's Fort. At this time the disease had obtained such an influence over my senses, that days and nights were passed in delirium, and a mental struggle to ascertain whether the impressions my mind received were true or false . . . When I gazed on Bent's Fort, the buildings seemed completely metamorphosed; new towers had been erected, the walls heightened . . .[53]

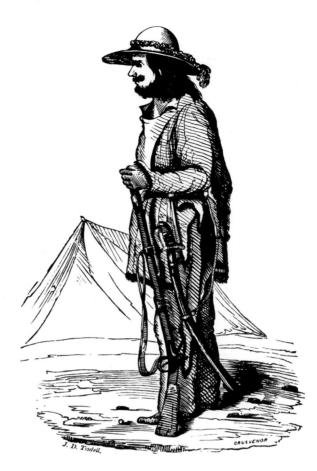

2.9 Disease, rather than Mexican sabres and bullets, caused most of the American casualties of the Mexican War. This volunteer was likely to have suffered from "dysentery," and possibly malaria, sometime during his service.

In addition to Abert, twenty-one sick volunteers as well as "a number of dragoons and teamsters . . . ," about sixty men in all, were left at the fort when the Army moved south.[54] Francis Parkman, visiting the Fort at the time, noted:

> Bent's Fort does not supply the best accomodations for an invalid . . . The sick chamber was a little mud room where he [Parkman's "friend," a Missouri volunteer nicknamed Tete Rouge] and a companion attacked by the same disease, were laid together, with nothing but a buffalo-robe between them and the ground. The assistant-surgeon's deputy visited them once a day and brought each a huge dose of calomel . . . In spite of the doctor, however, he eventually recovered.[55]

3 INDIANS AND SOLDIERS

An important but dangerous occupation . . . is that of the medicine man . . . When an Indian is to be treated for sickness a small wickiup, or medicine tent, is erected . . . and the doctor and his patient repair there for the healing . . . If a cure is not effected and the patient and his friends believe that the medicine man is not trying to cure . . . they may take the unlucky [doctor's] life.

V.Z. Reed (1893)[1]
(Regarding the Ute Indians of Colorado)

WHEN WE THINK OF THE prehistoric inhabitants of ancient Colorado, we think of the Anasazi. Even they were not the first Coloradans, however, and even in Anasazi times there were other Indians in Colorado—on the Eastern plains and in the Great Basin. It is Anasazi remains that are available however, because of their remote location, their numbers, and the preservative effects of southwestern climate. So it is the Anasazi to whom we turn when we want to study "the ancient ones."

The ancestors of the Anasazi, in the centuries before Christ, lived in caves and rock shelters, foraged and hunted for food, and wove watertight baskets. By around A.D. 450, the Anasazi were living in pit houses and had learned to farm. Much of their diet came to consist of corn, squash and beans. Their tools, pottery, and art work became more sophisticated, as did, presumably, other aspects of their culture. Towards the end of their era, the Anasazi moved from the mesa tops to the canyons where they built spectacular, multi-family and multistoried dwellings into the cliff walls. Shortly before 1300, and for reasons which remain unclear, the Anasazi suddenly left their homes. They are believed to be the ancestors of some of today's southwestern peoples.

Just as Anasazi culture has been reconstructed from their artifacts, the little that we know of Anasazi medicine has been derived from human remains. The Anasazi carefully placed their dead in burial pits, caves, and discarded storage areas. Bodies were folded into a flexed position and wrapped in skins. A basket was often placed over the deceased's face, and various mortuary offerings—sandals, beads and ornaments, pottery, and other items—placed alongside. If the care of their dead reflects their concern for the living, one would expect the Anasazi to have had a significant system of medical care. Some of the burials contain many bodies. Apparently "buried" at the same time and without any signs of warfare, it has been suggested that such multiple burials represent local "epidemics." Unfortunately, the amount of medical information which can be derived from bones and mummified remains is limited, and as the distinguished archeologist, H.M. Wormington, has said, " It is rare that the cause of death can be determined."[2]

Colorado's Mesa Verde is the most extensive site of Anasazi culture. Many of its mesa top pits and cliff dwellings have been carefully excavated and hundreds of burial sites uncovered. These have provided a modest amount of information of medical interest.[3] The Anasazi were short (men averaged five feet, four inches, women five feet) and not heavily muscled. Their average life expectancy was less than thirty years, a figure influenced by a very high rate of infant and childhood mortality. Women in the reproductive years of life also had a high mortality rate. Examples of flattened skulls suggest the use of infant cradle boards. Dr. James S. Miles, an orthopedic surgeon, examined hundreds of burial sites and some 40,000 bones from Wetherill Mesa, one of Mesa Verde's more recent excavations.[4] Dr. Miles found a number of specific bone and joint lesions and diseases. Virtually all adults showed evidence of degenerative arthritis by the age of 35. In a few individuals, a specific type of skull lesion suggested the possibility of an inherited form of anemia. Both of these findings have been seen in Anasazi remains from other sites. There were no bone changes suggestive of chronic malnutrition or vitamin deficiencies such as rickets, or of other metabolic or genetic diseases. Although a few lesions suggested the possibility of tuberculosis, there was no definite evidence of this disease. A variety of fractures was found but not enough to suggest an unusual frequency of trauma in the everyday life of Wetherill Mesa or to provide evidence of warfare. Dr. Miles concluded from his study of Anasazi remains that "our osseous evidence . . . indicates a surprisingly healthy population, one that 'wore' poorly, but one that was capable of great physical independence."[4]

A few medical prostheses have been found at Mesa Verde. A pair of child's crutches has axillary supports well padded with yucca fiber and covered by sewn leather—an indication, perhaps, of an ancient physician's concern for his patient's comfort. Another device appears to be a corset, laced in front and made of aspen bark. This may have been used by an Anasazi with a "slipped disc."[4] Other sites have yielded well-made wooden splints and hollow devices which may have been used to draw out pathogenic spirits or, in more practical fashion, to aspirate abscesses and wounds.[5] Such findings suggest that a fuller knowledge of Anasazi medicine would make an interesting story indeed.

Utes, Arapahoes, and Cheyennes

In more recent times, many Indian tribes passed through Colorado's eastern plains and around its fringes. The Utes occupied the central mountains and the western basin from ancient times. By the nineteenth century, the eastern plains had become the home of the Arapahoes

and their cousins, the Cheyennes. Both the Utes and the Plains Indians were renowned horsemen and warriors, but they were also very different from each other. The Utes were mountain people, hunting and foraging over high trails and familiar with the innumerable nooks and crannies of the great ranges. They tended to be short and stocky, dark skinned, and, like other people isolated from the mainstream, perhaps a bit moody. The Arapahoes and the Cheyennes ranged the plains and depended on the buffalo for food, clothing, and implements. They were tall and thin, but muscular, light-skinned, and had the "Roman" nose profile so beloved by Anglo artists. The Ute language was of Shoshonean origin while the Cheyennes and Arapahoes spoke a language of Algonquian derivation. Ute and Plains Indian territories bordered each other along Colorado's Front Range. Ute buffalo hunters ranged into the plains, while Cheyennes and Arapahoes sometimes trespassed into the mountain parks. They were enemies, and warfare between the two groups was frequent.

In the early years at least, the Utes in their mountain fastness were somewhat isolated from the white man's diseases. The Plains Indians, however, were exposed early to traders and trappers and, ultimately, to hordes of overland travelers and settlers. In 1849 the California gold rush brought a mass migration of whites across the plains, and cholera soon followed. That year, what the Indians called "the big cramps" was said to have wiped out two hundred Cheyenne lodges, perhaps half of the tribe's population.[6]

Cholera raged across the plains well into the 1850s, when it was joined by smallpox. The Indian agent at Bent's Fort, wrote in 1858: "A few years ago, the cholera and smallpox breaking out in the village of the Arapahoes swept them off by hundreds . . . ."[7]

By 1855 the Arapahoes were so debilitated by disease that they were unable to hold their annual buffalo hunt. Instead, they attempted to avoid starvation by stealing sheep and cattle.[8] The Indians, while not necessarily afraid of the white man, did fear his diseases, a fact which some of the whites used. When a family of homesteaders on the Purgatory River in southeastern Colorado was visited by a band of uninvited Indians in the 1860s, the wife pretended to have smallpox.[9] The Indian visitors gave the family some medicinal herbs and advice and promptly left. In 1862 the situation was reversed when smallpox broke out among the Cheyennes. The *Rocky Mountain News* announced:

There is no longer any doubt that smallpox rages among the Cheyenne . . . near Fort Wise. There

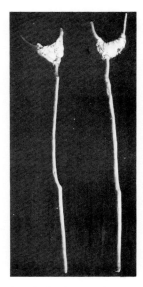

3.1 A child's crutches from Mesa Verde. (Dr. James Miles)

is no telling how soon they may bend their steps this way. To guard against this danger, our citizens should take precautions . . . Those who have not been vaccinated should be, at once.[10]

Even the U. S. government showed some sympathy when smallpox broke out among the Indians. In 1863 the government sent a special agent, Dr. H.T. Ketcham, to vaccinate the tribes.[11] Ketcham wrote from Fort Lyon that the Arapahoes were "suffering terribly from smallpox. Many are badly pitted. All are anxious to be vaccinated." He managed to inoculate 1,100 of them, but, in addition to smallpox, he found the Indians to be malnourished and "sick with erysipelas, whooping cough and diarrhea." In addition, venereal disease and alcoholism were rampant, and even their respected chief, Little Raven, was drunk much of the time. The prevalence of venereal disease among the Arapahoes had been commented on a few years before by Agent Miller:

> At this time venereal [disease] is gradually but surely thinning them out, and in a few years this once powerful and warlike people will cease to exist . . . for there is scarcely a family which is not . . . afflicted with this terrible disease.[12]

Attempts to limit the Cheyennes and Arapahoes to a reservation north of the Arkansas River were unsuccessful and a succession of raids on white settlers was followed in 1864 by the infamous Chivington massacre. By 1869 the Plains Indians had been expelled from Colorado, mainly to reservations in the Indian Territory, present-day Oklahoma.

The Utes' mountain home provided them with only temporary shelter from the white man's diseases. In 1854 an outbreak of smallpox occurred among the Utes. The whites were blamed and, in retribution, a Ute war party massacred the inhabitants of Fort Pueblo.[13] By the 1860s, the health of the Utes had degenerated. An early visitor provided a dismal portrayal of Ute health and disease:

> Coughs are frequent, and dyspepsia; sickness and deaths are quite common among the children. The incongruous mixture of white man's food and raiment and life with their own . . . is sapping their vitality at its fountains . . . The sugar they gobble up . . . and such unnatural food such as this and fine flour breed diseases and weaknesses that are already destroying the race . . . To make matters worse, they have got hold of our quack medicines.[14]

Unfortunately for them, the Utes' San Juan Mountains contained gold and silver. In 1879 some members of one Ute band brutally massacred their government agent and his co-workers, took several white women captive, and killed a number of soldiers. The prospectors and developers took avantage of the Meeker massacre to expel all of the Utes from their valuable mountain property. Most were sent to reservations in Utah. A few were allowed to remain on the Southern Ute and Ute Mountain Reservations along Colorado's southwestern border.[15] They had left their mountains behind but not the white man's diseases. Although other diseases took their toll, smallpox remained the most feared. In 1883 an outbreak of smallpox killed fifteen Utes at the Agency, and outbreaks continued into the twentieth century.[16]

Like other Indian tribes, the Utes, Cheyennes, and Arapahoes did not distinguish health and disease from other aspects of Nature. Man was as one with the world—the earth and water, the animals and plants, the sky and the universe. One's destiny was in the hands of spirits, and "Medicine" encompassed all. Good medicine, in this holistic sense, included physical, mental, and spiritual well-being and health. Bad medicine included injury and disease. The Cheyennes believed that disease might enter the body in the form of tiny arrows shot by hostile forces.[17] The Utes included among the causes of disease, ghosts, an enemy's evil thoughts, the violation of taboos, and bad dreams.[18] The shaman, or medicine-man, was the mediator between man and the spirits, and as such, he also served as a physician. Whether in treating a war wound, a difficult labor, or pneumonia, it was the medicine-man's job to placate or, if need be, to exorcise evil spirits and to substitute good Medicine for bad.

3.2 A white observer described the medical efforts of Washington, an Arapaho medicine man: "Whatever the diagnosis, his remedy is invariably the same, and consists of beating upon a tom-tom, yelling hideously, and dancing wildly about the patient, until he is either frightened to death or recovers by natural processes." H.R. Lemley. "Among the Arrapahoes" Harpers Weekly 60:494, 1880.

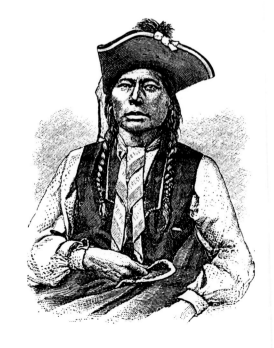

Among the Cheyennes, a young man might achieve the spiritual power of a shaman through a dream or a vision, but he still had to learn the secrets, formulae, and invocations from one who already was a medicine-man. "The doctoring of human beings," concluded George Bird Grinnell, was "elaborate and full of ceremony."[19] The father of a sick child, for example, would signal his request for medical assistance by offering a smoking pipe, stem foward, to the doctor. If he accepted, the medicine-man next proceeded to purify himself and his patient. The purification and the healing itself might include the burning of certain leaves, the shaking of rattles and gourds, the chanting of prayers and songs, the distribution of offerings, the smoking of pipes, and the application of balms, salves, and various medicines. The medicine-man sometimes tried to draw spirits out of the body by sucking at the affected part.

Josephine Meeker was one of the few Anglos to witness the efforts of an early Ute medicine-man. The medicine-man had been called to treat a sick child, and Josephine, who was considered one of the family, was allowed to remain in the tent and participate in the chanting. She observed:

> The medicine-man kneels close to the sufferer, with his back to the spectators, while he sings in a series of high-keyed grunts, gradually reaching a lower and more solemn tone. The family join, and at intervals he howls so loudly that one can hear him for a mile; then his voice dies away and only a gurgling sound is heard . . . The child lies nearly stripped. The doctor presses his lips against the breast of the sufferer and repeats the gurgling sound . . . Sometimes the ceremony is repeated all night. The sick-bed ceremonies were strange and weird.[20]

In 1927 the Durango Public Library acquired a Ute medicine-man's kit or "medicine bundle," providing a unique opportunity to examine Ute medical paraphenalia. The kit included whistles, owl and eagle feathers—including an eagle feather fan—strings of beads, and rattles.[21] Many of the kit's contents were decorated or embellished with such items as porcupine quills or bird claws.

The successful medicine-man was respected, feared, and well paid. Sidney Jocknick, a western Colorado pioneer, wrote that "when a man establishes a reputation [as a shaman], he is believed in implicitly, and many fees of blankets and horses are paid to him for his services."[22] On the other hand, it was also a dangerous profession. The shaman who could cure disease might also create it, perhaps paid to do so by

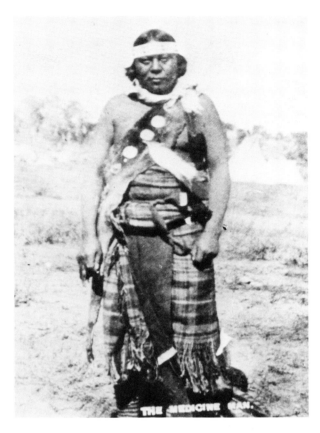

3.3 Rare photo of a Ute medicine man.

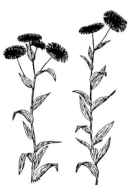

3.4 The Cheyennes boiled the leaves and stems of the column flower *(Ratibida columnaris)* into a solution which they applied to rattlesnake bites.

one's enemies. One early observer knew of "two instances where so called bad medicine men . . . were killed . . . In one case, a chief held the victim while his throat was cut by the father of the boy who had been bewitched."[23] Jocknick recalled that "if ever a hint or suspicion is raised that the medicine man is a 'quack,' as for instance, he fails to make good his work after contracting to cure 'his case,' his life must pay the forfeit."[24] The Ute chief, Tamouchi, was said to have killed a medicine-man who failed to cure his wife.[25]

Like their white counterparts, Indian physicians relied heavily on plants for their medicines. Various leaves, flowers, roots, and barks were dried, ground, pounded, boiled and burnt to provide teas, chews, balms, poultices, salves and lotions. The Cheyennes had a long list of such remedies.[26] A tea was prepared from the root of the sweet flag (*Acorus calamus*) to treat intestinal pain and an infusion of boiled wild mint leaves was drunk to prevent vomiting. Wet bearberry leaves were rubbed on a sore back, a poultice of ground wild garlic was applied to carbuncles, and skeleton weed was used to induce lactation. The Utes used the sandpuff for intestinal problems, *Lithospermum pilosum* as a diuretic, grindelia for cough, and the squaw weed for all sorts of medicinal purposes.[27] Boiled sagebrush was used for colds, and fresh mint leaves were applied to bee stings.[28] Not all remedies were

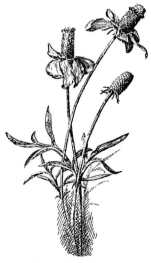

3.5 The daisy was also boiled, and the inhaled steam used to treat dizzyness, various aches and pains, backache, and drowsiness.

botanical. Skunk grease was used as a skin mois-
tener, and horse urine was used to relieve itching
and to treat skin infections. The treatment of
wounds was an important part of Indian medical
care. Cauterization was used to stop bleeding
and to seal wounds. When the Arapaho chief,
Black Coal, lost two fingers in battle, he applied
hot ashes to the wounds.[29] The Utes poured
animal fat or sugar into a wound to suppress
bleeding.[30]

Sweat houses or lodges were used by many
Indian tribes. A description of an Arapaho
"sweating lodge" appeared in *Harper's Magazine*
a century ago:

> A bower of willow wands thrust into the ground
> over which is stretched a skin or canvas. [It is]
> about three feet high and 8 - 10 feet in circumfer-
> ence. Several red hot large stones are in the center
> and around them are crouched a dozen or so In-
> dians. Water is slowly poured on the stones releas-
> ing hot air and vapor. After profuse perspiration
> they jump into an adjoining stream or wallow
> naked in the snow.[31]

In addition to sweat lodges, Colorado's Indians had the benefit of its many springs (Chapter 14). Springs were considered the re-
spositories of the "Gitche Manitou"—the spirit
of good medicine. Visiting the area of present-
day Manitou Springs in 1847, George Ruxton
commented, "The Indians regard with awe the
medicine waters of these fountains, as being the
abode of a spirit who breathes through the transparent water, and thus by his exhalations, causes
the perturbation of its surface."[32]

Less than thirty years later, the Indians
evicted, Manitou Springs was being developed
by the white man as Colorado's premier health
resort. Dr. S. Edwin Solly, one of the major
proponents of Manitou's benefits, described the
spring's medical uses by the (now departed) Indians:

> Believing as they did that the Good Spirit breathed
> into the waters the breath of life, they bathed and
> drank of them, thinking thereby to find a cure for
> every ill . . . It has been found that they thought
> most highly of their virtue when their bones and
> joints were racked with pain, their skins covered
> with unsightly blotches, or their warriors weakened
> by wounds or with mountain sickness . . .[33]

Most of Colorado's springs were in the Utes'
territory, and they fought to protect their birth-
right. The springs at Pagosa were the site of
many battles with the Navajos.[34] The last battle
was said to have been in 1867 between Indian
Agent Albert Pfeiffer representing the Utes and
a young Navajo warrior. Pfeiffer's bowie knife

ended the duel and the Utes retained possession
of the spring. According to legend, the spring
at Pagosa had been a gift from the Great Spirit.
In ancient times, a terrible plague had befallen
the Utes, all known medicines had failed, and
the tribe was dwindling. As a last resort, a great
council was held, with dancing and chanting
around the huge fire. The next morning, where
the fire had been, there was a "Pagosah," or
spring of healing waters. The Utes bathed in it
and drank its waters and were restored to
health.[35]

Even more beloved by the Utes were the
springs and vapor caves at Glenwood. An early
Glenwood Springs physician described its medical use:

> The Utes are said to have come from far and near
> in search of health at this natural sanatorium, and
> when a patient was pronounced as fit . . . by his
> wise medicine-men, the following method was em-
> ployed: Across two long poles a blanket was
> stretched and fastened, on which the victim [i.e.
> patient] was laid. His comrades then . . . raised
> and carried him to the hot pool in which he was
> immersed. A cry of agony, or the length of endur-
> ance, was the signal for the 'bath attendants' to
> lift him out of the water, and with brief intermis-
> sions, this procedure was repeated as often as the
> patient could stand it.[36]

The Indians regarded menstruation, pregnancy,
and childbirth with the same holistic attitude
that they regarded everything else in their lives.
The menstruating Ute woman was sequestered
for several days in the menstrual hut, where she
would while away her time with friends.[37] It
was believed that if she touched her hair or teeth
during this time, they would fall out. She was
considered bad luck to any man who chanced
upon her and intercourse was forbidden.
Cheyenne attitudes and practices regarding
menstruation were similar.[38] Pregnancy was
also associated with a variety of taboos. Among
the Utes, for example, beaver were avoided, lest
they "build a dam in the woman, and her waters
would not break."[39] When the time for delivery
approached, a birthing hut was built. The husband and the woman's mother were present,
possibly accompanied by another old woman
or, if there were problems, a medicine-man. The
Cheyenne woman was similarly assisted, and
sometimes the procedure was aided by various
medicines.[40] In general, Indian women delivered in a squatting or kneeling position.

The Ute father lived in the birthing hut until
the umbilical cord fell off about ten days after
delivery. The mother remained there for about
a month, and both practiced various taboos.[41]

Twins were considered bad luck, deformed babies were allowed to die, and hermaphrodites were tolerated—if not particularly welcomed. The newborn baby was washed with yucca soap, wrapped warmly, and breast fed from birth. The Cheyenne newborn was dried with powder made from the prairie puffball before being wrapped.[42] The mother was given medicines to stimulate lactation, while, in the meantime, the baby was fed by other mothers who were already nursing. Arapaho mothers wrapped their infants in fine deerskins and used buffalo chips to keep them dry and prevent rashes. Colostrum was often aspirated to expedite lacation.[43] In general, Indian parents treated infants and young children with a great deal of love and affection.

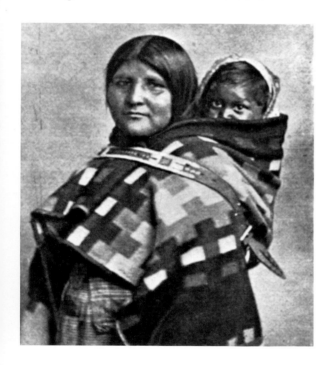

The white man's attitude towards Indian medicine was as varied as his attitude towards the Indian. On the way to Colorado with the Long expedition in 1819, Dr. Edwin James commented on the overall good health of the Plains Indians and that "their catalogue of diseases . . . is infinitely less extensive than that of civilized man."[44] In 1859 two physician-prospectors were said to have been killed by Utes near present-day Georgetown.[45] In the 1860s, the problem was with the Cheyennes and Arapahoes, and Colorado's physicians were as fearful and hostile towards the Indians as were the rest of her citizens.

There is no indication that the Cheyennes and Araphoes had received any organized medical care before their exile from Colorado. The Utes, however, did receive such care, both professional and non-professional. The so-called Denver Utes who "hung around" the city in the early

days were assigned a physician by their agent.[46] The Ute Agency at Los Pinos had a physician, but apparently Nathan Meeker's White River Agency did not. Meeker had come equipped with a textbook of obstetrics, but there is no record of his having participated in any deliveries. Mrs. Meeker and, later, daughter Josie, served as "physicians" prior to the infamous massacre of Agent Meeker and others at White River in 1879.[47] Even during their capture, Mrs. Meeker was allowed to treat the infant son of Chief Douglas.[48]

The flamboyant Ute chief, Colorow, had encounters with a number of Colorado physicians. On his frequent trips to Denver, Colorow often visited with Dr. Frederick Bancroft. Bancroft was said to have been a great friend of the chief's and on one occasion vaccinated several of Colorow's "wives."[49] Other physicians were also visited by the chief. In Leadville, one day, Colorow went to a doctor's office to ask for some medicine. The doctor was out and, in his absence, a non-medical prankster gave the chief a dose of epsom salts—which didn't make him feel any better.[50] In his later years, Colorow used to hang around Glenwood Springs, once part of the Utes' vast domain, regaling the tourists and health-seekers with anecdotes. Eventually, he developed "dropsy" and recurrent ascites. Saguache's Dr. J.T. Melvin removed the fluid periodically.[51] One day Colorow

3.6 Ute mother and child. In general, Indians took great care of their children.

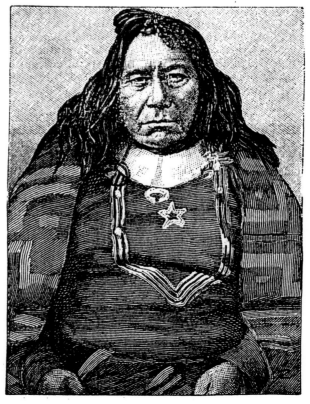

3.7 Colorow's death has been attributed to his efforts to drain abdominal fluid from his own abdomen.

used an unsterilized knife in an attempt to relieve himself of some of his ascitic fluid. He perforated his intestine, developed peritonitis, and died soon afterward.

If Colorow was "flamboyant," then the Utes' Chief Ouray was "statesmanlike." Even as he was dying of renal failure, Ouray was trying to resolve the aftermath of the Meeker massacre. In August of 1880, in the midst of negotiations, and after having been treated by the agency physician, Ouray became so ill that he could not attend an important council. Another physician was sent for from Animas City, and eventually there were three white physicians in attendance. Eventually, Ouray dismissed the doctors and called in his medicine-men, who began their more traditional measures. The *Gunnison Review* reported "the wildest wailings and moanings and other strange orgies which seemed to be both religious and medical. To onlookers from the Agency, it was a wonder he [Ouray] survived so long."[52] Ouray died a week later. One white pioneer ascribed his death to "Bright's disease, which was unduly hastened by the malpractice of his medicine-men."[53] It might have been more accurate to state that the nineteenth century white doctor's ability to treat renal failure was no more effective than that of the Ute medicine-man. Nor had Ouray's political efforts on behalf of his people been particularly successful. Most of the tribe were expelled to reservations in Utah and the remainder relegated to a strip of land along Colorado's southwestern border.

As time went one, tuberculosis became an increasingly serious problem among the Indians. Dr. H.R. Bull, physician to the U.S. Indian School at Grand Junction, Colorado, in the 1890s, reported on "the large mortality from tuberculosis in this institution."[54] The doctor was surprised at his charges' susceptibility to tuberculosis, despite their "changed condition of life . . . from teepees to dormitories, from nakedness to clothes and regular meals." In his monumental study of disease among the southwestern tribes, Dr. Alex Hridlicka reported the status of Colorado's Southern Utes.[55] The transition from the days of the "hunter and free rover" was not going well, new habits were being adopted "slowly and unwillingly," and although there had recently been some improvement, the whole life of the Southern Utes showed a "transitional degradation." Illness was common, sanitary conditions were poor, and alcoholism and tuberculosis were rife. Early in the 1900s, the Utes began to seek solace in the hallucinatory plant, peyote. The problems of Colorado's Utes were not unique. Similar problems had become the heritage of Colorado's expatriated Utes in Utah and her exiled Cheyennes and Arapahoes in Oklahoma.

Soldiers and Forts

Private John Cooley, Troop G, 3d Cavalry
Purgatory Creek, Colorado Territory, Oct. 3, 1866:
Arrow flesh-wound . . . on left side of thorax. Treated in post hospital at Fort Garland, Colorado; Recovered and returned to duty.
                    Surgeon General's Office (1871)[56]

The land cession which followed the Mexican War added the last section to future Colorado. Soon afterward, concerns over Indian hostilities led to the establishment of two forts in the area. The first, Fort Massachusetts, was built in 1852 in the south-central part of the state, near the junction between Ute and Navaho lands. It had a complement of three officers and 125 men. An assistant surgeon was assigned to the garrison, and the following year an army inspector reported that the fort's "hospital and medicines [were] well conducted."[57]

Dr. DeWitt Peters, Kit Carson's biographer, was the assistant surgeon at Fort Massachusetts in 1854. Peters's major complaint was the monotony of life at the small, isolated post. The major excitement, he recalled, came on Saturday nights when his orderly filled a vinegar barrel with hot water for his weekly bath. Warfare at Fort Massachusetts appears to have been limited to fighting mosquitos, "torments so thick . . . that you can almost cut them up with a knife."[58]

In 1857 Fort Massachusetts was replaced by Fort Garland, a larger adobe compound built a few miles away. Fort Garland's hospital had two wards with twelve beds, a dispensary, kitchen, and dining room.[59] There was no bathing facility and the hospital's "water-closet" was a "small wooden building standing over a deep pit." Unfortunately, when the hospital was constructed, the adobes were improperly dried, and when the walls began to settle, the building's supporting beams broke. Nearly twenty years later, an inspector reported that the damage had yet to be repaired; the roof was sagging, the walls caving in, and the whole building kept standing by "supports."[60]

In the meantime, on the eastern plains, the Cheyennes and Arapahoes were becoming increasingly aggressive. Colonel Bent had moved his establishment thirty miles down river on the Arkansas, and the army decided that it would build a fort next door to guard the Santa Fe

Trail. Fort Wise, constructed in 1860, included an adobe hospital with twenty-six beds.

With the coming of the Civil War, Camp Weld was established on the South Platte River near Denver to house recruits. The camp's hospital director was Dr. J.F. Hamilton, one of Denver's pioneer physicians. The hospital consisted of two stories, including a fifteen-bed ward.[61] There was something of a festive air about Camp Weld. Far from any battlefields, it was often the site of social events and visits from Denver's ladies. It's major medical event occurred in October 1861 when an entire scouting party was stricken by snowblindness. Young Mollie Sanford came out from Denver to visit the boys in blue:

> There are about 21 of the soldiers lying there . . . I went to all of the stores to find some dark green goods to make [eye]shades, but found none, so took my green silk parasol and made them. So I feel as if I had done something for my country.[62]

After the war, increasing Indian "troubles" resulted in a large part of the nation's peacetime army being stationed in the West. Its medical needs were provided by several hundred physicians, some regular army doctors, others civilian or "contract" doctors.[63] An applicant for a regular army position had to pass a rigorous examination to be eligible for the most junior position, assistant surgeon—the equivalent of first lieutenant. The successful applicant was likely to be stationed in some isolated post for a few years, with little opportunity to spend his $120 a month salary. In ten years, if he advanced to surgeon, his salary would jump to $215 a month. Still, in a country overpopulated with physicians, army appointments were coveted, and there were long waiting lists. While they waited, many applicants became "contract surgeons," civilian physicians employed by the army. In his reminiscences, Dr. B.J. Byrne recalled his days as a contract surgeon at Fort Lewis in southwestern Colorado. When his contract was up, he left the army "started a drugstore and put out my sign" in the nearby town of Cortez.[64]

In addition to the forts already mentioned, Colorado had Fort Sedgwick in the northeast near Julesburg (established 1860), Fort Lyon, when Fort Wise was renamed and relocated in 1867, Fort Reynolds east of Pueblo (1867), and Fort Crawford on the Uncompahgre south of Montrose (1880). Each of these facilities had a doctor and a hospital. The hospital, like the laundry and stables, was usually located away from the central facility.

Fort Sedgwick's hospital was fairly typical. The *Surgeon General's Report* of 1870 described it as

. . . adobe, L-shaped, 28 feet front by 100 feet deep, with a wing . . . 200 yards to the rear of the parade ground. [It contained] a ward of ten beds . . . , a dispensary, . . . no bath or wash-room and no water closet connected. It is warmed by stoves. The wing portion of the building was erected as a ward, but at present is occupied as the surgeon's quarters. The hospital, in size, is sufficient for a four-company post, but its construction is faulty; improvement in this particular has been sought but not yet accomplished.[65]

The same report described a much more elegant hospital at Fort Lyon—complete with an indoor bath room and water closet and a covered porch around the building.[65]

Regardless of whether he was an army or a contract surgeon, the post physician's duties were generally the same. He was responsible for the medical care of all personnel, as well as families and civilian employees. In remote areas he might be called upon to treat travelers, homesteaders, and even Indians. If he was fortunate, he had the assistance of a steward and, in the larger hospitals, of a wardmaster or nurse. Generally, the steward served as combination medic, nurse and orderly. The doctor was responsible for the daily sick call. This was an important job, the commanding officer expecting his doctor to be able to distinguish the malingerer from the truly ill and to provide a duty roster sufficient to carry out the post's military activities. The doctor ordered and procured the medical supplies (often a difficult task in some of the more isolated locations), kept financial records, and submitted a quarterly report to the surgeon general.

The physician was also in charge of public health at the fort—sanitation, food inspection, and the like—and was the post's weather man, keeping the meteorological records. Finally, the doctor, especially if he was an army man, was expected to share in some of the non-medical administrative duties of an officer—serving on courts martial, for example.

For many army doctors, like Dr. Peters, the major features of post life were tedium, boredom, and loneliness. They were isolated from the company of other physicians, away from intellectual stimulation, and subject to the regimentation and social mores of military life and to the frus-

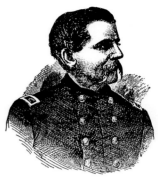

3.8 Dr. Peters complained of the boredom at Fort Massachusetts; however, he did meet Kit Carson there and later wrote the great scout's biography.

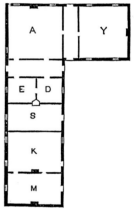

3.9 The hospital at Fort Sedgwick was fairly typical of a military hospital at a small post. It included a ward, dispensary, steward's room, kitchen, dining room, and surgeon's quarters

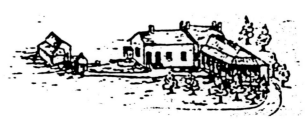

3.10 The hospital at Fort Lyon.

trations of the federal bureaucracy. Some sought solace in alcohol. Others took advantage of their surroundings and published a number of important studies on the natural history, geology, and Indian ethnology of the West. Dr. Elliot Coues, one of America's great ornithologists, did much of his early work while stationed at several western forts. Coues, in fact, seems to have paid much more attention to birds than to his patients, much to the chagrin of his commanding officers.[66]

Trauma was, of course, one of the major medical problems at the military posts. The other major problem was infectious disease. Prior to the Civil War, cholera and malaria had predominated in the western forts. Later, in addition to the usual nineteenth century litany of infectious diseases, including the perennial venereal diseases, military physicians had to deal with the consequences of inadequate sanitary conditions. Poor sanitation seems to have been a way of life at many military posts. At Fort Sedgwick, "offal and refuse material were conveyed some distance from the post and thrown on the prairie."[67] Fort Lyon, despite its modern hospital, had no sewage system. The excuse at Fort Lyon was that "the men detailed to ditch-digging would . . . fail to see the future benefits to be enjoyed . . ."[67] The surgeon general's report described the fort's water supply:

> Water is obtained from the Arkansas River, and is carried in water-tanks on wagons and daily distributed. The Arkansas water is very palatable [except] from April to August, when it has a great deal of mineral and organic matter . . . and affects some persons, causing diarrhea.[67]

Scurvy

Scurvy was a common problem in the western garrisons. Traditionally regarded as a disease of the open seas, it was equally common in any population whose diet was devoid of fruits and vegetables, and, as we now know, vitamin C.[68] In the West, this included some of the early explorers and the immigrants on the overland trails. With a diet consisting of "wild meats and about three ounces of hard bread per day," it is not surprising that the Long expedition suffered from the disease.[69] The mountain men and Indians appear to have been familiar with the antiscorbutic effects of wild onions, cactus juice, and berries. With his diet often limited to bacon, salted beef, biscuits, beans, grease, and coffee, however, the nineteenth century American soldier was a prime candidate for scurvy. This was especially true in the West where fruits and veg-

etables were scarce. Early on, the army was still using potash and citric acid as antiscorbutics, which they are not.[70] By the 1850s, the army was providing dried vegetables and urging post commanders to maintain vegetable gardens.

Colorado's forts were listed by the surgeon general as being susceptible to scurvy,[71] and Fort Garland's Dr. Peters ate pickles to prevent the disease.[72] When an outbreak of scurvy occurred at Fort Sedgwick, the doctor had those who were still well gather prickly pear cactus. After the spines were removed, the cactus was cooked into an "apple sauce" and fed to his scorbutic patients with good results.[73]

In 1875 the surgeon general reported that "at all posts where there are no company gardens, the officers are urged that vegetables . . . be added to the ration." Unfortunately, the report added, " [There] probably will always be a few posts to which it is impossible to furnish fresh vegetables . . ."[74] Not surprisingly, the soldiers resisted attempts to make them tend vegetable gardens and, besides, they preferred their bacon and hardtack to fruits and vegetables. Nevertheless, there must have been some success in implementing the antiscorbutic campaign at Fort Garland since only one case of scurvy was reported in a year.

Indian Wars

The medical routine of the Western military posts was periodically broken by the threat and, occasionally, by the reality of Indian attacks. The Indians were not foolhardy enough to attack the posts themselves. Typically they would fall upon a courier, a work crew, or a hunting or scouting party. The fort would respond by sending out a rescue party or a punitive expedition and sometimes a battle would result.

Arrow wounds were a specialty of the western army surgeon. Private John Cooley, Troop G, Third Cavalry, received an arrow wound on Purgatory Creek in October 1866. Cooley was fortunate; his wound was minor and he soon returned to duty. Three days later, another soldier in Troop G was herding horses near Fort Stevens when he was attacked.[75] Acting Assistant Surgeon Joseph Kugler reported the incident:

> An arrow entered the right side of the thorax between the first and second ribs. It was forcibly extracted by the patient, who stated that a great gush of blood followed. After being conveyed by ambulance over a rough mountain road, he was admitted to hospital at Fort Garland [six days later] in a very weak condition.[75]

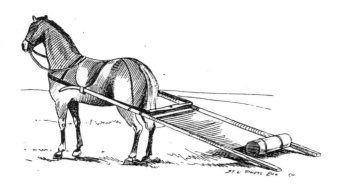

Dr. Kugler found that the soldier's right lung was collapsed and the pleural space was filled with blood. He applied "hot fomentations to the wound" and gave his patient "stimulating expectorants." Two months later "the effusion in the right pleural cavity was diminishing and air entered more freely into the lung." Four months after being wounded, the soldier was returned to duty.

Arrow wounds and their treatment were the subjects of several papers written by western army surgeons.[76] Flesh wounds were of little concern, except for the infections which might follow. Chest wounds, especially those which pierced the lung, were more serious and often fatal. Penetration of the intestine resulted in bacterial peritonitis and was almost always fatal. It was said that the Indians made an effort to score such "gut shots." An arrowhead impacted in bone was especially difficult to remove. After a skirmish near Fort Sedgwick in 1865, one soldier used a blacksmith's pliers to remove an arrow from the "hip bone" of his fellow.[77] Unfortunately, simply pulling on the shaft might break the arrow and leave the point. Since the shaft might be the only way of locating the point, it was often left in place during evacuation. Multiple hits were common, and it was not unusual to see a wounded soldier being brought in to the post with several two-to-three foot long arrows protruding from his body. The surgeon might then use any one of a number of recommended procedures to remove them, such as using a wire loop to snare the point.[78] Often, a direct approach was taken: "cut down upon the arrow-head and remove it with forceps—for the surgeon should not work in the dark."[79] Dr. Coues, the surgeon-ornithologist, noted a "tendency to despondency" among arrow wound victims. In dealing with such situations, he recommended that, "however serious the wound," the surgeon should "make light of it to the patient."[80]

While stationed at Fort Lewis in the early 1880s, Dr. Byrne treated "the last white man

shot with an arrow."[81] One evening, while the doctor was dressing for a game of whist with his fellow officers, the tent flap was suddenly thrown open. A wounded man was brought in, an arrow protruding from his chest. The arrowhead, having penetrated a lung, was wedged between the man's ribs. There was a howling storm that night, and the wind blowing into the tent made it impossible to keep the lamp lit. The doctor decided to wait until morning to operate, but when dawn came, the man was found dead. Dr. Byrne removed the portion of the chest wall containing the arrow and sent it to the Army Medical Museum in Washington, where it presumably remains.

During the Civil War the Cheyennes and Arapahoes increased their attacks on the plains. Mutilated bodies of travelers and homesteaders

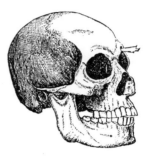

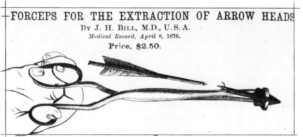

FORCEPS FOR THE EXTRACTION OF ARROW HEADS
By J. H. BILL, M.D., U.S.A.
Medical Record, April 8, 1876.
Price, $2.50.

3.11 The army adopted the Indians' travois to transport wounded men.

3.12 Arrow wounds were a major topic of medical interest on the frontier.

3.13 This arrow extractor was designed by Surgeon J.H. Bill, author of a major paper on the treatment of arrow wounds.

3.14 "Too late." Note the two-to-three foot long arrows.

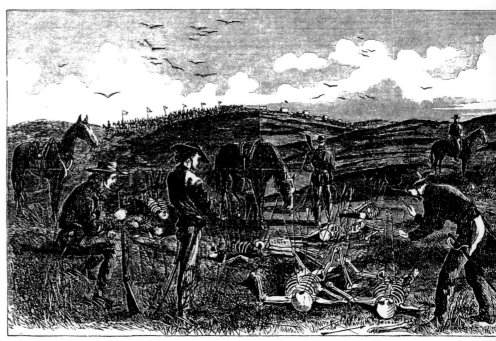

were being brought into Denver, and there were rumors of an impending attack on the city itself. A body of volunteer militia was hastily assembled and, accompanied by a few regular troops, marched out under the command of a minister-soldier, Colonel John Chivington, to punish the hostiles. At Sand Creek, they surprised several hundred Cheyennes in camp, attacked, and slaughtered them. Most were women and children. Variously designated a "battle" or a "massacre," Sand Creek has been the subject of debate for more than a century, and it will undoubtedly continue to be so. A congressional investigation revealed that wounded Indians had been killed and bodies mutilated, and Chivington was eventually censured.[82] The hearings also included a few items of medical interest, especially the testimony of Assistant Surgeon Caleb S. Birdsal. Dr. Birdsal reported that he treated thirty-eight wounded soldiers, some of whom had been shot by their own fellows in the chaos. The doctor converted some of the Cheyenne lodges into hospital tents, and his time "was occupied that day and night and the next day caring for the wounded." There is no comment as to the nature of the soldiers' wounds. He did note that he had no blankets to cover the wounded (the battle was in late November) and that he had to requisition some from an Indian trader. One justification for the attack was that the camp had contained some of the Indian marauders. A number of scalps were found in the Cheyenne lodges, and Surgeon Birdsal was asked to state his opinion as to whether they had been taken from whites and whether they had been taken recently. He replied that some of the scalps were from white persons and that "one or two of them were not more than ten days off of the head." As to the treatment of wounded Indians, there was little for Dr. Birdsal to do. The few wounded Indians were carried off by their comrades, some of them dying away from the battlefield and, therefore, not included in Chivington's body count of four or five hundred. Nine soldiers had been killed.

In 1868 the Cheyennes, Arapahoes, and Sioux were still attacking settlers, railroad workers, and travelers on the plains. The army chased them, but the Indians refused to stay put and engage in conventional warfare. On August 29, 1868, the army tried an experiment. Fifty irregular troops, scouts, trappers, and hunters were sent out on the equivalent of a Viet Nam "search and destroy" mission. Under the command of Major George Forsyth and with Lieutenant F.H. Beecher and Surgeon John H. Mooers, the party left Fort Wallace, Kansas, and headed

west into Colorado. A little more than two weeks later, they found their quarry south of present-day Wray, Colorado. Forsyth and his men had stumbled on an encampment of several thousand Indians. Soon discovered, the soldiers beat a hasty retreat to a sandbar in the middle of nearly dry Arickaree Fork.[83]

Lieutenant Beecher was among the first to die, bequeathing his name to "The Battle of Beecher Island." Major Forsyth was wounded three times. The first was a flesh wound in his right thigh, "the most painful wound I have ever received." This was soon followed by a bullet through his left leg, "breaking and shattering the bone midway between the leg and ankle." Finally, he recalled,

> A bullet struck me just on the top of my soft felt hat . . . knocked me almost senseless . . . and a large bump swelled up almost at once. I took little heed of the intense headache that for a short time half blinded me. A month later the surgeon's probe disclosed the fact that my skull had been fractured and he removed a loose piece of it.[84]

The major was in the same pit as Doctor Mooers. The doctor had "been doing splendid service with his rifle" and had just shot another Indian. Forsyth recalled that as the Indian fell dead, the surgeon remarked, "That rascally redskin will not trouble us again." The next thing the major heard was

> the peculiar thud that tells the breaking of bone by a bullet. Turning to the doctor, I saw him put his hand to his head, saying "I'm hit" . . . I saw at once that there was no hope. A bullet had entered his forehead, just over the eye, and the wound was mortal. He never spoke another rational word, but lingered three days before dying.[84]

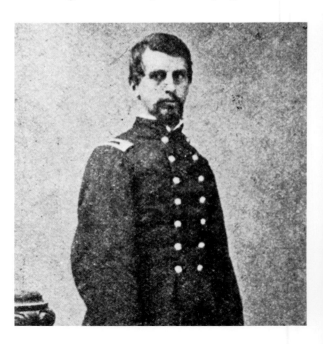

3.15 Dr. Mooers was among the first to die in the Battle of Beecher Island.

On the third day, Major Forsyth managed to send a courier to Fort Wallace. By then there were two more dead, eight badly wounded and ten slightly wounded—out of his original command of fifty men. In his plea for help, he noted: "My surgeon having been mortally wounded, none of my wounded men have had their wounds dressed yet, so please bring out a surgeon with you." The wounded included "Howard Morton [who] lost one of his eyes by a bullet that lodged just behind it, but wrapped a handkerchief around his head and fought on steadily."[84] Another man had an arrow point lodged squarely in his frontal bone. It was dislodged "when a bullet ploughed across his forehead . . . the two falling together to the ground. He wrapped a rag round his head and, though covered with blood, fought to the very close . . . ."[84]

As the days wore on, the situation on the sandbar grew worse. The summer heat and insects, the delirious cries of the wounded and the taunts of the Indians, the sickening stench of decay (animals as well as men had been killed), and the hunger, thirst, and fear were enough to have depressed even John Wayne.

The bullet embedded in Forsyth's thigh was causing him a great deal of pain. His surgeon dead, the major

> appealed to several of the men to cut it out, but as soon as they saw how close it lay to the artery, they declined . . . However, I determined that it should come out, as I feared sloughing, and then the artery would probably break anyway; so, taking the razor from my saddle pocket, and getting two of the men to press the adjacent flesh back and draw it taut, I managed to cut it out myself . . .[84]

Finally, after nine days, the cavalry arrived. The rescue party included Dr. J. A. Fitzgerald.

The doctor must have been awed by the medical problems he faced, not the least of which was Major Forsyth's shattered leg. From the sound of the injury it is surprising that the doctor did not amputate on the spot—that certainly would have been the case a few years before on any Civil War battlefield. Instead, Dr. Fitzgerald cut down the only tree on the sandbar, a young cottonwood, stripped the bark, lined a section of it with cloth, and, as the Major later recalled,

> placed my shattered leg in it. In that way I rode in an ambulance over a hundred miles to Fort Wallace. Here we met Surgeon Morris J. Asch . . . and it was owing to the unremitting care and splendid surgical ability of these two officers that I am now alive.[84]

In 1879, this time in western Colorado, a medical-military event reminiscent of the Battle of Beecher Island occurred. Major Thomas Thornburgh and his troopers were on their way to rescue the Meekers and other whites at White River Agency when they were surrounded by a band of Utes. Thornburgh was killed and, although he himself was wounded, Surgeon R.B. Grimes managed to care for the other forty-three wounded soldiers until their rescue.[85]

When we hear about army doctors in the old West, we tend to think about alcoholics and misfits. In that light, Major Forsyth's comments, made after many years of military service and long after the Battle of Beecher Island, are worth noting. In terse military prose, the old soldier commented:

> I wish here to put on record my unqualified admiration of the medical department of the U.S. Army. The ability, training and devotion to duty of these officers is worthy of all praise.[86]

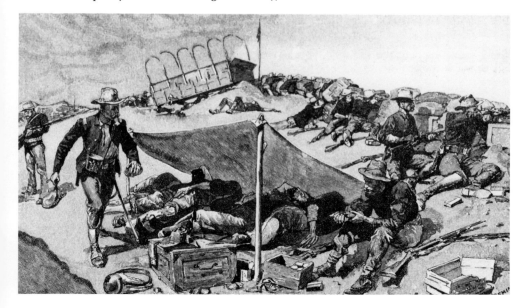

3.16 Surgeon R.B. Grimes was kept busy treating more than forty wounded soldiers trapped by the Utes in 1879.

4 GOLD FEVER

Those who had [gold] fever took a relapse, and they had it bad. It was a raging epidemic, and spread faster than the cholera in Egypt.

A.P. Hill, 1884[1]

IN THE 1850s, WITH THE exception of a few small Hispanic settlements in the lower San Luis Valley and an occasional trading post or military garrison, Colorado's only inhabitants were the Ute, Cheyenne, and Arapaho Indians. In 1858 there was a dramatic change. That winter, some intinerant prospectors found a few flecks of gold in Cherry Creek, in the vicinity of what is now downtown Denver. Word of the discovery soon went east, and the following spring saw a huge migration of of fortune seekers, on foot and horseback, by stage and wagon, wending their way across Kansas and Nebraska to what had become known as the Pike's Peak diggings. In all, it has been estimated that one hundred thousand people left their homes and headed for Colorado. Some had barely started out when word came back along the trail that the whole thing was a "bust," that the little bit of gold in the creek had been harvested, and there was no more. Thousands of disappointed overlanders returned to their homes, many before they had even come close to the mountains. Then, there was new word. True, there was little gold to be found in Cherry Creek, but not far beyond, in the mountains, gold had been found in abundance. All that was needed was a pan or a pick and shovel, some pluck, and a little luck in the new diggings. There were Russell and Gregory gulches near Central City, Jackson's Bar near Idaho Springs, the hills above Georgetown, and, for the truly adventur-

ous, the more distant camps in California Gulch near present-day Leadville and in South Park. At least that was the story being circulated by word of mouth, by eastern newspapers, and by the merchants in trailhead towns in Missouri and Kansas. The first wave of emigrants had crested high and ebbed quickly; the second was the beginning of a migration that would last for decades, even as the deep ruts of wagon wheels were replaced by steel tracks.

Most of the fifty-niners were unprepared for the arduous and difficult journey across the plains. The more than seven hundred miles between the last supply points in western Missouri and eastern Kansas and the terminus at Denver City alternated between bitter cold and searing heat. They were devoid of shelter and stingy in their supply of water and nourishment. Incidents of cannibalism were reported. Under the best of circumstances a traveler might make the trip in a month; a loaded wagon would take much longer. Malnutrition, dehydration, heatstroke, frostbite, accidents, even such exaggerated dangers as rattlesnakes and Indian attacks, all added to the normally high toll of nineteenth century disease.[2] For the men, women and children who made the slow, laborious passage it was truly "survival of the fittest."

Dr. Charles Clark was one of many physicians who crossed the plains in those early days. At the age of twenty-five, Clark had left Chicago and joined a party heading for Colorado's goldfields. Young, healthy, and relatively well prepared for the journey, the doctor was shocked to find that many of his fellow travelers were

> of a different stripe [and] not fitted for the undertaking. Some had come from the enclosures of a shop or office, with physical powers far below the ordinary standard . . . unprepared for the hardships of crossing the plains. There were some even in the decadence of life—men decrepit with the burden of years, with shrinking muscles and shaking nerves, who were tottering on to the gold fields.[3]

At the other end of the spectrum were the infants and children. One traveler sent this example of gold fever to his hometown newspaper:

> The man was driving an overloaded wagon, while the woman was hauling their sick child in a hand-cart, carrying the medicine in her hands. In their hurry to reach the land of gold they could not stop long enough for their invalid offspring to recover its shattered health.[4]

Another overland physician, Dr. George Willing, was amazed at the large number of women on the trail, commenting, " How they make out is a marvel to me. It is hard enough on a man."[5] He encountered a young woman, who, widowed two days before, "was brought to bed of a baby. I never witnessed such distress in my life, and pray I never may again." On the trail a week later, the doctor

> passed a little hillock of sand by the roadside. Beneath it are the remains of the little infant . . . it died yesterday, of starvation, I fear, for it never nursed and no proper food could be procured for it. Another sorrow for its unfortunate young mother.[5]

In 1859 nearly a score of guidebooks were published to assist the gold seeker over the trails to the Pike's Peak diggings. They tended to paint a rosy picture for the prospective traveler. Kan-

sas and Nebraska, through which the overland trails passed for much of their way, were, according to Redpath and Hinton's guidebook, "pronounced by pioneers to be the healthiest of Western countries."[6] Another guidebook, Gunn's, described Kansas' climate as "one of the healthiest to be found on this continent."[7] Dr. Willing, who unlike many of the guidebook authors, had actually crossed the plains, offered an opinion which was both succinct and contrary: "The boasted healthfulness of the plains I hold to be humbug."[8] Dr. Clark's opinion was similar, though more detailed:

> Sickness often visited the emigrant. The prevailing diseases were bilious fever, which often assumed a typhoid character, pleurisy, pneumonia and scurvy, besides there were many other incidental ailments which were excited into action by exposures, insufficient and improper food and over-exertion. . . . Diarrhoea and dysentery were prevalent.[9]

The guidebooks offered all sorts of advice on food. Although generally more attuned to the preservation of food than to nutrition, several of the guidebooks did recommend the inclusion of dried fruit or pickles to prevent scurvy.[10] Reed's guidebook warned the traveler against any temptation to gorge himself on buffalo meat: "I would advise you, from sad experience, to commence the use of it very gradually, as it is almost sure to create a diarrhea when used to excess."[11]

Milk was an especially valuable commodity on the overland journey. One traveler noted that "many of the emigrants yoke in milch cows with their oxen . . . providing themselves with a rare luxury, for even in the border towns . . . milk commands 40 cents a gallon, while whiskey sells at 22 cents."[12] The desire for milk led to some interesting entrepreneurial endeavors. One traveler reported a "wagon, drawn by six cows, bearing the label, in flaming characters, 'Female Express—Milk for Sale'."[13] A frontier newspaper reported that

> Messrs. Jones and Russell [of Leavenworth, Kansas] . . . sent out . . . eighty milk cows, with all the appliances for an entire dairy at each station along the road.[14]

Water was a serious problem on the trail. Not only was it scarce, but what water there was was often unpalatable. One fifty-niner wrote that upon finally reaching the Platte:

> My throat was so dry and swollen that I could not drink at first . . . but I kept trying, and at last succeeded. I thought it the best water I ever had

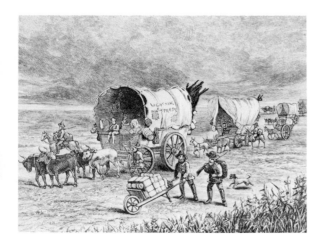

4.1 Most of the 1859 guide books provided little medical advice to the gold seekers.

tasted. I dream of it in ecstasy to this day. It did not rob us of a bit of the satisfaction when we discovered . . . it was full of dead and decaying buffalo.[15]

The guidebooks were inconsistent in their advice about drinking prairie water. Redpath and Hinton noted that

> little pools collect in different places, which although the surface is green, are perfectly healthy and afford refreshing water in the hottest months.[16]

But Marcy warned that

> water taken from stagnant pools, charged with putrid vegetable matter and animalculae would be very likely to generate fevers and dysenteries if taken into the stomach without purification.[17]

Marcy suggested a number of ways by which the traveler might purify such scummy water, e.g. through the use of charcoal or the leaves of the prickly pear cactus.

Neither author, however, realized that the source of disease was not the algae or other visible materials which made such water unpleasant but the invisible and as yet undiscovered bacteria which made even the most pellucid water potentially lethal. The usual sources for the microorganisms of typhoid and dysentery were human excrement, and since the basic principles of sanitation were of little interest to the gold seekers, such "filth" diseases were common on the overland trails. An 1860 traveler's diary describes a typical scene:

> We passed a handcart party of four men. Three of them were drawing the cart containing their whole outfit and the fourth member of the company, quite low with dysentery. Mr. Hopkins—a merchant from Dubuque . . . died of the same disease . . . and was buried by the roadside . . . seventy-five miles east [of Denver].[18]

A member of Dr. Willing's party, a Mr. Alexander from Missouri, having died of "bilious fever," came even closer to his destination and was buried "beneath the shadow of the Peak he had toiled so anxiously to reach."[19] Dr. Clark commented:

> Seldom a day passed that we did not see one or more graves beside the road. They were often visited by the traveler—flinging a shadow o'er his heart, and reminding him that Death held his court there as well as in the crowded city.[20]

Other hazards were to be found on the trail. Having taken the southern route, Dr. Willing was subjected to "hordes of mosquitoes" which he found to be in "incredible numbers and fero-

4.2 Deaths and impromptu funerals were common on the overland trail.

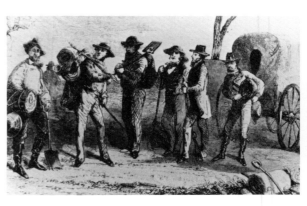

ciously savage. Smoke is my only protection," he complained, "and a pipe my sole consolation."[21] Marcy warned that although "it is seldom that any person is bitten by [rattlesnakes] . . . this is a possible contingency, and it can never be amiss to have an antidote at hand." Although he recommended the classical approach—ligate above the bite, incise the puncture sites, and "suck out the poison, spitting out the saliva," and such remedies as hartshorn and cedron—he commented: "Of all the remedies known to me, I should decidedly prefer ardent spirits. It is considered a sovereign antidote among our Western frontier settlers . . ."[22]

Far more common than rattlesnake bites were accidents of various kinds, particularly from firearms. Wary of Indian and fellow traveler alike, the overlander tended to keep his gun near at hand. Tierney's guidebook cautioned

> emigrants against the dangerous practice of placing a loaded gun, with the cap on, in any of their wagons. More accidents occur on the plains from this practice than from any other[23]

Marcy, noting "that the chief causes of accidents from the use of firearms arise from carelessness," reminded the traveler, "Always look to your gun, but never let your gun look at you."[24] One unfortunate overlander did not heed this sound advice, having

> accidentally shot himself through the hand in pulling his rifle out of the wagon muzzle foremost . . . The wound had reached the gangrene stage, and they halted [our party] to ask surgical aid from our doctor.[25]

For the seriously ill or injured traveler, an "ambulance" such as the one which carried Dr. William Street's wife across the plains, could be used. Actually, Dr. Street's ambulance was a wagon fitted with springs, "fitted up to be very comfortable and . . . drawn by two large horses."[26] For a party "without ambulances or wagons," Marcy's guidebook provided specific instructions on the construction and use of horse litters, hand litters, and what must have been

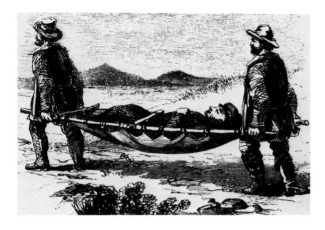

the most uncomfortable conveyence ever devised by man, the Indian's horse-drawn travois.[27] The last was essentially a litter, "one end [of which] is made fast to the sides of the animal, while the other end is left to trail upon the ground," subjecting the victim to every bone-jarring undulation of the trail.

The few guidebooks that suggested a medicine kit were quite conservative in their recommendations. Parson's guidebook, for example, proposed that "a few simple medicines, such as any physician might direct, would be convenient."[28] Nevertheless, according to Dr. Clark:

> Every man had a package of drugs and nostrums, with written directions for use, sometimes consisting of blue pill, a little ipecac and opium, together with a bottle of peppermint, pain killer and somebody's sovereign remedy for all ills.[29]

Dr. Clark was concerned about the availability of such medications to "those who are totally ignorant of their nature and of the indications that call for their use" and advised " all who contemplate taking this trip to leave . . . drugs behind."[29]

Drs. Willing, Clark, and Street were but three of the many doctors who came overland in those early days. When all was well among his party or wagon-train, the overland physician's day might be just as mundane as that of his non-medical companions. On such a day, Willing wrote in his diary: "Have been variously employed during the day, doctoring cattle, mess-furniture, and bed clothes. Can't say which were most benefited by my skill."[30] On the other hand, a doctor's medical talents were often needed but, as Dr. Clark noted:

> The services of a doctor could not at all times be obtained [on the trail]. Although there were many of the profession en route, they were continually on the move, like the rest, and it was difficult to tell where to find them.[31]

The Gold Fields

The doctors were in as much of a hurry to get to the gold fields as everyone else. Once there they found prospecting and mining to be tedious, backbreaking, and generally unrewarding. They also found large numbers of fellow physicians. One doctor's experience was probably typical: "Having tried mining, he found that it was hard work . . . and he'd be d----d if he wasn't going back where he could practice medicine for a living."[32]

Descriptions of the earliest mining camps provide an interesting paradox—unhealthy living conditions and healthy inhabitants. Gunn's 1859 guidebook states that "reports from the gold mines all concur in saying that among the miners sickness is literally unknown."[33]

Many of the early immigrants were impressed with the salubrious effects of Colorado's climate. One newcomer wrote home: "I think the country is remarkably healthy. I have not been ill an hour since I left home."[34] Another remarked on the women and children in a camp near the Gregory diggings: "They all appear . . . thanks to this salubrious air, to be endowed with excellent health."

Dr. Clark was one of those who soon found "a miner's life to be a hard and laborious one." At work, he complained, miners were subjected to "constant exposure to heat and cold [and] standing in mud and water to their knees." When not working, the miner "lived in a tent or rude shanty." His bed consisted of a "blanket or two on the ground, or on a frame of poles." Meals were a monotonous fare of "pan-cakes, made from flour and water, with the addition of a little soda and cream tartar, a strip or two of fried bacon, and a cup of tea or coffee." Under such conditions, Clark found that the previously healthy miners would "soon lose a portion of their constitutional stability" and would soon be "suffering often from sickness."[35]

Despite Colorado's dry climate, the miner often found himself soaking wet. He was warned, "when your work is finished, your clothing is . . . saturated with moisture, either from water or perspiration [and] you feel chilled, cold and eventually, more or less rheumatic."[37] Joint pains, or "rheumatism," was one of the most common complaints. Those who worked the gold fields near Idaho Springs made use of the springs to relieve their aching joints. Doctors were of little help, although one prospector, Luke Tierney, provided a testimonial for a Dr. Wilcox (who "practically" cured him of

4.3 Marcy's guidebook did provide some medical information—including suggestions on medical evacuation.

rheumatism) in the pages of the *Rocky Mountain News*.[38] The mysterious "mountain fever," discussed later in this chapter, was much feared in the camps. Pneumonia was another common problem and was ascribed to dampness, cold, and the high altitude. Eventually, pneumonia replaced mountain fever as the bane of the mining camps. In addition, the miners brought with them diseases which they had acquired "back home"—malaria, venereal diseases, tuberculosis, and other chronic infectious diseases. Accidents were frequent. A misjudged blow from a hammer or pick, a flying particle lodged in a miner's eye, a delayed blast from black powder—these were just a few of the potentials for serious injury or death.

Even more important, perhaps, as the camps grew and their populations increased, sanitary conditions progressively deteriorated. Marcy warned about the harmful "effect of crowding men together in close quarters," so clearly demonstrated in faraway "Hindostan."[38] Dr. Clark found the diggings at Gregory Gulch to be

> surrounded by dirt and filth that is constantly accumulating, and which, in some localities that I have seen, is breeding disease and propagating vermin.[39]

There were serious outbreaks of typhoid and other "filth" diseases. The *Mountaineer*, a mining camp newspaper, reported such an outbreak in 1860: "Typhoid fever of a peculiarly obstinate and malignant species is quite prevalent in both the diggings and the valleys."[40]

No longer could it be said that "the water of the creeks in the mining region is pure, sweet, and wholesome."[41] Not only were there pathogenic bacteria in the water, there must have large quantities of minerals as well. In addition, there was concern over mercury poisoning. Mercury was used to separate native gold from other particulate matter. In Central City, the miners' demand for mercury had, according to one wag, driven up the price of calomel, a mercury-containing medication used to treat syphilis and other illnesses.[42] Mercury poisoning was a real concern, however, and Burt and Berthoud, in a chapter entitled, "Chemistry for the Gold Miner," warned that "care is taken that the fumes of the mercury do not escape, since they may produce salivation and other distressing symptoms."

Some attempts were made to institute rudiments of public health into the early mining camps. The *Laws and Regulations of Clear Creek's Union District* warned that "any person who shall cause any nuisance affecting the health of the people . . . shall be sued for the same in the miner's court."[44] In the Nevada District near Central City, a person could be fined for fouling the water, e.g. by slaughtering an animal within a mile of a stream.[45] Such laws, although well intentioned, were difficult to enforce. These men had endured terrible hardships in their search for gold, and they were not about to be distracted by some namby-pamby rules and regulations. They had not come west to be told where they could "take a ----." Thus, as in the Gregory Gulch diggings:

> Men became utterly indifferent to their personal appearance. There was no system, no rules, no discipline to enforce comparative cleanliness. The camp work was done hurriedly, carelessly . . . with the result of extreme untidiness—if so mild a term can be construed to present the actual condition . . . In any other part of the world, the abuses committed by the heedless multitude . . . would have brought a pestilence . . .[46]

A painful, if not a serious consequence of such living conditions, was described by Dr. Clark. A party of miners were sitting arround their campfire—occasionally scratching.

> At every bite one would reach for the invader . . . bringing out a big louse about the size of a grain of wheat, casting it away while he kept on talking. The sight was one calculated to disturb a healthy stomach . . . yet it was one extremely common in the mountains . . . for the reason that men pay so little attention to personal cleanliness, going from week to week without ablution or changing their clothes.[47]

Mountain Fever

Mountain fever was the mystery disease of the early mining camps. To this day we aren't sure of the nature of mountain fever, or whether the term referred to one disease or several. Whatever it was, mountain fever was regarded as a serious problem. In 1859 Henry Villard, visiting the diggings, reported that "the so-called mountain fever [claimed] many victims and caused many more to abandon their work and seek the plains."[48] The following year, Dr. Clark found the camps near Central City to be

> the locality of much sickness, the endemic malady, mountain fever, prevailing to considerable extent. At the time we passed through, there were several persons lying dangerously ill with it, and one or two had died the day previous.[49]

Villard ascribed mountain fever to "intense rainfall and excessive moisture [which], together with general exposure, scanty and ill-prepared food, the free use of bad water and worse whisky," all resulted in a "disease of typhoid character."[50] A relationship to typhoid was also suggested by a mining camp newspaper in 1860:

> The "mountain fever," as it is termed for want of a more specific name, is somewhat prevalent . . . In all but a few instances, it has assumed a typhoid form.[51]

These outbreaks may, indeed, have been typhoid. An apparently different disease was described as mountain fever by Dr. Irving J. Pollok, one of Colorado's earliest medical pioneers.[52] In 1860 Pollak encountered what he diagnosed as mountain fever in McNulty's Gulch, a mining camp above 11,000 feet in the Ten Mile District, not far from present day Kokomo. The miners had brought a number of dogs and cats with them to the camp. Within three months, after a mysterious illness characterized by constipation and "tetany," all of the pets had died. Dr. Pollak autopsied the animals, but all he could find were some focal areas of intestinal inflammation. Soon afterward, a similar disease began to appear among the men, women, and children of the area. Dr. Pollak described the clinical picture in a miner,

> a young man [who] complained of obstinate constipation and abdominal pains. He was found nearly helpless and was brought down [from the mine] . . . Spasms of the voluntary muscles and and tetanic symptoms appeared. I found a doughy abdomen, pulse 90 and feeble, tongue furred with a milky white coating, vomiting constant, and a haggard expression, with a cramping of the muscles of the lower extremities and back.[52]

Pollak's treatment consisted of

> an infusion of sinipsis thrown up the rectum through a . . . tube, passed up as far as possible. I found in passing up the tube it met with a resistance as if the gut was filled with soft putty, or pushing the tube through a loaf of unbaked bread.[52]

The doctor suspected that mountain sickness might have been due to lead poisoning. The camp's drinking water was obtained from melting snow which ran in rivulets through ground rich in lead-bearing ore. Another consideration was the altitude and, after the death of a thirteen year old, Pollak advised the populace to move down the gulch to the Arkansas River valley. The camp's women and children followed the doctor's advice and had no further problem with mountain fever. The men, however, chose to remain near the mines and continued to suffer from the disease, even after changing their water supply. The next winter a number of sick miners had to be carried out by "a party on sledges and snow-shoes." Two of them died soon afterward.

By the early 1870s, Pollok had moved to the Clear Creek Mining District. He soon found that here, too, there were "many and persistent cases" of mountain fever. When forty miners came down with the disease at the Stevens Mine near Montezuma, the miners renamed the disease "Stevens gripes." Another outbreak occurred at the nearby Belmont mine at an altitude above 13,000 feet. The prevalence of the disease made it difficult to recruit miners, the owners were becoming desperate, and "the frequency of patients seeking aid . . . again called my [Pollak's] especial investigation for the cause . . ." He soon eliminated one possibility when he found that

> the sources of drinking water were different in the Stevens and Belmont outbreaks, a spring in one case and melted snow in the other. Pollak analyzed the water supplies for lead, found inconsequential levels, and discounted his earlier theory. He found that the recently employed [were] as liable [to develop mountain fever] as men at work longer— the top or surface miners no more exempt than the deep shaft worker, the abstemious and the toper alike affected.[52]

Finally, Pollak noted, "I have seen no case of this disease that orginated below timberline." Noting that "almost everyone who has crossed our mountain ranges [has] experienced exhilirating effects, something akin to the effects of a brandy sling," he proposed that the cause of mountain sickness might be the altitude and dryness of the mining camps.

Mountain fever continued to be diagnosed in the mining camps, but some physicians began to question the its diagnostic validity. Dr. David Dougan, a physician in Leadville, was quoted in 1886:

> The term mountain fever has, by long-continued and frequent use, almost established itself in the nomenclature of disease in the mountain districts . . . Whether or not its use is proper as designating a separate and distict type of fever, a pathologic entity, may well be questioned.[53]

Towards the end of the century, most physicians had come to regard mountain fever as a variant of typhoid or even of a postulated "typho-malarial" fever,[54] and by the turn of the century a paper entitled, "Mountain Fever, So Called," pretty much laid the issue to rest.[55] If mountain fever did, indeed, exist as a distinct disease, it appears to have disappeared, and it is unlikely that we will ever know its true nature.

Digging Doctors[56]

Most of the gold rush doctors came to Colorado, not to practice medicine, but to find gold. Not unexpectedly, the majority had to fall back on their profession when gold proved hard to find. One doctor wrote home from the "Spanish Diggins" near Idaho Springs "I believe I make more practicing medicine than in mining. I make no prescription for less than $5 and if I give medicine from $8 to $10."[57] Another doctor reported that his fees had been paid in gold dust, nuggets, buffalo skins, dried venison, jerked buffalo, and bear meat.[58]

An early visitor to the mining camps commented on the large number of physicians. In response to the question, "Who should go?" to the Pike's Peak gold regions, Henry Villard answered:

> Common laborers are likely to be in good demand, merchants are likely to find a lucrative opening, [but] doctors are already plentifully supplied and not much demanded.[59]

Dr. Clark found the medical profession well represented in the camps. Although many of the immigrant doctors had "thrown physic to the dogs, having served an unappreciative public,"

> others, with an eye to practice, had their names inscribed in big letters on their establishment—the ominous M.D. having a two-fold significance, not

only implying that he was a Doctoris Medicinae, but that "Money Down" was required.[60]

The first of Colorado's "digging" doctors was Levi J. Russell. Levi and his brothers Green and Oliver had been raised in the gold mining district of northwestern Georgia. After he and his brothers had spent a couple of years prospecting in California, Levi decided on a more dependable livelihood. He graduated from medical school in 1856, but two years later, he and his brothers were again searching for gold. By June of 1858, the brothers were in Colorado, panning Cherry Creek. Levi helped build the first cabin in the townsite of Auraria, later incorporated into what became downtown Denver. He was also listed as a physician in Denver's first business directory.[61] As Cherry Creek's gold gave out, the brothers moved to the nearby mountains. They soon made one of the big strikes of the early days, Russell Gulch near Central City. With the coming of the Civil War, the Russells' Confederate loyalties brought them back to Georgia. They never returned to Colorado. Years later, another pioneer recalled Levi as "a peculiarly winning kind of man . . . gentle, humane, kindly . . . and quiet in his ways, but who could be positive and determined enough when necessary. All of us liked him."[62] For six years Levi practiced medicine in his home state. In 1868 he moved to Texas, where he farmed, doctored, and raised a family. He retired to Arizona, where he died in 1908.[63]

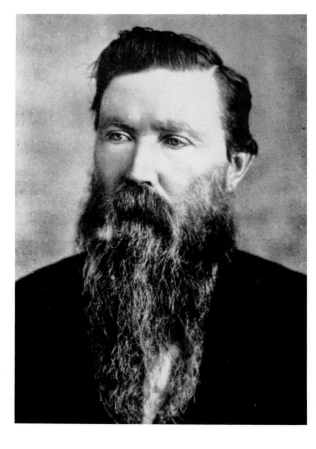

4.4 Dr. Levi Russell in his later years.

4.5 The Russells' cabin also served as Dr. Levi's office—the first doctor's office in Denver.

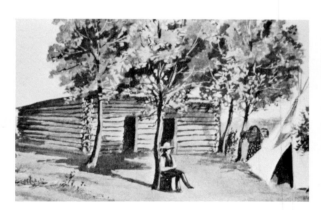

Unlike Drs. Clark, Willing, and Russell, all of whom left the territory, some of the digging doctors remained in Colorado. Dr. Pollok, whom we encountered in our discussion of mountain fever, hadn't even planned to come to Colorado. He was a member of a party of English sportsmen hunting on the plains in 1858 when the group encountered the Russell brothers. The brothers, on their way to Colorado, pursuaded Pollok to join them. During the next few years, Pollok prospected in Russell Gulch. Later, he left the Russells and moved to California and Mosquito Gulches (where, as we have seen, he investigated mountain fever), served in the territorial legislature, and, when the Civil War broke out, joined the Second Colorado Cavalry as its surgeon. In 1869 he married and moved to Georgetown, where he remained to practice medicine.[64]

Another early physician, Dr. John Parsons, came to South Park in 1859 to prospect. Parsons did not distinguish himself as either a doctor or a miner but established a mint in the mining camp of Tarryall. For two years, while the South Park camps were booming, Parsons' mint turned out gold coins which are now among the most coveted of collector's pieces. As the camp declined, Parsons moved to Denver and, over the next two decades, engaged in a variety of business, agricultural, and mining enterprises.[65]

The dual role of the physician-miner was stated clearly and succinctly on Dr. A.F. Peck's professional card. Published in the *Rocky Mountain News* on April 23, 1859, (the newspaper's very first issue), the advertisement stated that the doctor might be found at Cache la Poudre "when not professionally engaged or digging gold."[66] Peck was said to have been staked to his Colorado venture by another kind of bonanza. Back in Omaha, he had been asked to perform an autopsy on a horse thief who had been lynched. In addition to the man's broken neck, the doctor's major finding was $300—in the horsethief's pocket. This was, apparently, Dr. Peck's first and last success in finding gold.[67]

A. F. PECK, M. D.

PHYSICIAN AND SURGEON,

Cache-a-La-Poudre, Nebraska.

WHERE he may at all times be found when not professionally engaged or digging gold.

n1tf

Searching for gold could be dangerous. Dr. J.L. Shank and his party of prospectors were killed by Indians in South Park.[68] In 1860 Dr. E.A. Arnold, a Harvard graduate and president of the Territorial Council of Colorado, joined a group of prospectors from Mountain City. Their scalped and mutilated bodies were found several days later.[69] Most of the physicians remained within the relative safety of the mining camps

or nearby towns. There they practiced some medicine, did a little prospecting nearby, and, perhaps, found some other work in order to make ends meet. Dr. C. A. Roberts of Mountain City (near Central City) was a mining claim adjustor and recorder, prosecuting attorney, and for a while editor of the *Central City Gold Reporter*.[70] One pioneer physician recalled some of his early colleagues. In Black Hawk and Central City there were:

> Dr. Reed, the Indian missionary, with his little drug store, . . . and Dr. H.W. Allen . . . conducting a drug store and practicing medicine. Drs. Judd and Toll were further up the gulch above Gregory Point. Near [the mining supply town of] Boulder Dr. Goodwin . . . practiced from . . . his ranch [while] Dr. Gurney was a kind of peripatetic . . . making his home wherever night overtook him.[71]

The miner's attitude toward doctors might be described as mixed—and was probably not very different from that of the rest of society. Lawrence N. Greenleaf, Colorado pioneer and poet, expressed his feelings in 1868:

> A myriad shams, on every hand we see;
> Doctors grow rich although they disagree.
> While one prescribes a liberal dose for all,
> That of another is minutely small.
> One showers with water, packs in ice;
> Another calls this practice an enormous vice;
> One lets you eat whate'er your palate craves;
> Unless you nearly starve another raves . . .
> Betwixt the doctors, doses large and small
> The wonder is, that we survive at all![72]

In the more remote camps, a sick or injured miner might die alone, away from the care of a physician and the love of a family. One pioneer recalled:

> How often in my own experience in the mining camps I have seen men die far away from the tender and loving care of mother, wife, and sister.[73]

The few women in the camps often provided the only medical care available. Long before he became Colorado's leading silver king, H.A.W. and Augusta Tabor lived in several different primitive mining camps. During their stay at Payne's Bar, near present day Idaho Springs, Mrs. Tabor cared for a miner who had come down with mountain fever:

> For four weeks he lay, very ill, at the door of our tent in a wagon bed, I acting as physician and nurse. A miner with a gunshot wound . . . was also brought to my door for attention.[74]

The same year, 1859, "Aunt" Clara Brown, a black woman, settled in Central City. She often

4.6 Dr. Peck's professional card appeared in the first issue of the *Rocky Mountain News*, April 23, 1859.

[]

nursed the sick miners, worked as a midwife, and even turned her home into a makeshift hospital on occasion.[75]

Central City's Hospital

There were no hospitals in the early mining camps. The seriously ill or injured miner would recover or die in his cabin or perhaps, in a room in a boarding house or the doctor's home. In 1868 Central City's Catholic priest, Father Riverty, recognizing the need for a hospital in the growing mining camp, called for a donation of $10 from each of its citizens.[76] He was unsuccessful and, although Bishop Machebeuf continued to give consideration to the project, the Church ultimately decided to build its first hospital in Denver.[77]

A more successful effort was made by Central City's Episcopalians. In 1870 they opened St. Luke's Hospital "for the care of the sick and afflicted without regard to creed, color, nationality, age, sex or *former life*."[78] Dr. E. Garrott was the physician-in-charge. A "ladies committee" was appointed to "visit each ward for two days each week . . . and to provide watchers and see that each patient is made as comfortable as possible." The costs of operating the hospital, $150 a month, seemed exorbitant, but the *Central City Register* editorialized that "we have seen the figures and know that every item is necessary." The hospital called for donations, including "old sheets that will do to strip into bandages, old comfortables, and rubber blankets." The weekly charge was $6, but those who could not afford to pay were admitted anyway. Such a liberal admissions policy was not conducive to fiscal health and the hospital soon found itself in financial straits. St. Luke's Hospital closed in 1871. Ironically, Central City, the first mining camp to have its own hospital, never had another one.

5 MINES AND MINING CAMPS I[1]

At no place, perhaps, within the domain of civilization, can be found a people living . . . under such disadvantageous hygienic surroundings [as in Leadville]. First, we may notice the great exposure entailed by the employment of the miners . . . When the day's work has ended . . . cleanliness is disregarded to an astonishing degree, the bed a pallet of hay without sheets, the blankets scarcely ever aired . . . Conditions such as these predispose to disease . . .

D.H. Dougan, M.D. (Leadville), 1880[2]

FOR A WHILE, IT LOOKED AS though Central City and some of the other early gold camps were played out, but newer, cheaper, and more efficient methods of extraction led to their resurrection in the late 1860s. It was not until the late 1870s, however, that Colorado's mining boom really took off. This time it was a succession of silver bonanzas that led the way and brought thousands of immigrants to Leadville, Aspen, Lake City, Breckenridge and many other smaller towns and camps throughout the mountains. At about the same time, the Utes were evicted, and the gold and silver of the San Juans led to boom times in Ouray, Telluride, and Silverton. In the 1890s Creede joined the silver camps, and Cripple Creek, the richest of all the gold districts, was born.

From the point of view of health and disease, Lake City was a fairly typical example of the newer mining camps. The *Rocky Mountain News* described Lake City's medical status in 1877—and it was not a particularly healthy one:

> The climate of Lake City is not the most salubrious in the world . . . Sick men are to be found everywhere—in wagons and tents, log cabins and dug-outs . . . Bilious complaints are common . . . [as is] the dreaded mountain fever . . . Measles and erysipelas have joined hands and taken the town by storm . . . Pneumonia is prevalent and persons subject to heart disease or weak lungs should think twice before coming here. The graveyard . . . is developing into respectable proportions.[3]

As the mining camps grew, some of them into cities, they became more unsanitary and unhealthy. The miner's meager wages paid for a bunk, grub, whisky, tobacco, and the occasional company of a woman. The mine owner's profits went into great mansions, investments, and bank vaults. Neither was interested in pure drinking water or adequate sewer pipes. It was not surprising, therefore, that typhoid was prevalent in the mining camps. Filth was everywhere and bathtubs were rare. Animal carcasses were left to rot in streets and alleys. In wet weather, the streets were mud; when the weather was dry, the air was filled with dust. The mines were both dangerous and unhealthy. The streets were unsafe, the food was impure, and the air was polluted.

Leadville was the queen of the silver camps. In the early 1860s gold had been found in California Gulch, near present-day Leadville. When the gold played out, the area was virtually abandoned. In the 1870s, the dark rock which the gold prospectors had ignored turned out to contain not only lead carbonate but silver as well. Leadville was established in 1877, and within two years there were ten thousand people in the town and its nearby mines. Nearly two miles above sea level, it was given the picturesque nickname of Cloud City, but, like the other mining towns, its growth was totally haphazard, with no thought given to sanitation, clean water, or sewage. From its very beginnings, Leadville

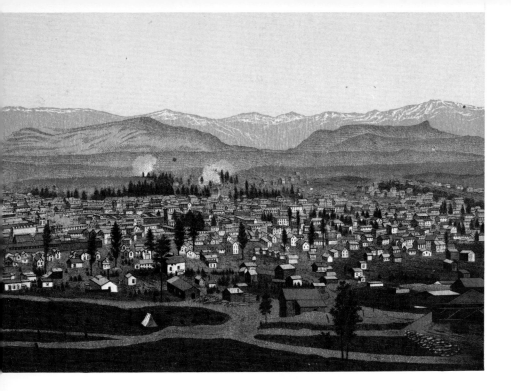

5.1 Despite this idealized view, Leadville was called the "city of the dead" because of its alleged unhealthfulness and high mortality rate.

was accused of being an unhealthy place to live. The *Ouray Times* called it "the suburban city of the dead" where five or six deaths deaths occurred every day.[4] In 1880 there were nearly eight hundred deaths in Leadville. One observer blamed the town's high death rate on the bad habits of its citizens:

> Much has been said about the unhealthfulness of Leadville, because a good many people have died there from intemperance, exposure, etc., as well as from natural causes . . . Care and cleanliness have been . . . neglected in this magic city, and she pays the penalty by an undeserved reputation for unhealthfulness.[5]

The next year, Leadville's city physician took pride in reporting a marked reduction in the town's mortality rate. In addition, he noted, "the general condition of the streets and alleys have received attention, and last summer the city was

probably cleaner than ever before."[6] Nevertheless, sanitation and public health remained a matter of concern and discussion. The *Leadville Chronicle* described the animal carcasses, piles of garbage, and offal collecting in the rear of homes and hotels.[7] In 1886 Leadville finally installed a sewage system, but in 1900 the city's unsavory reputation was reestablished by a massive outbreak of typhoid (Chapter 17).

Prospectors and Miners

In the early days, prospectors and miners were one and the same. Later, those who looked for gold and silver were distinguished from the thousands who came to mine the many lodes which the prospectors had discovered. The prospector generally lived an isolated existence, sometimes snowed in for an entire winter in his cabin above timberline. If he became ill or was injured, he either recovered or died, without any medical care. Periodically, with spring thaw, there would be reports of the decomposed body of a prospector being found in his cabin. Such was the case with "Old Man" Walter, found dead in his cabin at the Molas mine near Silverton in 1898.[8]

The miners were a different breed. They were men who were looking, not for bonanzas, but for a day's work. Many were native Americans, Irishmen, Scots, or Cornishmen. Others were from Germany, Italy, Scandanavia, Austria-Hungary, or the Slavic countries and spoke little or no English. Most were single, although in later years, wives and children were added to the mining camps. When he was not working, the miner was likely to be found in one of a camp's many saloons or sleeping in a bunk bed.

5.2 The miners worked under unhealthy and dangerous conditions.

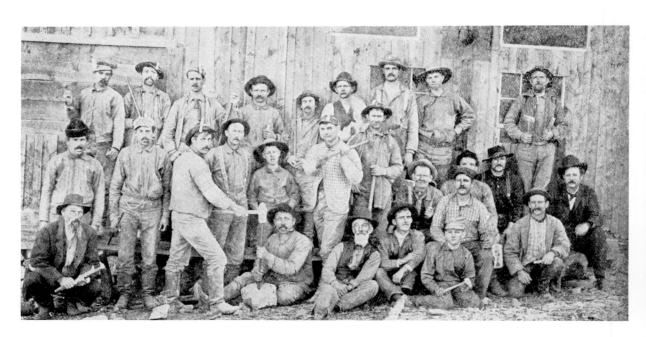

Leadville's Mammoth Sleeping Gardens had five hundred bunks. The bunks were stacked in tiers, and the miners slept in shifts, at fifty cents a shift.

Many of the miners lived in boarding houses at the mines themselves, sometimes at altitudes of more than 12,000 feet. Often conditions were no less crowded, dirty, or poorly ventilated there than they were in town, and such sites were often isolated for the winter. In addition, drinking water was even more likely to be contaminated at the mines than in town. Often a mine's outhouses and stables were located above its water source. The State Board of Health urged the mines to build protective walls around their wells to prevent their being used "as cesspools for garbage, boots, shoes, dead dogs, etc."[9] The board also reminded mine foremen that they were responsible for the cleanliness of the boarding houses and that they should arrange "for the disposal of slops and refuse matter."[10] Such advice, instructions, and warnings were, however, generally ignored. At the huge Camp Bird mine and mill near Ouray, raw sewage was routinely dumped into the nearby Uncompahgre River. Not surprisingly, an outbreak of typhoid at the Camp Bird was followed by one downstream in the town of Montrose.[11] When the *Leadville Herald Democrat* charged that living conditions in the boarding houses at the Mary Murphy mine were unhealthy, the mine's superintendent responded that their doctor, "an upright gentleman and first-class physician," had examined his men and found them all to be in good health.[12]

In general, the miners were well fed, the mine owners apparently understanding the relationship of caloric intake to energy and work. At one mine, for example, it was said that

> The food is surprisingly good and plentiful. Bread and pies are baked daily . . . The workers wolf their food and have no inclination to conversation.[13]

Personal cleanliness varied considerably. In town, the miner might spend two bits for a bath every once in a while. In Leadville, having been paid his monthly wages, the miner could repair to Costello's Bath House. There he could luxuriate in hot water, wash himself with bar soap, dry himself with a Turkish towel, and make use of a variety of toilet articles. The State Bureau of Mines deplored the fact that

> [Although many miners] are cleanly . . . some are not, and a few filthy men injected into a bunk house soon infect the whole . . . The condition of the bunk house is almost a sure index to the class of men employed.[14]

One miner summarized his impressions:

> The life of a miner above timber line is one of hard labor, privation and danger. It might be called self-imposed slavery. Working in the caverns of the earth, deprived of daylight and sun, and only getting a whiff of fresh air when walking from the mine under a snow shed to the boarding-house, was a sacrifice to normal life.[15]

The work was hard and the day was long. For twelve hours in the early days, then ten hours as reforms were introduced, the miner

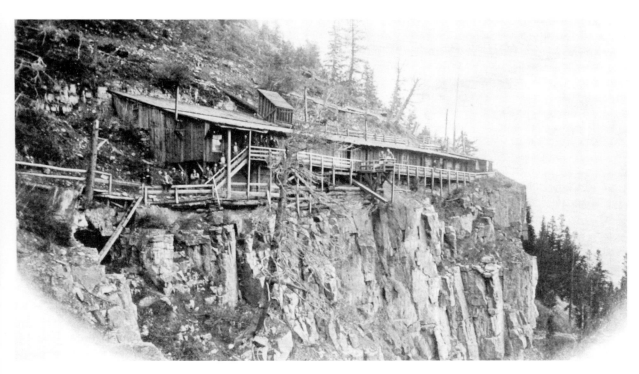

5.3 Their living conditions were not much better than their working conditions. Boarding houses were crowded and unsanitary, sometimes perched, like this one, in precarious locations at high altitudes.

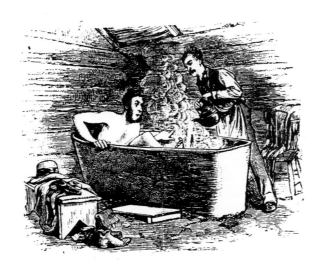

5.4 The miners were not known for personal cleanliness. It cost this Leadville miner two bits for his bath.

endured cold, dampness, dust, noise, stench, darkness, and danger—all at altitudes of up to 13,000 feet. Some worked seven days a week, often for long stretches without a day off. Under such conditions, a man became "worn out . . . his vitality exhausted, his surplus energy used up . . . he lost his recuperative power," and he became susceptible to pneumonia and other diseases.[16] The editor of Ouray's *Solid Muldoon* wrote of the miners at the Virginius:

> Men who delve in the bowels of the earth at an altitude exceeding 10,000 feet . . . are in no condition to stand the ravages [of disease] . . . The very complexion of the miners on the Virginius, who come down to attend the funeral [of a comrade], tells too plainly the condition of their lungs and liver.[17]

It was no wonder that, after the age of thirty-five, the mortality of miners was nearly four times greater than that of a comparable population of men.[18]

The mining camps were subject to the same infectious diseases as other nineteenth century communities. Venereal disease and alcoholism were common, and the lack of sanitation bred typhoid. Mountain fever was being diagnosed less frequently than in the early days and had been replaced as the scourge of the mining camps by pneumonia. In addition, the miners were susceptible to what was called "rheumatism," lead poisoning, and, if they lived long enough, silicosis.

The danger of avalanches loomed over some of the camps. Inside the mines, accidents—falls, cave-ins, fires, floods, and explosions—claimed many victims. Eyes were ruined by flying particles and ears by deafening noise. Reverend Darley officiated at the funerals of many miners, and he succinctly referred to the list of dead miners in his pastor's register as a "hard roll."[19]

Before considering some of these hazards, it

should be noted that there were many other workers in the mining industry besides miners. In the mines, there were also teamsters, timbermen, tram drivers, trammers, cagers, nippers, and others. Each occupation had its hazards, with the miner having more than his share. Mill and smelter workers were exposed to still other dangers. The noise of the massive stamps was literally deafening, the dust destroyed lungs, and the machinery could crush bones as well as rock. The smelters were filled with the noxious and toxic gaseous effluvia of roasting ores and chemicals.

Pneumonia

The people of the mining camps were tough. There was little that they feared. They were afraid of pneumonia, however, the disease which could strike and kill even the healthiest, strongest, and toughest miner. The San Juans' Reverend James Gibbons described a typical spring in his district:

> Pneumonia is much feared at the mines . . . and when the first symptoms of the dread disease appear, the sick miner at once seeks a low altitude and enters . . . the hospital . . . That spring, pneumonia was prevalent in the San Juans, and many of the boys crossed the range for the last time. Deaths and funerals became so common![20]

The newspapers and medical journals tersely reported periodic outbreaks: "Pneumonia has been epidemic in the San Juan country. The Ouray Miners' Hospital is full of patients and a number of deaths have resulted."[21]

The physicians of the mining camps were all too familiar with pneumonia's clinical presentation. Cripple Creek's Dr. Carl Meyer described a typical case in 1896:

> A young, strong miner, about twenty-five years old, never sick before, complains one day of a little headache, drowsiness, loss of appetite, has a little dry cough, is tired, does not like to work, but goes on as well as he can. To improve his condition he takes a few drinks in the afternoon. [That night] he gets a chill, has [chest] pains, excessive . . . cough, very high fever . . . This is the typical pneumonia . . . feared by the physician as well as the general public . . . Sometimes the patient feels better, gets up . . . [and then] drops dead. So it happens . . . on the street, in a saloon, in a dancing hall . . .[22]

Leadville's reputation as an unhealthy locale was based, to a large extent on the prevalence of pneumonia. One author wrote that Leadville was considered a "deathtrap," and that "the impression in the East is that a holocaust of pneumonia victims die daily."[23] That impression was reinforced when, in 1880, two nationally known figures died of pneumonia in Leadville: "Texas Jack Omohundro," Buffalo Bill's buddy, and Charles Vivian, founder of the national fraternal order, the Elks.[24] The same year, the *Denver Tribune* reported that, "so prevalent and generally fatal is pneumonia at the present hour in Leadville, that it has come to be regarded by many as an epidemic almost as formidable as cholera [or] yellow fever."[25] Leadville's city fathers resented what they regarded as an undeserved stigma. Some of the charges, they suggested, were made by other mountain towns in order to build up their own reputations at Leadville's expense:

> The lie is circulated that everyone that visits Leadville is sure to contract pneumonia . . . Such reports are fallacious and unworthy of consideration . . . the dread disease exists no more in Leadville than it does in other localities.[26]

Why was pneumonia so common in the mountains? Several reasons were offered. Some blamed the altitude. Silverton's Dr. J.W. Brown pointed to "the rarefied condition of the atmosphere [and] the deprivation of oxygen."[27] Others felt that the situation was more complicated. Ouray's *Solid Muldoon* noted that "men who delve in the bowels of the earth . . . are in no condition to stand the ravages of pneumonia . . ." —hence, the high mortality rate in the mining camps.[28]

Central City's Dr. George McMurtrie had definite feelings about those who developed pneumonia, especially in Leadville:

> The men . . . are of the worst class, broken down by exposure, rum, and an irregular mode of life. In such a class the slightest exposure was sufficient to bring on the disease, and they died like rotten sheep.[29]

The combination of alcoholism and pneumonia was considered to be especially lethal. One doctor commented that "all drunkards died in Leadville if they had pneumonia."[30] One miner recalled that in the San Juan country, if a man had pneumonia, the first question asked was:

> "Is he a drinking man?" If the answer was "Yes," the advice was . . . "Roll him in blankets and put him in a tram bucket and send him down" . . . If the answer was "No, we are quite sure he never drinks any liquor," then "Give him a pint of whiskey, roll him in a blanket, put him in a tram bucket and send him down" . . . Fellows who were addicted to alcoholic stimulants had very little chance. They usually died. The sober fellows had a good chance to get well.[31]

There was really very little a physician could

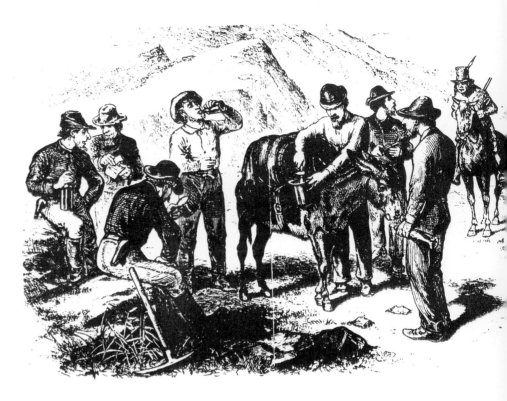

5.5 Alcohol was readily available, even at the most remote mines. The combination of alcohol and pneumonia was frequently lethal.

do for a patient with pneumonia in the pre-antibiotic era. A few still phlebotomized their patients; Silverton's Dr. Brown induced sweating to break the fever, and others used opium and chest splints to relieve any pleuritic pain.[32] When possible, the patient was sent to a lower altitude. Dr. Charles Gardiner recalled that he was in charge of fifty men working in a silver mine at 13,500 feet:

> Pneumonia was fairly frequent . . . and when a case occurred I would at once wrap him in blankets, tie him on an improvised sled made of snowshoes [i.e. skis], and have him dragged over the snow-field to a town of 9,000 feet altitude. Almost invariably this produced a prompt improvement in the patient's condition.[33]

If a physician would certify the need, the railroads would allow a patient with pneumonia reduced fare to Denver. As a result, sick miners would often arrive, penniless, at Denver's County Hospital.[34]

Rheumatism

"Rheumatism" was a common complaint among Colorado's miners. Aching, painful joints were blamed on the altitude, the frigid dampness of the mines, and the cramped and bent positions of the miners. Silverton's Dr. W. W. Wilkinson specialized in the treatment of rheumatism, and his office-residence-hospital included a "Russo-Turkish bath room."[35] Wilkinson felt that the disease was due to an "autointoxication" related to the miner's excessive intake of meat, smoking and drinking, "defective oxygenation from working in bad air," and "altitude, strong sunlight, positive electric conditions . . . and daily extremes in [atmospheric] temperature".

The true nature of miner's "rheumatism" is unclear. In some patients it seems to have been an acute febrile arthritis affecting multiple joints, and the patient was severely ill. Wilkinson ruled out the possibility of gonorrheal disease, and rheumatoid and gouty arthritis were unlikely. Rheumatic fever is associated with arthritis, and some of the cases of the acute multi-joint variety may have due to this disease. The more chronic form was probably osteoarthritis, the degenerative, so-called "wear and tear," disease of joints. Dr. Wilkinson treated his patients with steam baths and large doses of sodium salicylate, the nineteenth century equivalent of aspirin.

Many "rheumatic" miners made use of the natural springs near some of the mining camps. Silverton's miners took advantage of Trimble Hot Springs, north of Durango.[36] Reverend Gibbons described the springs as "a fountain of perpetual youth [to which] the miner repairs to invigorate his system impaired by hard work . . . and [by] the high altitude of Silverton and its neighboring mines." Ouray's miners favored Mother Buchanan's Bath House. Mother was from the "old country," Donegal, and had a "heart full of sympathy and good humor." At her establishment

> many an afflicted miner had the rheumatism dislodged from his bones in the big pool of hot water which bubbles fresh from the earth. The water was hot enough to boil eggs.[36]

Lead Poisoning

At Missouri's lead mines, lead poisoning was known to be a problem for decades. In the early

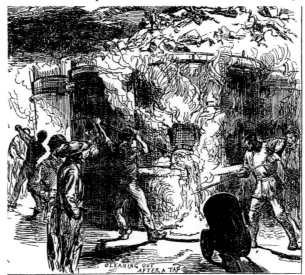

5.6 The smelters, with their noxious fumes and other hazards, were as dangerous as the mines.

1860s, Dr. Pollak had wondered about lead as a cause of mountain fever in Colorado's mining camps but had subsequently discounted the possibility. With the coming of the silver boom, which was based on silver-rich lead carbonate ore, lead poisoning became a major concern. As the president of the Colorado Board of Health pointed out in 1880, "little was heard of lead poisoning in Colorado before the discovery of the carbonate of that metal in the mines of Leadville."[37] In the early 1880s, a prominent Leadville physician, Dr. F.F. D'Avignon, complained that nearly all of his patients were suffering from lead poisoning.[38] By that time, there was no doubt that "the mineral deposits of Leadville . . . carry a large proportion of lead . . . [and that] workmen in the mines and smelters are alike subject to lead poisoning."[39] In the three years from 1880 through 1882, Leadville's St. Vincent's Hospital recorded 162 miners and 605 smelter workers with lead poisoning.[40]

There is little mention of lead poisoning in Colorado's medical literature, however, and it is difficult to determine its significance as a medical problem in early Colorado.

As for treatment, one non-medical observer suggested that, for Leadville's miners, at least,

> Nature has provided a remedy for the disease near at hand. The mineral springs at Cottonwood Canon . . . are a specific in almost any stage of [lead poisoning]. All the patient has to do is to lay off a few days or weeks . . . bathe and drink freely of the waters . . . to get the lead out of his system . . . and go back to his work rejuvenated.[40]

The Mines

The mines were even more unsanitary than the mining camps. The miner who needed to relieve himself during his ten or twelve hour shift simply picked a convenient spot to do so. Ventilation was poor in the closed spaces of the mines, and the miner must have welcomed the distracting aromas of burning fuses and exploded powder. During its early years, in one of its infrequent considerations of health problems in the mines, Colorado's Board of Health reported that the mines were virtual cesspools where human and animal refuse collected, often draining down from one level to the next.[41] The board recommended "cleaning out the tunnels occasionally and cutting trenches [which would] lead to cesspools or vaults excavated for that purpose." The mine owners were unlikely to support any such diversion of mining activity at their expense. The Bureau of Mines was more conservative, simply recommending that "when meals are eaten underground, the scattering of slops and refuse should not be permitted" and that abandoned sections of the mine should not serve as "[water] closets."

The medical profession did not pay much attention to sanitation in the mines either. In 1896 Dr. J. W. Exline pointed out, at a meeting of the Colorado State Medical Society, that the sanitation of mines

> is a subject likely to be overlooked by medical gatherings of this kind . . . I cannot recall a single instance in which [this topic] was made the topic of a single paper.[42]

Dr. Exline went on to state that "the principal cause of ill health [in] the mining class is attributable to the atmosphere in which they work. This is not strange," he added, "for the air of the mines is . . . unfit for the purposes of respiration." As the mines became deeper, ventilation became less and less effective, and the air progressively poorer. Prior to the introduction of electrically powered blowers, ventilation was primitive. The atmosphere was filled with dust and noxious gases generated by explosives. The mines were at high altitudes and the air, relatively "thin" to begin with, was soon depleted of oxygen. Sometimes it was not even enough to sustain the miner's candle or oil lamp. Miners often passed out in the "bad air," a phenomenon known as "miner's con."

In addition to pneumonia, other respiratory problems were common among the miners. Chronic laryngitis was ascribed to the effects of the pneumatic drill, so that "with every stroke of the hammer, the miner expels air with a rasping noise, which irritates the vocal membranes."[43] Chronic bronchitis was believed to be due to a combination of mouth breathing, inhalation of dust, and the cold air used in pneumatic drilling—all resulting in a "chronic catarrhal condition of the bronchi . . ."[43]

The stagnant air of the mines was also responsible for "powder headache," one of the most discomforting, though not one of the more dangerous, aspects of hard rock mining. Men who were exposed to giant powder often developed intense headaches in which "every heartbeat caused a throbbing pain in the head and a humming in the ears."[43] This was accompanied by tearing and bloodshot eyes, nausea and vomiting, muscle twitching, and a staggering gait. On at least one occasion, an affected miner was thought to be drunk on the job and fired. Giant powder is derived from nitroglycerine, and powder headache has been ascribed to the nitroglycerine—perhaps the result of its ability to dilate blood vessels, the same property which has been used in treating angina

pectoris.

Working in the mines led to minor as well as major illnesses. Sudamina was one of the minor ones, a dermatitis which was common in those miners who worked in overheated environments. In this condition, the sweat glands became blocked, forming small blisters. The skin was described as rough or "pebble-like," and the lesions generally dried up and rubbed off.[43] Another was "miner's nystagmus," lateral oscil-

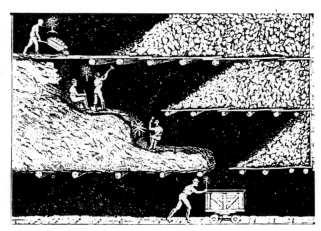

5.7 Despite the mines' increasing depth and complexity, adequate ventilation and safety measures were virtually non-existent.

lations of the eyes said to be due to the poor light provided by candles.

Silicosis

Gold and silver are found in "hard" rock, i.e. in association with silica. The drilling, blasting and milling of hard rock results in silica dust which, unless precautions are taken, is inhaled into the lungs. There the silica particles remain, chronically irritating pulmonary tissue and, over a period of years, resulting in its replacement by scar. Normally, with each breath the lungs expand, air enters the pulmonary tissue, and oxygen diffuses into the bloodstream on its way to the body's tissues. If precautions are not taken to prevent the inhalation of dust, the lungs of a long-term hard rock miner become nearly as hard as the rock he mined. Such lungs are virtually unexpandable and the little oxygen that does get to pulmonary tissue is blocked from entering the bloodstream. In addition, patients with silicosis have an increased susceptibility to pulmonary tuberculosis. Corresponding to this pathologic picture were the human detritus of the mining camps, middle aged and elderly men who, after some twenty or more years in the mines, were no longer able to work and, in the latter stages of the disease, were using much of their energy just to breathe and stay alive.

Silicosis was known by a variety of names: miner's consumption, miner's phthisis, calcicosis, fibroid phthisis. It was uncommon in the early days of surface mining, but when the mines began to become deeper and more complex and powerful drills and blasting powders were developed, adequate ventilation became impossible, and the miner worked in a perpetual cloud of dust. Both miner and mine owner were more concerned with the quantity of ore produced than with the amount of dust in the air. To the miner, dust was simply an annoyance. He did not know it might eventually kill him. The invention of hollow drills through which water could be sprayed, thereby reducing the amount of dust, was met by resistance on the part of both owners and miners, and many mines continued to use solid drills until well into the twentieth century. It was for good reason that these solid or "dry" drills were called "widow-makers." Inadequate ventilation remained a problem until the introduction of electricity made the use of exhaust fans possible. In addition, in the early years, there were no laws requiring minimal safety and health standards and practices in the mines. When such laws were

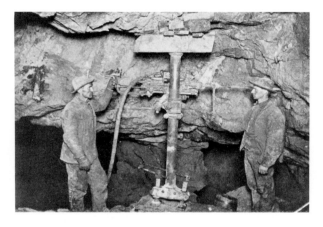

5.8 Silicosis was a common long-term complication of hard-rock mining and milling. Non-water lubricated or "dry" drills were known as "widow-makers" because of the vast clouds of silica dust they created.

introduced late in the nineteenth century, they were vague and rarely enforced.

Although Colorado's physicians showed ample courage in dealing with such public health problems as smallpox and typhoid, there is, with rare exception, little mention of silicosis in the state's medical journals or in the published transactions of its medical societies. Many of the mining camp doctors were, of course, under contract to the mine owners. "Big city" and country doctors, on the other hand, were not terribly concerned about the mining camps. By the turn of the century, there must have been tens of thousands of active or former workers who had been exposed to silica dust in Colorado's mines and mills.

In 1899 an article on calcicosis pulmonum (silicosis) was published in the *Denver Medical*

Times. Of interest is the fact that the article, virtually the only one on silicosis found in Colorado's early medical literature, was written, not by a Coloradan, but by a physician in Salt Lake City and dealt with his experiences with hard rock mill workers in southern Utah and Nevada.[44] He could have been describing any one of many Colorado mills when he stated: "In and about the mill the air is filled with an impalpable dust. In portions of the mill it is so dense that one cannot be recognized a few feet away, and an electric light is in evidence by a spark." The paper, presented at a meeting of the Rocky Mountain Inter-State Medical Association, led to some heated discussion. One physician, having also seen the results of breathing silica dust in miners and mill workers, suggested that

> there is but one remedy, and that is prophylactic . . . There are methods that have been devised for removing this dust . . . but it costs money . . . So long as human life is regarded of less value than gold, so long will these lives continue to be sacrificed . . . The most effective remedy to be devised would be the vigorous application of the strong arm of the law.[45]

Colorado's Dr. J.N. Hall echoed this sentiment: "It seems to me if the strong arm of the law does not take hold of this matter, it will be a shame."[45] These remarks were answered by the physician who was employed by the mill cited in the paper. His analysis, he reported, showed that mill workers who had "used proper caution" in their work did not die of silicosis. He pointed out that he had urged the workers to protect themselves from dust with "large sponges worn over the face provided by the company" and that "when they felt the dust was overcoming them, they should go outside and rest awhile." He assured his colleagues that, "when you speak of the strong arm of the law taking hold of the owners of the mill, you are not doing any more than the owners are trying to do. Nobody at first realized what the danger was . . ." and the owners had increased ventilation and taken other measures to improve the situation. Unfortunately, he concluded, there was not much that could be done about the problem.[46]

In one study, nearly one-third of Colorado's hard rock miners were found to have silicosis at autopsy.[47] The problem continued. In 1929 Dr. T.E. Beyer described the 124 cases of silicosis he had diagnosed at Denver's Municipal Tuberculosis Dispensary. Seventy years after the Gold Rush, Dr. Beyer charged, the state still lacked adequate protective laws, and he reminded his colleagues that

> upon the medical profession falls the grave responsibility of awakening public sentiment and initiating legislation which will bring about a condition of industrial hygiene in Colorado mines.[48]

Thirty years later and a century after the Gold Rush, Dr. Beyer acknowledged the introduction of federally enforced safeguards. He also reminded Colorado's doctors of the embarassing fact that "the contribution of the medical profession toward the control of occupational diseases [such as silicosis] was, perforce, negligible."[49]

Mine Accidents

Mining is not only an unhealthy occupation, it is a dangerous one as well. What is true today was even truer in the "old" days. On the way to, and into, the mines during his workshift and on his way out again, day after day, the miner risked a variety of injuries. Until the late nineteenth century, there were no rules to encourage, let alone ensure, safety in the industry—whether in the mine, mill, or smelter. Those laws which were finally enacted, first by the state and later by the federal government, were often unenforced and ignored by owners, superintendents, foremen, and even the miners themselves. Every day, the worker's well-being was dependent, not on laws, but on management's sense of responsibility, the experience and common sense of his foreman, his fellow workers, and himself, and, for want of a better word, luck. The miners had their own list of safety "do's" and "don'ts"—some based on facts, some learned from the mistakes of others, and some derived from supposition or even superstition. Union demands for safety measures were usually rejected by the owners as too expensive. By 1895 mining accidents had become so common that Colorado established a State Bureau of Mines. One of its major responsibilities was stated in its first *Bulletin*:

> To inspect and determine the safety of devices and methods used in mining . . . and take necessary measures to make them safe. On receipt of notice the Bureau shall inquire into the cause of accidents.[50]

Even though minor and even major non-fatal accidents were often unreported, the number which was reported was impressive. In the eighteen months between June 1895 and late November 1896, there were 154 fatalities and 162 serious and often disabling injuries among Colorado's 16,000 miners and 9,000 mining in-

dustry workers.[50] To put it another way, over an eighteen month period, a mine worker's chance of being crushed, asphyxiated, burned, blasted, drowned, or similarly maimed or killed, was more than one in a hundred. If you worked in the mines for twenty years, your overall risk increased to more than one in five. This was in addition to the non-traumatic medical problems that the mine workers faced.

Mine injuries were both terrible and common. Reverend Gibbons described one of the many accident victims he attended in the San Juan country.[51] In the pre-dawn darkness, he recalled, "I received a message from the Yankee Girl mine announcing that C---- had fallen 140 feet down a shaft, and was lying, broken and crushed, at the point of death." After a long and hair-raising journey over a narrow, snowpacked mountain trail,

> we reached the Yankee Girl and found poor C---- in a sad plight. Most of his bones were broken, and he lay on his bunk, suffering intense agony, but still retaining his senses. It is inspiring to witness the rare patience with which the hardy miner endures pain.[51]

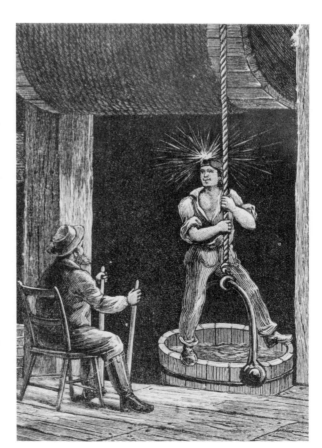

5.9 Riding the ore buckets was a high-risk way to get to work.

Eventually, the miner was evacuated to Durango, "where the doctors decided that it would be necessary to put him in a plaster of paris cast to keep him together." The Reverend

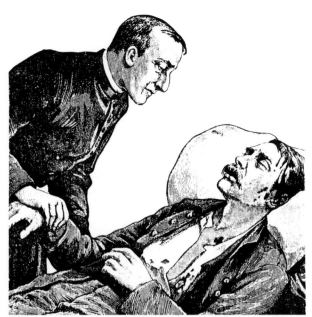

5.10 Sometimes the injured miner was attended to by a clergyman before the doctor could get to the scene.

did not indicate whether "poor C----" survived his injuries.

Accidents sometimes occurred on the way to and from work, especially among those who rode the ore buckets. The buckets swung their way up and down the slopes on ropes suspended between tram towers. Equally courageous, or foolhardy, was the miner who rode the huge ore wagons, fully loaded and picking their way along steep shelf "roads" hugging sheer canyon walls. Having arrived at the shaft house, the miner was lowered down the shaft in an ore bucket or cage, often several hundred feet, to his working level. The shafts themselves were often poorly lit and unguarded. A Bureau of Mines report is eloquent in its brevity:[52]

5.11 Many gravestones in Colorado's mining camp cemetaries attest to the dangers of mining—and to the bravery of many miners. This one is in Telluride.

> Stefan Wienewski, attempting to get into the bucket, fell to the bottom of the shaft in the Cashier—fatal. January 13, 1895.
>
> Dolphice Collins was caught between the cage and the shaft wall in the Independence—fatal. December 15, 1895.
>
> Edwin Judkins became dizzy and fell down a shaft at the Little Annie—fatal. April 16, 1896.

Once down to his level, the miner had to contend with moving tram cars, steam lines, electric wiring, machinery of various types, and the heavy, hot, and massively vibrating drills. Again, from the Bureau of Mines report:[52]

> Frank Cooney fell into a rock crusher at the Tomboy—fatal. September 30, 1895.
>
> S. Olevetta took hold of a live electric wire at the Revenue—fatal. July 18, 1896.
>
> George Reynolds was struck by the hammer while drilling at the Tomboy—fatal. May 30, 1896.

Shafts, tunnels, drifts—all were supported by

timber which had been positioned by teams of "timbering men." If poorly positioned, or if the wood become water-soaked and rotten, or with minor shifts in the earth's crust, tons of rock would suddenly fall, trapping or crushing the miners. Such cave-ins were common:[52]

> Eight men were killed in a cave-in at the Anna Lee. January 4, 1896.
>
> Ten men were killed when a cave-in trapped them, thereby cutting off air circulation, in the Belgian Sept. 26, 1895.

The mine's structures, from the shaft house to the supports within the mine, were wood, and fire was a constant threat. In the mines themselves fires were dangerous mainly as a result of their smoke, the poor ventilation resulting in asphyxiation:[53]

> Twenty-four miners were killed by smoke when the wooden structure at the entrance to the Smuggler-Union caught fire and, in the panic, nobody thought to close the door at the tunnel entrance. November 20, 1901.

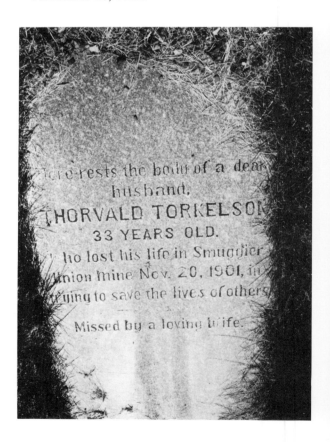

Although hard rock mining was not associated with methane and the other explosive gases found in coal mines, the miners would occasionally enter a pocket of "carbonate gas," apparently a mixture of carbon dioxide and nitrogen. This mixture, although inert and non-flammable, could infiltrate the area and replace what little oxygen there was. The situation was analogous to being in an airless room. If the miner was unaware of the situation, he might pass out and be asphyxiated. The *Rico Sun* reported such an incident. A miner, as he descended in an ore bucket to the bottom of the 300 foot shaft of the Silver Glance mine, was suddenly overcome by "a body of gas [which] had forced itself up through the broken formation and filled the shaft."[54] He died, but another miner who had gone down to rescue his buddy, though overcome, survived. Miners knew that, when their candle was snuffed out, is was likely to be due to such a deadly pocket of carbonate gas, and they exited quickly. Gas pockets were especially common in the volcanic bed of the Cripple Creek Mining District. It was said that, on awakening in the morning, the district's miners would look for low-lying clouds among the surrounding mountain peaks. From bitter experience, the miners had learned that low-lying clouds foretold the possibility of carbonate gas deep in the mines. Such clouds, apparently, are a sign of low barometric pressure which, in turn, tends to draw gas out from the rock and into the drifts and shafts of the mines.[55]

Explosions

Hard rock mining was a fairly simple procedure. Holes were drilled into the rock face, explosive charges were placed into the holes, the rock face was blasted away, and the debris hauled off. The cycle of drilling, blasting, and clearing was repeated with each shift, sometimes throughout a twenty-four hour day. The black powder used by the early miners was replaced by the more powerful nitroglycerine derivative, giant powder. Unfortunately, giant powder froze at relatively high temperatures, and, when frozen, it was unusable. Frozen giant powder had to be thawed if it was to be used—a very tricky operation since heating and thawing made giant powder highly unstable and liable to explode.

Dr. Exline was dismayed to find that "the laws of Colorado are mute on the subject of explosives . . . Even the most incompetent and reckless may be entrusted with . . . these powerful agents."[56] The Colorado Bureau of Mines did provide specific recommendations for the handling of giant powder, advising the miner, for example, not to carry the explosives "in their bootlegs or elsewhere about their person."[57] Apparently Jim Walsh, a miner at the Virginius, did not think much of such bureaucratic cautions. One day, the powder he was carrying in his pocket exploded and blew Jim to bits.[57]

The bureau also recommended that giant powder be thawed in a steam bath and that dry heat was unsafe. Unfortunately, such recommendations may not have reached some miners, many of whom spoke little English. Again, others simply ignored the recommendations. Some miners, direct men with straightfoward solutions to simple problems, used the most convenient source of heat available to them—their cabin stove. Reverend Gibbons commented:

> It is an unfortunate custom of miners to take giant powder into their cabins, hold it by the fire and thaw it out. When frozen it will not explode, but when thawed it is one of the most dangerous and powerful explosives.[58]

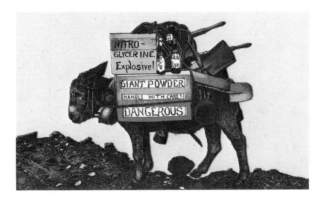

5.12 Explosives were not always treated with the respect they deserved.

Billy Maher was so engaged when "all of a sudden, eight sticks of the powder went off. The result was appalling . . . The stove went through the roof, the cabin was demolished [and] Billy was horribly mangled." He was brought to St. Joseph's Hospital in Ouray where he died.[58] Similar events were frequently reported in the mining camp newspapers. In the *Aspen Times* of Christmas Eve, 1888:

> Charles Gordon was killed by an explosion of giant powder while warming it in a stove oven. The accident occurred at the west end of Hyman Steet.[59]

The *Report of the Bureau of Mines* was even more succinct:[60]

> J.D. Sullivan, Cleveland Mine, Lake County. Five years a miner. Thawing powder in oven of cook stove. Lost right hand.

> H.R. Morris, Little May mine, DuBois mining district. Powder warming on blacksmith forge. Probable loss of both eyes.

Even the small charge contained within blasting caps was dangerous. In St. Elmo, miner H. E. Johnson's little girl was playing with a blasting cap when it went off, amputating her hand.[61]

Most accidental explosions occurred in the mines, however. Having drilled multiple holes

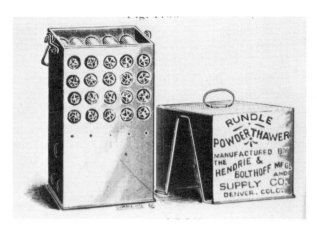

5.13 Some miners preferred to thaw their giant powder on the stove rather than in an apparatus such as this one, approved by the Colorado Commissioner of Mines. The result was sometimes lethal.

ginius Mine at two A.M. one winter night:

> The [powder] had gone off decapitating Robinson . . . Maloney's . . . brains were oozing out. Big Paddy Burns, had received . . . a shower of rock in the side of his head. He thought he was killed and bellowed lustily for the priest. The men who were around gave him a stimulant to keep him alive. The poor fellow was seriously hurt.[62]

Thanks to Dr. Rowan and the sisters at St. Joseph's Hospital, where it took six months for him to recover, Big Paddy survived. His recovery was not uneventful, however:

> During that time a splinter now and then worked its way out of his skull—to the great amusement of the boys and the dismay of Paddy. Finally, he left the hospital and the mountains too, and went back to the north of Ireland . . .[62]

In general, accidents were blamed on God or the miner. According to the bureau, it was the old timers who were especially to blame, those who "from long practice have become reckless."[63] Such attitudes on the part of the mine owners, the courts, and government agencies, continued well into the twentieth century.

in a rock face, the miner filled each with a charge of giant powder. Sometimes the explosion failed to detonate one of the charges. When he was aware of such a "missed shot," the miner would try to find and remove it. Often, however, he was unaware of the problem, and drilling was resumed. Either situation was likely to result in an accidental explosion. This scene was described by Reverend Gibbons who, with Dr. W. W. Rowan was called from Ouray to the Vir-

6 MINES AND MINING CAMPS II

Seven new physicians have gone to Cripple Creek . . . The rush to Cripple Creek seems to continue.

Colorado Medical Journal, 1896[1]

IN MAY 1877 DR. JOHN LAW left his practice in Alma, joined "the human driftwood" crossing 13,000-foot Mosquito Pass to Leadville, and become the booming new camp's first doctor.[2] Dr. Law was soon joined by others and, within three years, there were fifty-eight physicians in town.[3] Throughout the mountains, as some camps boomed and others went bust, whole populations drifted from camp to camp. It was said of the mining camp doctors that they "were as roving as their patients."[4] Dr. Law was a bona fide M.D., but since there was no state licensing law until 1881, and since even after that date it was impossible to monitor the more remote camps, the professional legitimacy of some mining camp doctors is questionable. Rosita's Dr. Perry, for example, was described as "a free genius, untrammeled by the prejudices of the old school, or, for that matter, any other school of medicine."[5] Many physicians advertised by placing their "card" in the local newspaper. The *Rico Democrat* of November 6, 1891, carried three such "physician's" cards, but only one of the names was followed by an M.D.[6] Among the eighty-nine doctors who lived in Clear Creek County from 1865 to 1895, fully one-third had not attended medical school.[7]

The folks in Silverton said that Dr. J. O. Parker had originally come to town as a veterinarian. Finding it hard to make a living he went off to a diploma mill, paid for his degree, and returned to hang a brand new shingle in his office window—"J.O. Parker, M.D." The townspeople were tolerant of a man's trying to better himself, and although

they chuckled at the quick transformation . . ., as he was a good fellow they closed their intelligence

to argument, feeling perhaps that the doctor wouldn't do any more harm than the average follower of Aesculapius. The doctor had a good practice.[8]

When Dr. Law arrived in Leadville, he had already had experience as a mining camp physician and knew what to expect. Others were newcomers to the mountains and the miners enjoyed testing their mettle. Dr. Lewis Lemen, twenty-three years old and just out of medical school, was put to the test soon after arriving in Georgetown. Thirsty after his long trip, Lemen visited one of the town's many saloons. He was soon approached by a "Cousin Jack," one of the tough Cornish miners. Bolting the saloon's door behind him, the miner turned to the new arrival and declared,

'We miners have a rule that every new doctor . . . has to set up the drinks for the Cousin Jacks.' The patronizing and insolent manner of the miner angered Dr. Lemen. He replied: 'is that so! Now I drink when I want to and I treat a friend when I want to, but I'll be ------- if I'll set up any drinks under compulsion.' With his six foot three, and his 225 pounds, he turned to the door. 'Unlock that door,' said Lemen . . . Sizing up his man, the Jack decided that it would be best to comply [and] Lemen strode out of the saloon.[9]

New doctors faced a lot of competition. Georgetown, with little more than 3,000 people in 1880, had a dozen physicians.[10] As a new doctor in Leadville, Dr. David Dougan waited twenty-nine days before a patient walked into his office.[11] On his arrival at the new camp at Crested Butte, Dr. Charles Gardiner found that two physicians had already preceded him.[12] With fifteen dollars in his pocket and a brand

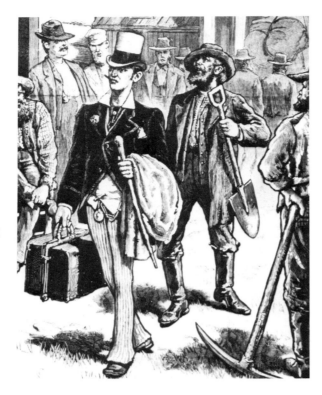

6.1 The newly arrived dude, possibly a doctor, was carefully scrutinized by Leadville's oldtimers.

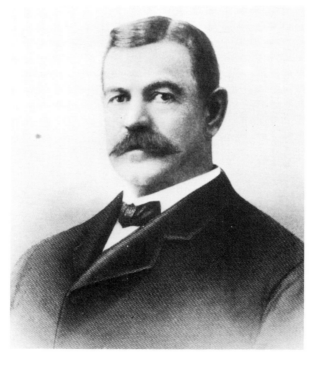

6.2 The newly arrived Dr. Lemen was not about to be intimidated by Georgetown's "cousin Jacks."

a great deal from their wives. Dr. Jacob Campbell was the only doctor in Ward when he arrived with his new bride. Mrs. Campbell soon got used to waking up alone, her husband having been called out in the night to attend to an injured miner. Life was difficult in the camps, she recalled, but she came to enjoy the gratitude and respect which the miners showed her and her husband.[13]

Any new mining camp doctor would give his eye teeth for the position of "surgeon" with one of the big mines. By signing a contract to provide medical service to one or more mines, the doctor ensured himself of a livelihood. Some were paid a salary and actually lived at the mine. Others were "on call" and were paid a fee for service. Creede's Dr. Biles was paid a dollar a month for each working miner.[14]

Dr. Russell J. Collins and his son, Dr. William R. Collins, were fairly typical of the mining camp physicians. Together, their practices spanned much of Colorado's mining boom, from 1866 to 1912. The elder Dr. Collins had received his M.D. in 1851. After ten years of small town practice in the Midwest and four years as a Union army surgeon in the Civil War, Dr. Russell decided to move west. In 1866 the thirty-eight year old doctor brought his wife and children overland in a covered wagon.[15] Originally headed for California, the family was exhausted by the time they reached Denver. That city had more than enough doctors, but they heard about the need for a physician in the mining camp of Empire, near Berthoud Pass. After a difficult journey over mountain trails they finally arrived, only to discover that the town was already in decline. The following year the family moved to nearby Georgetown where, for thirty-five years, Dr. Russell maintained a successful practice. One of the townspeople later recalled the doctor as a large, jovial man, smoking a cigar, and wearing a heavy beaver overcoat in winter. He was also remembered for his honesty and generosity, often "forgetting" to bill his poorer patients and sometimes even leaving them money to pay for medicines.[16]

Dr. Russell's son, Dr. William, started out as a writer for Georgetown's *Colorado Miner*. Eventually, he decided on a medical career, and at the age of thirty-six graduated from St. Louis University's medical school. The following year, 1885, saw him begin a remarkable twenty year journey through a succession of mining camps: Aspen, Leadville (twice), Cripple Creek, Idaho Springs, Georgetown (twice), Victor, and Empire, as well as Butte, Montana, and in Alaska.[17] Finally, in 1902, Dr. William returned to

new diploma, Gardiner decided to tough it out. He bought some board and nails and built himself an office on Main Street. Like many new physicians, Gardiner included dentistry and veterinary medicine in his practice. Many physicians operated a drug store out of their offices, and some added a few rooms for inpatients, thereby designating their establishments as "hospitals."

Most of the early mining camp doctors were single. Those who were married had to expect

Georgetown, and when his father died the following year, he took over his practice. Dr. William remained in Georgetown for ten years. When he retired in 1912, he ended a combined mining camp practice that had begun in 1866.

The mining camp physicians were a varied group, and some were as rough and ready as their patients. Ouray's Dr. W.W. Rowan is an example.[18] Having arrived in town in 1880, the doctor and Reverend Gibbons often worked as a team, providing for the miners' medical and spiritual needs. They frequently travelled together, often over treacherous mountain trails in the middle of the winter, to care for a sick miner or to the scene of a mining disaster. Dr. Rowan claimed that his "special" pills could cure most anything; if they didn't, the miners joked, the next step might be a trip to what was referred to as Dr. Rowan's "ranch," i.e. Ouray's cemetery. Dr. Rowan served Ouray for many years, as its hospital director, superintendent of schools, mayor, and legislative representative.

Some doctors managed to bring some culture and refinement with them, even to the most remote camps. Dr. Alexander N. Simpson, camp physician at the Amythest Mine near Creede, maintained a veritable museum in his home and proudly displayed his collections of coins, minerals, and natural history specimens.[19] His office reception room was described as "both tasteful and artistic, [proving] the doctor to be a connoisseur [of beauty]." In addition to his cultural activities, Dr. Simpson was quite active professionally. He was the local surgeon for the railroad and physician for a number of mines besides the Amythest.

The mining camps, especially the smaller and more isolated ones, also attracted some rather unorthodox and unusual members of the medical profession. Dr. John Francis McGowan certainly fit into that category. Born in Ireland and a bona fide M.D., McGowan came to Tin Cup, Colorado, in 1882. Many years later, Dr. Nolie Mumey interviewed a number of oldtimers who still remembered Dr. McGowan.[20] They portrayed the doctor variously as shy, withdrawn, uncouth, blunt, uncaring, unpleasant, and always dirty and nearly always drunk. A nurse in town refused to work with him, fearful of the "germs" in his long, black beard. It was said that Dr. McGowan's formulary consisted of three prescriptions and a linament that he, himself, had concocted. Another was more positive, recalling of Dr. McGowan that "no individual was of more help to the miners . . . He cheered them when they were discouraged and assisted them through sickness back to health."[21] Appar-

ently the only thing McGowan feared was the humiliation of being picked up by the town's "drunk cart." His death in 1918 was as tragic as his life. Having moved to the nearby mining camp of Pitkin, he was found after a night of drinking and smoking in bed, severely burned and incoherent. Apparently his beard had caught fire. He died several days later.

Alcoholism was a major problem among some of the mining camp physicians, particularly in isolated communities where there was little to do but drink. A Dr. Herzog, formerly a surgeon in the German army, slept during the day and spent his evenings in Silverton's saloons.[22] His office was said to be the street, his clientele the demimonde, and his favorite prescription—"Get drunk and you'll feel different." It has also been suggested that a number of physicians were drug abusers. This is difficult to document, but it was reported that the sudden death of Dr. F.F. D'Avignon, a respected physician in Leadville, was due to his alleged addiction to chloroform.[23] Some physicians even ran afoul of the law. Dr. George P. Johnston took out a great deal of insurance on his house in Silver Plume. When it burned down the doctor collected, and then promptly disappeared, leaving a long list of unsatisfied creditors.[24]

Some of the mining camp doctors were as uneducated as most of their patients. The "Dr." Perry alluded to previously as "untrammeled" by an M.D., attempted to impress the citizens of Rosita by giving a series of free lectures on "Hygiene." In those lectures, described as "both amusing and startling," the "doctor displayed a wonderful ignorance of the pronunciation of the most ordinary chemical terms, was perfectly at home among theories he did not comprehend, . . . scattered accepted theories to the winds and planted his own conclusions proudly on their ruins." The doctor did not do well in town, not necessarily because the camp didn't think much of his medical background, but because "it wasn't a good time for doctors anyway. Times were too hard to indulge in any sickness or other extravagance, . . . there was very little whiskey drunk and no killing going on."[25]

Dr. Harry Thomas was the antithesis of Drs. McGowan and Perry. The father of famed newsman and author Lowell Thomas, the doctor was described by his son as dedicated, well-trained, urbane, cultured, and a family man.[26] After working as a schoolteacher to earn tuition, Thomas received his M.D. from the University of Nebraska and practiced in Iowa. In 1900 he and his family moved to Victor in the Cripple Creek Mining District. Lowell Thomas recalled

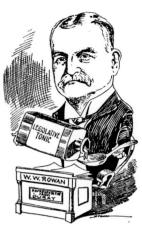

6.3 Ouray's Dr. W.W. Rowan served that San Juan mining camp for many years, not only as a physician, but as mayor and state legislator.

his father treating wounded strikers during the labor troubles of 1903-04, world famous opera house performers such as Lilian Russell, injured miners, and, as city physician, the camp's prostitutes. Dr. Thomas founded the town's literary club, enjoyed everything from music to mathematics, and took his son on mineral and fossil collecting expeditions in the mountains. Lowell recalled that any extra cash was spent on books, and the family's library contained three thousand volumes. The doctor kept up with medical advances by taking postgraduate courses at Johns Hopkins and other eastern medical centers. Gradually, as more and more of the district's mines closed, there were simply not enough patients to go around, and in 1918 the Thomas family left Victor and Colorado.

As in the earlier gold rush, some of the later mining camp doctors came to practice medicine, some to "mine," and some to do a little of both. One of the few "digging doctors" who found his bonanza was Dr. Abner Wright.[27] Wright's prospecting days went all the way back to the California Gold Rush of 1849 and his long list of adventures included a wrestling match with a grizzly bear. Finding no gold, he had returned to his midwestern practice. In 1860 Dr. Wright joined the Colorado Gold Rush, and again finding no gold, resumed his practice once more. Finally, in the 1870s, succumbing to the "fever" once again, he prospected in Chalk Creek Canyon near St. Elmo, Colorado. This time he hit the jackpot—the lode that became the Mary Murphy mine. Wright sold his claim for $75,000, and apparently having achieved his lifelong goal, settled down to practice medicine in Buena Vista until his retirement in 1895. Ultimately, the Mary Murphy produced more than 14 million dollars in gold, silver, and other minerals.

A few of the new generation of "digging doctors" continued to do their own prospecting. In 1891 in a news item entitled, "Mining Doctor," the *Rico Democrat* reported:

> Dr. John Dugan is working on the Printer Boy lode in Aztec Gulch. The doctor has been bothered by the ground caving, but he hopes to remedy that soon and feels sure of striking it rich before the summer is over.[28]

Most of the new breed, however, were more interested in the financial aspects of mining, and became mine investors, owners, or even managers. Notations such as the following are frequent in the biographical sketches of late nineteenth and early twentieth century Colorado physicians:

> Henry C. James, M.D. of Silver Cliff. He has been

> speculating in mining [and] owns the Empress Josephine mine.[29]

> J.J. Hendricks, M.D. of Kokomo . . . one of the discoverers of the John R. mine and one of the owners of the Ida L. mine.[29]

> Henry Paul, M.D. of Aspen . . . was selected as manager of the Consolidated Aspen Durant mine.[29]

The editor of the *Colorado Medical Journal* was concerned by all of this "mining speculation by medical men." Noting that

> since riches do not commonly come through the practice of medicine . . . it is not surprising that, in a mining region, many physicians are tempted to invest in [mining] stocks.[30]

Indeed, sniffed the doctor,

> We have met a great number of medical men . . . who have made mining investments of late and, curiously enough, we have yet to see one who has not already made money—or who is not absolutely sure he is going to do so shortly. Unfortunately, the prognosis in some of these cases seems likely to be as erroneous as some diagnoses are prone to be, when the case comes to autopsy, for the investigation of a mine and its ultimate outcome seem analogous to our diagnosis and the autopsy. We have all known cases in which they did not agree.[30]

The same volume of the *Colorado Medical Journal* reported:

> Dr. Hugo Mager is at present happy over some Cripple Creek mining investments.[31]

> The Henrietta No. 2 mine is owned by a number of physicians in Colorado Springs; it promises a great deal.[31]

> Dr. B.J. Perry has moved from Aspen to Denver and given up medicine to engage in mining interests.[31]

The mining camp doctors engaged in a variety of other activities besides medicine and mining. Some went into politics. The first two mayors of Empire were physicians, as were the mayors of Cripple Creek, Idaho Springs, Leadville, and other communities.[32] Some went into business, selling everything from shoes to Singer sewing machines.[33] Dr. Jeffrey O'Neal's drugstore in Idaho Springs was famous for having one of the most elegant soda fountains in Colorado.[33] Others worked as journalists, lawmen, or postmasters. Dr. Jacob Rice built a toll road over the 12,000 foot pass linking Twin Lakes and Aspen, the forerunner of today's scenic Independence Pass road.[34] Some physicians engaged in a remarkable variety of non-medical endeavors.

Dr. John A. Whiting was mayor of Cripple Creek, a land developer, director of the Gold Dollar and Mabel M. mines, and had a "practice among the largest of any physician in the state."[35] The champion doctor-entrepreneur, however, must have been Dr. G. F. Hoop of Idaho Springs.[36] During the four years between 1885 and 1889, Dr. Hoop was active as an investor and officer in numerous mining enterprises, owner of a real estate firm, loan office, drug store, and hotel, and a candidate for political office. In addition, he maintained an active medical practice. Today's medical-entrepreneurial types might well admire Dr. Hoop.

Health Care

The larger mining camps such as Leadville, Aspen, Ouray, and Georgetown had numerous doctors and even hospitals. They were served by the railroads, and cases requiring special care could easily be evacuated to Denver. A dollar a month was deducted from each mine worker's wages, entitling him to the services of a contract physician and, when necessary, to hospitalization. In some communities, medical services were provided by unions or fraternal lodges. In Leadville, for example, it was said that the lodges

> care for the sick and bury the dead. Hundreds of men coming to Leadville . . . were taken sick and would have fallen victims to the most horrible suffering, had not their connection with some order brought them kind and loving brothers who . . . smoothed the fevered brows and wet the parched lips and nursed them back to health.[37]

The unemployed and the indigent had to depend upon the charity of physicians and hospitals or, in some communities, on the services of a physician employed by the city or county. In 1881 Leadville's city physician treated 120 "poor patients."[38]

Some of the larger mines had on-site medical facilities. At the Tomboy mine, high above Telluride, the company provided

> two clean, well-lighted rooms in the boarding house . . . with a doctor, generally young in experience, in constant attendance. His equipment was adequate for minor accidents, burns, cuts, etc. All critical cases were sent down the hill as soon as an ambulance could work its way up from Telluride.[39]

In the more remote areas, resourcefulness was often a physician's most valuable quality. Alone in primitive surroundings, the isolated doctor had no choice but to take on some difficult and

even seemingly impossible challenges. Dr. George W. Compton of Ophir found himself in such a situation when he arrived at a mountain cabin "twenty miles from nowhere." He had come that distance to attend a pregnant woman who was hemorrhaging. The enlarged and bleeding uterus, he soon discovered, was not due to pregnancy, but to a tumor. He determined that the only way to stop the bleeding was to remove the tumor—at once!

> I longed for some assistance, but as there was none at hand, I took off my coat, rolled up my sleeves and went after it . . . I soon had the growth peeled out and the hemorrhage arrested . . . It [was] about two and one-half pounds. Today the patient is doing well and promises to recover.[40]

This was no mean accomplishment in an era when abdominal surgery, even in a hospital operating room, was still a risky procedure.

Dr. Finla McClure was visiting a saloon in Junction City (later Garfield), Colorado, when an altercation led to a miner having his throat cut.

> With no instruments or anaesthetics . . . [the doctor] called to the bartender for darning needle and twine and, with the help of four men to hold the patient down, he sewed the gash together . . .[41]

Such medical resourcefulness was not limited to emergencies. Silverton's Dr. W.R. Winters was called to treat a young man whose hip had been broken in a mining accident. Typically, when such a fracture healed, the result was a markedly shortened leg. Dr. Winters was determined to avoid this outcome. He went to the local hardware store and bought "pulleys, weights, rope and other equipment." Then he

> had a carpenter build a framework over the man's bed. He prepared the patient, set the bone and, with the tackle, he tightened and held the break in place. The edges knit, and when well, the man had a straight leg.[42]

Isolation did not necessarily prevent a mining camp doctor from practicing "modern" medicine. In 1879, for example, in the tiny mining town of Empire, Dr. T. Hartmann performed some remarkable ophthalmic surgery, creating an "artificial pupil" and restoring sight to an eye blinded by an injury suffered many years before. The *Georgetown Courier* hailed the event, noting that " . . . as far as we know, this is the first operation of this kind that has ever been successfully attempted in the state of Colorado."[43]

Resourcefulness was sometimes needed just to get to the patient. The problems of terrain, great distances, primitive trails, and mud or snow, sometimes required unusual and even exotic means of transportation. In the winter, the doctor's horse and buggy, and even the horse alone, were often useless. Dr. F. M. Ramey crossed Mosquito Pass during a blinding snowstorm one night on foot in order to attend to a patient in Alma, finding his way by following the line of telegraph poles.[44] Sleighs were often used and the more athletic physician might even resort to snowshoes or skis. Dr. Jacob Rice put together a remarkable contraption for his winter-time housecalls. It was described as

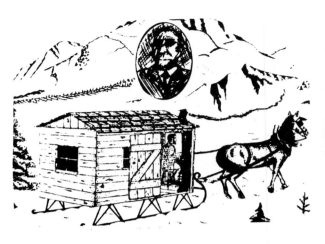

> a sleigh enclosed with a framework of boards, making a small house on runners. In the front . . . was a small stove with a little crooked stovepipe sticking out the top. He carried his supply of stovewood with him, so regardless of the weather, he was comfortably warm.[45]

6.4 Dr. Rice's "house on runners" must have been something to behold! The doctor practiced in Twin Lakes, on the eastern approach to the Independence Pass road, which he helped build. (Dr. Nolie Mumey)

Dr. Gardiner recalled a winter "housecall" to a miner whose face had been "mashed in" by a delayed blast.[46] Guided by the miner's brother, the doctor set out on snow "so crusted that they could not use snowshoes" and up ice-packed forty-five degree inclines to an altitude of nearly 14,000 feet. Because of the danger of avalanches, the guide walked ahead of the doctor lest they both be buried in a slide. Sure enough an avalanche hit, killing Gardiner's horse and breaking a few of his ribs. Whiskey eased the pain some, but the now unsteady physician nearly fell over a thousand foot ledge. By the time they reached the miner's cabin, Gardiner was virtually incapacitated by altitude sickness. He managed to give the injured miner a shot of morphine before he himself collapsed. The next day they used skis to put together a makeshift sled and managed to get the injured miner to town. In something of an understatement, Dr. Gardiner attributed the successful outcome of his excursion to the fact that "fortunately I was in good shape."

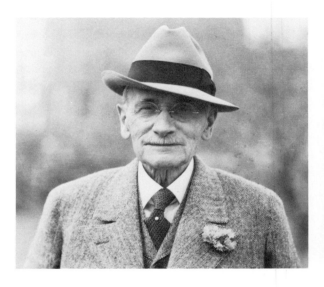

6.5 Dr. C.F. Gardiner spent his early professional years in Crested Butte. Some of his mining camp experiences are told in his classic account of early-day Colorado medicine, *Doctor at Timberline*.

Winter in the high country made the evacuation of sick and injured miners especially difficult. At the Mary Murphy a bobsled was kept at the upper level to facilitate medical transport.[47] When an injured miner was evacuated during a blinding snowstorm from St. Elmo to the hospital in Buena Vista, some of the party had to walk ahead of the sleigh with lanterns in order to light the way. It took the group eleven hours to cover twenty miles.[48] When a sick miner had to be evacuated from the Silver Lake mine above Silverton, he was put in an ore bucket and swung down the tramway. From the tramway terminal he was taken by sleigh to town.[49]

Even in the summer, housecalls could be dangerous in the mountains. Dr. John Law's mountain trek to a miner with pneumonia came to an abrupt halt when he encountered a pride of mountain lions. Not knowing what else to do, Leadville's pioneer physician let out "a yell . . . that would have done credit to any Sioux Indian." The big cats scattered and Dr. Law spent the next three days at the miner's cabin.[50]

Sometimes, a physician was simply not available. In *Digging Gold in the Rockies*, G. T. Ingham recalled:

> [We saw] many poor fellows sick and . . . entirely dependent upon strangers . . . There are no conveniences to help the sick in a new mining camp. There are no beds but the ground, no shelter but tents and rude huts . . . The food is unfit for the sick . . . Very frequently medical attendance cannot be had . . . Yet there are many noble acts shown by miners and others in the mountains toward those who are sick.[51]

Another visitor to the camps commented on how the miners cared for their brethren:

> The sick miner . . . has the most careful attention from his fellows. The hands that minister to his wants may be rough and toil-hardened and the voices about his bunk may lack the refinements of polite usage, but no lack of solicitous care or of nursing ever delays his recovery.[52]

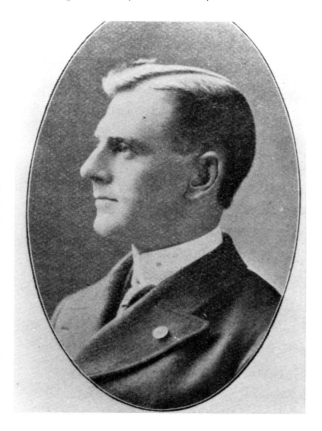

Ouray's Dr. Hamilton Fish had recognized the need to apply the principles of battlefield medicine to the more isolated mining camps.[53] The battlefield and the mine had a lot in common: the occurrence of massive wounds and the absence of immediate professional care. In both places, time was critical if lives were to be saved. In his campaign to introduce battlefield medicine to the mines, Fish trained mine foremen in the fundamentals of first aid: antisepsis, the control of hemorrhage, splinting, resuscitation, and so on. He designed a miner's first aid kit which contained an assortment of dressings, bandages, splints, antiseptics, anaesthetics— and a pint of whiskey. Fish also invented a harness which could be used to carry an injured man up or down a ladder and a special stretcher designed for use in tunnels. He also devised a horse-drawn conveyance, based on the Indian's travois, which could be used where "wheeled vehicles would be inadmissable and [which could] be used in deep snow by substituting a man on snowshoes [for the horse]."

Hospitals

As early as 1878 it was clear that Leadville was here to stay and that the growing community would soon need a hospital. The town's Catholic priest, Father Henry Robinson, appealed to the Sisters of Charity in Leavenworth, Kansas, for help. In December three sisters arrived after an adventurous trip from Denver.[54] Caught in a blizzard and wrapped in buffalo robes, the sisters had been transferred from their stagecoach to an improvised sleigh and finally arrived in Leadville during the night. The *Leadville Chronicle* devoted its front page to describing their welcome to the Cloud City:

> [The sisters] had heard that up here on the world's mountain top was sickness, sorrow and despair, and they came to comfort . . . [Seeing the sisters], the rough crowd . . . fell back in respectful silence, and many a rough, long-bearded, coarsely apparelled miner uncovered his head.[54]

The sisters must have been reassured by the sight of Father Robinson, although he himself was only just recovering from pneumonia.[55] They soon set to work, secured a donation of land, and collected funds, "nobody refusing assistance to the Sisters in their work of charity."[56] Even as construction proceeded, the unfinished hospital admitted its first patient, a frostbitten prospector who had tried to cross Mosquito Pass in mid-winter. The sisters pursuaded the workmen to board up the windows in one room for their unexpected guest. The prospector was beyond help, however, and four days later Father Robinson administered last rites.[57]

On March 1, 1879, St. Vincent's Hospital was officially opened. Located on what was then the outskirts of town and surrounded by a field of sage brush and pine stumps, the two story frame building had two wings with four wards and twelve private rooms.[58] There was enough space for forty to fifty beds, and cloth partitions allowed some privacy. The paint was hardly dry when twenty-seven cases of measles were admitted in one day. In addition to the usual ailments and injuries, the hospital cared for the terrible traumas associated with mining accidents. The sisters worked day and night and even Bishop Machebeuf commented that "they are overburdened with work."[59] During the first year, about a thousand patients were treated, of whom 100 died.

The hospital survived a town fire, but the sisters soon faced another threat. A railroad depot was to be built a few blocks away, and with their property now valuable, the sisters began to receive letters urging them to move the

6.6 Dr. Hamilton Fish left a successful practice in Denver to work with the miners of Ouray.

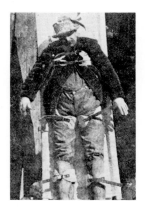

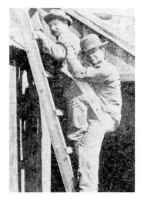

6.7 In his effort to bring "battlefield" medicine to the mines, Dr. Fish taught the foremen first-aid and devised evacuation devices and procedures for the miners.

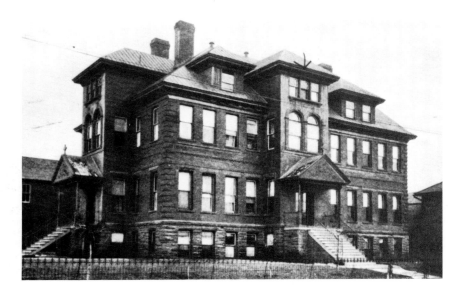

6.8 Leadville's St. Vincent's Hospital was an impressive structure.

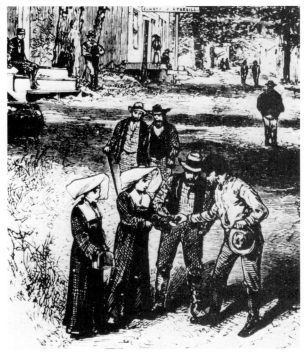

6.9 To keep the hospital financially solvent, St. Vincent's sisters scoured the mining camps to solicit funds.

hospital to another site. Eventually, armed volunteers were called upon to guard the hospital, and a shooting resulted when some "lot-jumpers" tried to tear down the hospital's fence.[60]

St. Vincent's was always in need of money, and the sisters, not busy enough with nursing, laundry, cooking, cleaning, and religious devotions, also served as fund raisers. It was said that they even "went down the mineshafts" to solicit donations from the miners.[61] By 1895 a number of improvements had been made, and the hospital was described as " large and commodious and fitted out with all the modern improvements." The sisters were especially proud of their new operating room, which was described as "bright and cheery, the floor being tiled most artistically, while the walls have an enamel finish." The sisters had grown to a staff

of eight who, it was said, were "equally as zealous as the little band of '79."[62] By 1895 the hospital had admitted more than 8,000 patients, many of them, it was proudly noted, non-Catholic. In 1901 a new hospital, a formidable three story building of brick and stone, was built adjacent to the original wooden structure.

In the next fifteen years, various orders of Catholic nuns established hospitals in Georgetown, Durango, Breckenridge, Ouray, and Cripple Creek. St. Joseph's Hospital, in Georgetown, was described as being "entirely free from sectarian influence."[63] The sisters had "had long experience in nursing the sick," and a yearly subscription of ten dollars would "ensure hospital care, board, lodging, [and the] attendance of a nurse and physician."[64]

Durango's Mercy Hospital was founded by the Sisters of Mercy in 1882.[65] Bishop Machebeuf, recognizing the need for a hospital in the southwestern part of the state, asked the sisters to move from their storefront "hospital" in the tiny town of Conejos. Within four months, land had been donated and an eight bed wooden hospital constructed. Several years later, a smallpox epidemic decimated the sisters and the hospital was closed for five months. In 1885 the frame building was replaced by a two story sandstone hospital with twenty-five beds. Although a definite improvement over the original structure, light was still provided by kerosene lamps, coal stoves were used for heat, and there was no plumbing. In 1892 an addition provided private rooms, running water, and steam heat.

Breckenridge's original hospital was a makeshift affair jointly administered by the county and the Miners Protective Association. Gratefully, they turned the enterprise over to the Benedictine Sisters in 1886. The hospital, renamed St. Joseph's, remained inadequate. Operations were done on an ordinary table, and the *Daily Journal* complained:

> The old rookery is no longer able to fill the bill. There is but one room . . . Half a dozen patients, one perhaps crushed in a mine, another frozen, a third suffering from pneumonia, a fourth with disorders requiring private attention . . . should not all occupy one room . . . Operations are sometimes necessary that . . . cannot be successfully performed in the presence of other patients . . . To call such accommodations a hospital is a misnomer.[66]

Bishop Machebeuf was also responsible for Ouray's hospital. The railroad from Durango reached only as far north as Silverton, and the road from Ouray and the northern camps was treacherous and often impassable. At the bishop's request, the Sisters of Mercy opened St. Joseph's Hospital in 1887.[67] The building was substantial, white stone, two stories and a basement, with a thirty foot frontage and sixty foot depth. Patients were classified as private, mine subscribers, or county and charity. The first "subscriber" patient was an injured miner from the Terrible Mine. The sisters were described as "indefatigable workers . . . never tiring . . . constantly in the service of their patients."[68] Reverend Gibbons recalled that many miners were so impressed by the devotion and self-sacrifice of the sisters that they converted to Catholicism.[69]

By 1894 the Cripple Creek gold district had a huge population but no hospital. Once again, an order of nuns[70] was asked to step in, and that year the Sisters of Mercy opened a small hospital. The miners managed to save it from the fire of 1896, but it was replaced in 1898 by the new St. Nicholas Hospital. This was a truly impressive building—three stories of stone and brick, twenty-six rooms, hot and cold running water, steam heat, an operating room, fine furnishings and a wine cellar for the sisters. The cost was $12,000. The first patient was a miner who had fallen down a mine shaft. In 1902 the sisters added living quarters and a school. By 1918, Cripple Creek had become moribund and the hospital reduced to twenty beds. In 1924 the sisters sold it to a group of physicians and the name was changed to Cripple Creek Hospital.

Not all of the mining camp hospitals were church affiliated. In addition to St. Vincent's Hospital, Leadville had the Union Veterans Hospital, the Women's Christian Temperance Union Hospital, a county hospital and poor house, and a private hospital which catered to those who did "not care to patronize the public institutions."[71] The latter included ladies who wished to "avoid publicity." St. Luke's Hospital, an Episcopal institution, was opened in 1885.

At one time, Cripple Creek was said to have had ten hospitals, mainly in private residences. The Teller County Hospital, which opened in 1902, also served as a poor house and nursing home.[72] Nearby Victor had two hospitals. One, the Red Cross Hospital had originally been the Gold Coin, a miner's club. Jack Dempsey was treated there after an accident in the Portland Mine.[73] Also known as the "District" or "Miner's" Hospital, it was closed in 1928, and its equipment was moved to St. Nicholas Hospital in Cripple Creek.

The mining camps of Gunnison, Lake City, and Fairplay all had hospitals.[74] A hospital was

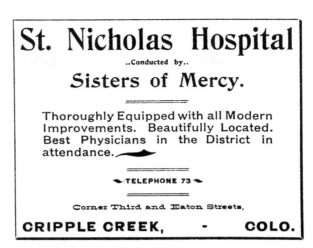

6.10 Cripple Creek's St. Nicholas Hospital advertised its modern facilities.

proposed but never built at Rico.[75] Sometimes there was a long interval between the proposal for a hospital and its construction. In 1883 the *Rocky Mountain News* reported: "Silverton is moving to erect a hospital for the . . . sick and wounded miner . . . The enterprise is a commendable one and should meet with hearty support."[76]

It was not until twenty-six years later, however, in 1909, that: "The Silverton Miners' Union Hospital was opened . . . well-built, two story and a half, basement of brick, with a capacity of thirty beds. It cost $30,000."[77]

In 1891, Aspen, always a classy town, celebrated the opening of its hospital with a grand ball on Hallam Lake. One hundred couples took the train from Denver to engage in the festivities. Aspen Citizen's Hospital was a community project and unaffiliated with any church. The hospital, on the north fork of the Roaring Fork River, was in "Queen Anne" style, brick, with two wards and four private rooms. Today's condominium buyer might wonder at its cost—$750 for the land and $20,000 for construction. The upper floor provided housing for nurses. In 1920 Citizen's Hospital was purchased by Dr. W. H. Twining.[78]

Telluride's Miner's Hospital was built in 1893, an impressive stone structure which is now a museum. In 1902 the Western Federation of Miners built the Miner's Union Hospital, which, the *Denver Times* reported, was to be the "best designed and most thoroughly equipped hospital in Southern Colorado." The three-story-plus-basement, brick and sandstone building contained four general wards and six private wards, an operating room, kitchen and dining room, a steam heating plant, and a union meeting hall. It became a focus of the miners' strike of 1903-04 and was closed, apparently by the National Guard.[79]

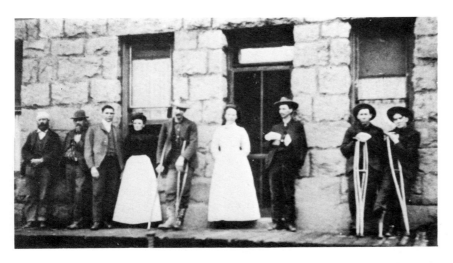

6.11 Miner-patients and nurses standing in front of Telluride's Miner's Hospital. (Nancy and Ed Bathke)

Fiscal insolvency is a chronic disease of hospitals, and then as now, hospitals were expensive to build and maintain. As construction progressed on Aspen's Citizens Hospital, costs increased and the *Aspen Times* called for donations. The town's 1300 miners were asked to donate a day's wages, three dollars,[80] and were reminded that the hospital would be "a great blessing to many an unfortunate miner."[81] The religious were reminded that "a hospital is entitled to the same consideration that a church is . . ."[82] The successful businessman was advised that if he would cut down from ten to five cigars a day he could "give the hospital fund $3.50 and be better off physically and just as well financially. No one would be the loser," said the *Times*, "but the cigar merchant and the government. Try it!"[83] A Hospital Day was held at the Mineral Palace, an extravaganza at which the Aspenite could see a variety of "deer, foxes, bear, flowers, minerals, horned toads, painting, shells, silver nuggets . . ." and many other fascinating exhibits. The *Times* reminded the townspeople:

> Don't forget to take a dollar for the hospital fund . . . Let the list [of donors] swell . . . You will never miss the dollar and it may be the means of saving several lives by good nursing in the palatial hospital building.[84]

The next morning, the *Times* was able to add thirty-three new names to the hospital's subscription list. By September $16,030 had been subscribed and a Grand Charity Ball was held to celebrate the hospital's opening. On that occasion, and with great civic pride, the *Times* commented that the opening of the hospital

> bears testimony to the intelligence, refinement, culture, humanity, progressiveness and liberality of the people of Aspen. It belongs to them, for the

entire expense . . . has been met by popular subscription . . . It is in every sense the peoples' offering for the good of afflicted humanity.[85]

Such an outpouring of public spirit was not evident in Silverton, where the need for a hospital had remained unfulfilled for decades. Years later it was recalled that

> An effort was made to obtain sizable donations from the people of the town, but in vain. It was expected that the big saloons who got so much money from the miners . . . would come forward, but no sizable subscription was made.[86]

The miner's union finally made Silverton's hospital a reality. It was said that, "without a grumble [they] practically did it all. With its membership it raised the entire sum."[86]

It was one thing to build a hospital and another to keep it solvent. The Catholic hospitals were expected to pay their own way, and the sisters spent a great deal of their time and effort nursing deficits as well as miners. Most of the hospitals had "health plans," a dollar a month from each miner's wages. This was not enough, however, and the sisters were a familiar sight in even the most remote mining camps, collecting for the hospital. One sister recalled traveling, " . . . as a poor beggar," on the mountain roads. She and her companions were returning from a "fund raiser" at the Hidden Treasure Mine near Lake City when their buggy overturned. They sustained serious injuries and the horse and buggy wound up in the river.[87]

In 1891 the sisters at Ouray's St. Joseph's Hospital were faced with a crisis when the mine owners established new rules for their workers. The miner's medical subscription of a dollar a month was eliminated, and the *Solid Muldoon* reported that the sisters were left with "practically no steady income at all."[88] In 1893 with the demonetization of silver, things became even worse. As the number of patients decreased, the sisters were assigned to other hospitals. Tom Walsh, the millionaire owner of the Camp Bird, persuaded the sisters to return and paid off the hospital's debt of $3,500. They stayed, even as silver and the town became less important. In 1900 Ouray held a fair which raised $1,000 for the hospital. Finally, in 1918 the hospital was sold and the sisters left.[89]

Things were no better in the other silver camps—once booming, they were now nearly deserted. Eventually, most of the mining camp hospitals closed their doors permanently.

7 DENVER

The city is well built; the houses are attractive, constructed of brick, stone, or wood. Denver has numerous public buildings, a theatre, a mint . . . , a college, schools and several newspapers, not to mention the churches . . . Denver has wide streets . . . planted with trees. Everywhere are stores, banks, hotels, saloons . . . The movement of life is everywhere.

Louis L. Simonin, 1867[1]

ALTHOUGH COLORADO'S Gold Rush began at what would become Denver, the few flecks of color in Cherry Creek were soon played out. The prospectors moved on to the mountains, but through the efforts of developer William Larimer, publisher William Byers, and others, the settlements at Cherry Creek were consolidated and Denver stayed on the map. Its early years were those of a rugged frontier town: log cabins, dirt streets, open sewers, and the like. Ministers, editors, and civic leaders vied with con men, saloon keepers, and "bummers" for control of the town. Denver's existence was threatened in the 1860s by flood and fire, Indian scares and Confederate rebels, and early mining industry doldrums and railroad snubs. Still, the town survived and grew.

Denver rapidly established a reputation for healthfulness. In an 1859 letter to the folks back home, a prospector wrote, "Universal good health prevails. I am getting so fleshy that my clothes are quite too small."[2] Denver's professional boosters agreed, one early publication proclaiming that "The salubrity of this vicinity is unquestionable. Indigenous maladies are entirely unknown."[3] This medically pristine environment was soon interrupted by the town's first death. General Larimer described the victim as a healthy and robust young man who, despite a "severe cold," had "gone up to the mountains to hunt . . . [He] got over-heated, took a sudden cold from the mountain winds, and died suddenly, with swollen glands . . ."[4]

The unfortunate young man might have been attended by any of a number of doctors in the area. Quite a few physicians had come overland with the gold seekers. Like their fellow travelers, most had come to prospect, and like their fellows, the great majority were unsuccessful in their quest, remained for a short time, and soon returned to their families and patients back east. Levi Russell had come to find gold but took the precaution of having his name included among the eight physicians listed in the town's 1859 directory.[5]

In 1860 the *Rocky Mountain News* reported what may have been the first major surgery performed in Denver, the amputation of a Mr. Johnson's gunshot-shattered arm by Dr. Drake McDowell and four other physicians.[6] The patient did well and the newspaper noted that "Dr. McDowell's operation is highly spoken of." Four days later, McDowell performed a "very delicate" operation for hare lip. A few months later, Dr. H.H. Beals operated on the daughter of Jim Baker, the famous mountain man and scout. According to the *Mountaineer*, the girl had been bitten on the lip by a spider. The wound became infected and had sloughed, leaving "a great gaping aperture which frightfully disfugured the face. The surgeon performed an operation which left no trace of the repulsive wound except a slight scar."[7]

Those were rip-roarin' days in early Denver. Both Drs. A. F. Peck and McDowell were in attendance at the infamous Whitsett-McClure duel, and Dr. S.E. Kennedy's office was the scene of a knife fight between irate patients.[8] Drs. Peck and William M. Belt were involved in a famous shootout at the Criterion saloon.[9] That fracas had included the proprietor of the Criterion, the notorious Charley Harrison. Harrison also had a run-in with another of Denver's pioneer physicians, Dr. O. D. Cass.[10] One day, Harrison's "woman" had become ill and he went to fetch the doctor. When Cass was indelicate enough to remind the saloon-keeper that his fee was twenty-five dollars in advance, Harrison "whipped out an ugly looking six-shooter," thrust it in the doctor's face, and told him, "Damn your fee; follow me, sir, and be quick about it." Cass recalled that Harrison "led me to the door of his cabin, opened it, pointed to the patient, and immediately disappeared in the darkness. I attended her for a week and cured her."[10]

Sometime later, Harrison reappeared at the doctor's office and placed twenty-five dollars in gold pieces on his desk. Fees were not always collected so easily. The fourth lawsuit in the history of Denver's District Court was brought by Dr. Peck against (later) Territorial Governor Alexander C. Hunt. Peck had cared for the Hunt family and their hired man for nearly two years but had been unable to collect any fees for his efforts. The court awarded the doctor the full amount, $139.50 plus costs.[11]

In 1859 Dr. McDowell attempted to establish a hospital in Denver. Negotiations were undertaken with the directors of the Denver City Town Company and property was assigned for the project. There is some evidence that Dr. McDowell found the property to be unsatisfactory. At any rate the plan for a hospital fizzled.[12] The following year saw several major, if short-lived medical milestones: the organization of the Jefferson Medical Society (Chapter 10), the adoption of a medical fee schedule and a Code of Ethics (Chapter 11), and the establishment of not one, but apparently, two hospitals.

There is reference to a hospital having been opened, at the request of Denver's officials, by Dr. A.R. Sternberger. Little else is known about it other than it was constructed of logs and "semi-public in character." It has been called the forerunner of today's Denver General Hospital.[13] There is more tangible evidence for the City Hospital directed by Drs. J.F. Hamilton and Cass and located on Sixteenth Street near Blake.[14] The City Hospital was staffed by a warden and nurses, and its officers and trustees included some of Denver's most prominent men. The *Rocky Mountain News* reported that, although

the hospital's census was down to four patients in the fall, it had had as many as sixteen during the summer.[15] One patient was the unfortunate Dr. J.S. Stone. Stone, a physician and judge of the Mountain City District Miner's Court, and L.W. Bliss, the acting territorial governor, had engaged in a shotgun duel, the result of "some personal language" used by Bliss "in presenting a toast."[16] Dr. Stone, severely wounded, lingered for months before he finally died.

Dr. Hamilton complained that the costs of running the hospital were becoming unbearable. Supporting the establishment from his own income and occasional contributions, he decided to move to a smaller building above Larimer Street.[17] The *Rocky Mountain News* commented, "The attention of the public should be called to [the hospital] and appropriation given for successfully carrying out the undertaking so nobly begun."[18] Dr. Hamilton was awarded recognition, if not remuneration, when the following month he was elected City Physician, an appointment in which he was "to serve without salary."[19] Hamilton continued in that role until 1861, when he joined the First Regiment of Colorado Volunteers as its surgeon and left for the Civil War.

The City Hospital did not survive Dr. Hamilton's departure, and the balance of the decade saw a haphazard series of arrangements made to house patients in Denver's poorhouse and in private homes at county expense.[20] In the 1860s only the poor went to hospitals, and little distinction was made between the hospital and the poorhouse. In these early years, Denver was part of Arapahoe County, and governmental complexities clouded the issue of who was responsible for the medically indigent—a theme which is familiar to observers of Denver's and Colorado's contemporary medical scene. In the 1870s, some progress was made, largely as the result of the efforts of two physicians, Drs. John Elsner and Frederick Bancroft. Despite their active private practices, both men served as city and county physicians and played major roles in the creation of what would become Denver General Hospital.[21]

In 1866 Dr. Bancroft proposed the establishment of a county hospital to the Board of County Commissioners, but no action was taken. In 1870 the new county physician, Dr. Elsner, rented a building, spent $250 equipping it, designated it as the County Hospital, and "collected the patients, [some of whom] were lying in the henhouses and barns . . ."[22] Next, in his annual report to the county commissioners, Elsner urged still "more commodious quarters for the

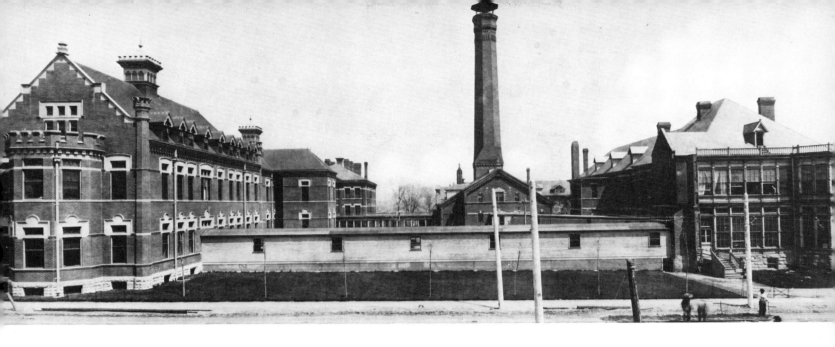

county patients." The commissioners responded by thanking the doctor "for his untiring energy" and tabling the proposal. Finally, in 1873 land was purchased at the corner of West 6th Avenue and Cherokee and the first building of a combination poorhouse-hospital was under construction.

Also in 1873, Denver's first private hospital, St. Joseph's, opened. The early '70s saw significant progress in Denver's medical environment. Two years before, Denver's doctors had established a medical society, adopted a code of ethics and a fee schedule, and began their efforts to organize a medical library.

As the years went on, more and more talented and well educated physicians came to Denver (many of them for health reasons), medical schools and additional hospitals were established, and efforts were made to enact public health laws and to improve the city's sanitation. By the 1890s, Denver was calling itself a medical center. The legitimacy of that self-designated title was enhanced in 1898, when Denver hosted the highly successful national meeting of the American Medical Association. At the same time, with increasing urbanization and the influx of large numbers of poor people from the East, typhoid and tuberculosis continued to be major problems, and the city's and the County Hospital's resources were perpetually tested and strained.

Denver General Hospital

Dr. Elsner stepped down as county physician in 1873, gratified that the position had become permanent and that a bona fide County Hospital had been opened. The new hospital was housed in a substantial brick building, 100 feet in length and costing $4,200.[23] In November 1874, the County Physician's *Annual Report* summarized the new hospital's activities during its first year:

During the year 189 patients have been received and treated at the hospital. Of these 18 died, 141 were discharged and 30 remain in the wards. More than half of these were foreign-born, Ireland alone furnishing 26 . . . For the seven months ending November 1, expenditures for the institution amounted to $2,175.[24]

Public hospitals have traditionally been the targets—sometimes justifiably, sometimes not—of individual physicians, medical societies, the media, politicians, special interest groups, and just plain angry citizens. They always seem to be involved in financial crises, professional scandals, and political fights. None so more than Denver General Hospital—from its very beginnings. The attacks began as soon as the dedication ceremonies were completed. The first barrage was fired by the Denver Medical Association and was directed against a broad front: the new hospital's architecture, organization, finances, and administration. Since the association had never been consulted in the hospital's

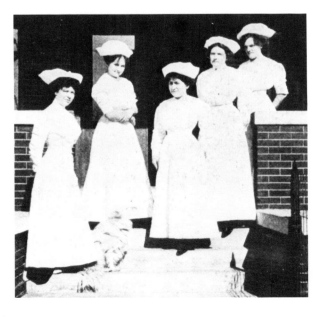

planning, it suggested that its members refrain from caring for the hospital's patients unless such care was reimbursed.[25] Not long afterward, the hospital's director was answering charges that the hospital was caring for patients who were not residents of the county. He responded by pointing out that the hospital had collected, that year, the [then] not insignificant sum of $1,500 in charges and reimbursements.[26] An attempt to build a separate structure for patients with contagious diseases was blocked by a county commissioner who commented that the hospital was just a poor house and was already big enough for its needs.[26] Despite such attacks, the 1880s saw significant growth and improvement—including an additional building, a downtown outpatient facility, and a pesthouse for contagious diseases. By 1889 another addition expanded the hospital's capacity to ninety-one beds, but this soon proved insufficient.

The County Hospital's horse-drawn ambulance, introduced in 1892, became a familiar site careening through downtown Denver in response to emergencies. Surgical cases, often on an emergency basis, constituted a major portion of the hospital's patient load. One surgeon, a professor at one of the medical schools, performed 127 major operations during his four month rotation at the County Hospital.[27] He was obviously a general surgeon as his work included orthopedic, neurosurgical, abdominal, and plastic surgery. In comparing his experience with that of today's Denver General Hospital, it should be noted that in four months there were only five stabbings and one gunshot wound. Infectious diseases, mental illness and alcoholism accounted for a large proportion of non-surgical admissions to the County Hospital. The *Annual Report* for 1891 cited tuberculosis (139 cases), pneumonia (123), typhoid (102), "insanity" (83), and delirium tremens (34). The hospital staff, that year, included two resident physicians, a druggist, thirty volunteer physicians and twenty-seven nurses.[28] In 1901 several

of the older structures were replaced by a new building.

The County Hospital grew despite continued challenges, scandals, and attacks. Politicians and the newspapers periodically charged the hospital with fiscal irresponsibility. On one occasion, it was claimed that the average cost of a week's hospitalization, six dollars, was twice what it should be.[29] An outbreak of typhoid in the hospital was traced to the contamination of refrigerated food by a misdirected hospital sewer line—but not before a doctor and the head nurse had died. An administrative impasse between Arapahoe County and the State Insane Asylum prevented the transfer of psychiatric patients to the asylum. Left in medical limbo, such patients were housed in the basement of the hospital, the nineteenth century equivalent of a medieval dungeon. The scandal broke when a patient was allegedly beaten to death by two attendants. An autopsy ascribed his "insanity" to acute meningitis and his death to trauma.[30] One of the staff surgeons charged that he had to operate under "the most septic and unsanitary conditions."[31]

In 1902 the city of Denver was administratively divorced from Arapahoe County and provided with county status of its own. As a result, Arapahoe County Hospital had its name changed to Denver City and County Hospital.[32] Unfortunately it took another ten years to complete the administrative transition. All sorts of staffing, equipment, and building needs remained unsatisfied, and Denver politics were superimposed upon county politics. In 1910 a report by Dr. Mary E. Bates' Board of County Visitors recommended extensive remodeling of the facilities, administration, and operations of the hospital.[33] The report pointed out:

> Various [department] heads whose appointments are dictated largely by "politics."
>
> "Chronics" and "regular boarders" who should be in the county home . . .
>
> Patients not apparently emergency cases received in the clerk's office where there are no provisions for their privacy or comfort while waiting . . .
>
> [Inadequate and outdated facilities and equipment] that practically compels antiquated styles of medical treatment and even serious neglect . . .

These comments were made during the administration of Mayor Robert Speer. Speer, in the tradition of other urban political bosses, combined minority votes with underworld connections and civic improvements with establishment connections. Unlike parks and boulevards, however, the City and County Hospital was not

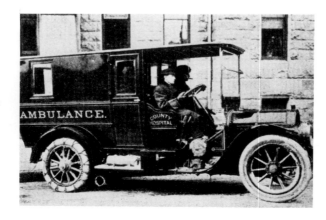

7.3 Denver General Hospital replaced its horse-drawn ambulance with a motorized one in the early 1900s.

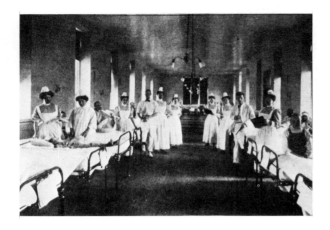

one of his priorities, and unlike other municipal facilities, it is hardly mentioned by Speer's biographers.[34] Ironically, one of Speer's early underworld buddies, gambling hall entrepreneur Vaso Chucovich, left a quarter of a million dollars in his will to create a memorial to his friend and protector. The money was ultimately used to build a children's wing at Denver General Hospital in 1941. In 1912 reformist efforts led to a complex series of political changes in the city's administration. Speer reemerged as mayor in 1917, but his death the following year saw continued instability until the election in 1923 of Benjamin Stapleton.

Throughout this era, political, administrative, and professional control of the hospital was dominated by two physicians, who served variously, as superintendent, commissioner of Health and Hospitals, and as Denver's mayor. These were William F. Sharpley and J. M. Perkins. Sharpley rose through the medical-political ranks from police surgeon to mayor and was in charge of the hospital no less than four times. Ms. L. C. Boyd, who was a nursing supervisor during those years, did not think much of Dr. Sharpley, noting that "under his regime there was always a steady decline in the management of the place . . . After the last time, 1919-1923, conditions were deplorable."[35] Another observer commented on the hospital's "rat-infested kitchen, beds without clean sheets, blankets too thin for warmth, confusion, dirt and poor food!"[36] The State Medical Society's journal referred to the County Hospital under Sharpley as a "a medico-political stronghold of malodorous maladministration."[37]

Although Sharpley was considered a villain by some, he was concerned with the welfare of the hospital and its patients. The *Denver Express* described Sharpley as angered by attempts to pare the hospital's budget while it remained a "scandalous death trap [with] wards . . . so crowded that beds are placed in the aisles."[38]

Two years later, the Denver Medical Society noted that a variety of improvements had been made at the hospital and gave credit to Sharpley, who, it pointed out, "in spite of considerable difficulty, has been responsible for the city's appropriation [to the hospital] and its efficient distribution."[39]

After several political shuffles, Sharpley was replaced by George Collins, a non-physician and a political hack and errand boy for the late Mayor Speer. To everyone's surprise, he turned out to be a devoted and effective hospital superintendent. As Ms. Boyd tells it, under Collins's leadership, the city's health administration was transferred to the hospital and many improvements were made in the hospital's facilities, personnel, and operations.[40] The State Medical Society concurred with Ms. Boyd's opinion, noting that "under Mr. Collins' supervision . . . [the Hospital] became as nearly a model of efficiency and economy . . . as was possible . . ."[41]

Over the years, much had changed at the Denver City and County Hospital—and much had not. Many of the patients could still be described, as in an earlier day's hospital report, as "usually very forlorn, suffering with dangerously acute, monotonously chronic, or seriously complicated conditions."[42] It could still be said that "towns and cities in Colorado . . . have shipped their paupers to Denver [and the hospital] in considerable numbers" and that Denver's private hospitals were not absorbing their fair share of indigent patients.[43] The hospital continued to be underfunded and regarded by many of Denver's taxpayers as an irrelevant and expensive burden which they, themselves, would never use.

The 1920s saw a civic media blitz which attempted to change the hospital's "poorhouse" image and attract the support of Denver's middle-class taxpayers. The first move was a name change—from County Hospital to the more elegant and inclusive Denver General Hospital. Newspaper articles and blurbs in the the city's slick house organ, *Municipal Facts*, emphasized that, "the hospital belongs to the people . . . of Denver . . . all classes of individuals—the poor, the defective, the insane, the middle class and the higher class . . . a cross-section of the entire population . . . ."[44] Another article recounted an average citizen's experiences while a patient at D. G. H.:

Until quite recently all that I knew about the [Denver General] Hospital was that it was situated at Sixth and Cherokee, that it had a very tall and

7.4 The surgical men's ward at Denver General Hospital, 1909.

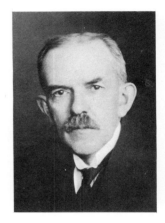

7.5 The controversial Dr. William Sharpley.

black smokestack, and that it was a place to avoid if possible. Then came a motorcycle ride one sunny day, and an unexpected crash with an automobile—and I suddenly [was] in another world.

> The Hospital is a democratic institution, receiving all classes of people. If Mrs. De Willoughby Smith-Smith smashes her electric brougham into a telephone post on Capitol Hill she may find herself in a bed next to Mrs. Flannigan, who set the uncorked gasoline bottle down on the stove for a minute . . . Every day the clanging ambulance rushes up . . . with injured men and women who, like you, never expected to see the inside of a hospital.[45]

After describing his experiences as a patient, the facilities, the hard working interns and nurses, and so on, the now initiated patient-reporter concluded:

> Visit your Hospital, Mr. Citizen. You will find there a separate world, a world of tragedy and laughter, of cheerful sacrifice and steady work, a world where pain and drowsy content lie often side by side, a world where each day sees the staging, with lightning rapidity, of many great acts in the drama of life.[45]

In today's era of sophisticated hospital marketing, this may seem a bit trite, but like all good marketing efforts, it contained an element of truth as well.

Urban Minorities

The fifty-niners were mostly of English and Scotch-Irish stock and native born. They were soon joined by Germans and Scots, and as the mines, smelters and railroads grew, by Welsh, Irish, Italians, Slavs, Greeks, Scandinavians, other Europeans, Orientals, Hispanics, and blacks. With the exception of the Southern Utes, Native Americans had been expelled from Colorado by 1880. Jews, mainly of German origin in the early days, were assimilated into the business and professional communities, if not the social circles, of Denver and the mining camps. Most of the Hispanic minority were descended from early New Mexican settlers and lived mainly in the southern San Luis Valley and the area around Trinidad. Blacks were a small minority in Denver and elsewhere in the state, some having arrived in the Civil War era. Some degree of discrimination was felt by the European minorities and much more by blacks and Hispanics, but no group was subjected to as much racial hatred in the early days as the Orientals, especially the Chinese. Originally imported as railroad workers, the Chinese were segregated into the Hop Alley districts of Denver and other

communities. Denver's one race riot was directed against the Chinese, in 1880.

As in the rest of the nation, most minorities were concentrated in the cities, and since Colorado's big city has always been Denver, the medical aspects of Colorado's minorities, with the exception of Native Americans (Chapter 3) and Hispanics (Chapter 8), are considered here. Unfortunately, little information is available on this topic. It is probably safe to assume, however, that the level of minority medical care was determined by two factors: 1) their socio-economic and educational status and, 2) the regard of the predominantly Anglo establishment. Both of these were generally low, and the level of medical care was presumably similar. As with all generalizations, there were, undoubtedly, gradations and exceptions. The poor Irishman was probably more likely to receive medical care than the poor Chinese, while the loyal black domestic was probably more likely to receive decent medical care than the vagrant and alcoholic Slav or Swede on Denver's skid row.

There is almost no mention of blacks in Colorado's early medical literature. In Denver the medical care of blacks was probably limited to the County Hospital, the free dispensaries run by the medical schools, the "back door" offices of white doctors, and the hard work of a handful of black doctors. One of the few published discussions of early Denver's black history states that blacks were denied admission to the private hospitals and the tuberculosis sanitaria.[46] The mortality rate for blacks was significantly higher than that of native whites and slightly lower than that of foreign-born whites.[47] Denver's few black doctors included two women, a Dr. T.G. Steward and the redoubtable Dr. Justina L. Ford.[48] Dr. Ford, who came to Denver in 1902, practiced for more than half a century. Her office-home was in a black section of town and she traveled by taxi to her patients' homes and to Denver General Hospital. Her practice was largely obstetric and she was said to have delivered more than 7,000 babies. When presented with a Human Relations Award at the age of eighty, Dr. Ford recalled how she had "fought like a tiger against the barriers of race and sex."[49] At least some degree of acceptance of black physicians by the medical establishment is indicated by Dr. Ford's membership in the county and state medical societies.

Published references to the medical aspects of Colorado's and Denver's Chinese usually refer to opium addiction, (Chapter 18), quack medicine (Chapter 21), their alleged disregard for sanitation, or as potential sources of exotic contagious diseases. There were only 850 Chinese in Colorado in 1902, half of them in Denver. The attitude of most Coloradans towards this tiny minority is indicated in that year's *Report of the Bureau of Labor Statistics*:

> It is probable that the most nauseating and disgusting features in connection with Chinese life in this city [Denver] will never be given to the world . . . A condition of immorality, vice, crime, and indecency that would cause the masses of people to rise up in righteous indignation and remove this plague spot from their midst.[50]

In the mining camps, it was commonly said that the altitude was too high for the Chinese and that, as a result, "their health is not good in that locality."[51] The miners of Ouray and Silverton were probably not thinking of the health of their Chinese brethren, however, when they evicted them from their communities.[51]

Denver's Dr. A. L. Bennett commented:

> The sanitary conditions of Chinatown on Wazee and Sixteenth streets, also of Chinatown back of Market Street, is bad. Filth collects in piles in alleys and yards . . . making a most fertile field for the growth of disease-producing germs . . . The Chinese are a peculiar people and need peculiar legislation to meet their Oriental disregard of filth and disease.[52]

Especially irritating to germ-conscious physicians was the practice of "spraying of clothing in Chinese laundries with water ejected from the mouth."[53] Not only was this considered a "filthy habit" but "by reason of the numerous diseases with which this race are affected, is said by physicians to be very dangerous to those who use the clothing thus laundered."[54] An order forbidding this practice was issued by the State Board of Health, printed in Chinese, and posted in each of Denver's Chinese laundries.[55] Such concerns led to the creation of the position of state inspector of Chinese, and two years later, the inspector "had reason to believe that the order [against spitting in laundries] has been practically barren of results."[56]

The inspector added that since the Chinese seldom sought the services of American physicians, it might be a good idea for him to examine the bodies of all dead Chinese in order to rule out the possibility of contagious diseases which might have been spread by the deceased prior to death.[57] There was particular concern over several exotic infectious diseases associated with the Orient. In 1878 in Denver, one Yee Chow Jung was reported to have died of leprosy.[58] That night his combination home and laundry was burned to the ground. It was said that the fire department had arrived *before* the fire started and that no attempt was made to save the building. Periodically, new rumors of this dreaded disease emerged, provoking near panic among Denver's populace. The discovery of a case in Denver's Chinatown in 1901 led to an "immediate absolute quarantine" and a request for assistance from Washington.[59] The man died before Washington got around to responding. Three years later, the inspector of Chinese was called upon to investigate a rumor of another case, but "after making a search, no sick Chinaman could be located."[60] In 1910 a leper named Yee Kee was discovered and deported to China. He subsequently committed suicide.[61]

By 1900 there were twenty-five thousand foreign-born people in Denver, nearly twenty percent of the city's population. Coming from a variety of countries, most were poor and uneducated, many spoke no English, and some were malnourished or chronically ill. They lived in crowded boarding houses and shacks and even in tents or makeshift hovels built from discarded crates.[62] In 1907 the *Journal of the American Medical Association* reported that there were thousands of "house tents" in Denver and that the police had ordered them removed. It is unlikely that the authorities were able to enforce their edict, and despite outcries from concerned citizens and service organizations, not to mention the board of health, thousands of "ethnics" continued to live in crowded, unsanitary, and unhealthy conditions. The Social Service Department of the University of Denver's School of Theology reported on the "housing problem in Denver":

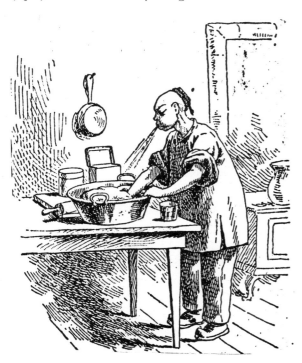

7.6 Spitting by Chinese cooks and laundrymen was specifically "forbidden" by an order of the Colorado State Board of Health. It was difficult to enforce.

The sections covered by the inquiry were the flat low-lying lands along the Platte River and Cherry Creek. They include . . . the 'squatter' properties and the 'jungles' [inhabited largely by Italians] and . . . a distinctively Jewish quarter . . . Both districts are subject to overflow by river water [and problems with] drainage, sewage, garbage disposal and the like. In many instances the garbage is simply thrown out . . . , [there are] large numbers of domestic animals, [and] ample provision for the breeding of the domestic fly . . . One fourth of the privy vaults were full or nearly so, and, in 21 instances, the contents leached into the soil.[63]

Denver's city health officer complained that, whether through "ignorance of the English language or "pure cussedness," the foreigners "disregard any precautions for the spread of disease."[64] He added that they totally ignored all quarantine restrictions and "even take their children in the desquamative stage of scarlet fever through the streets."

The patient population at the County Hospital provides us with a rough estimate of the ethnic composition of Denver's poor in the early 1900s.[65] The two largest groups were Irish and German, followed by Russians, Swedes, Austrians, and Italians. There were still quite a few English and Scots, and smaller numbers of Greeks, Bulgarians, Hungarians, Finns, Danes, Swiss, Norwegians, Bohemians, Poles, and Rumanians. Although most of the Jews were of Russian origin, others were included among several other nationalities.

Some of the ethnic groups were able to find doctors of their own nationality and language. There were, for example, quite a few German-speaking physicians in early Denver. The shingle hanging in Dr. Matthias Klaiber's office window, above Conrad Frick's shoe store on Larimer Street, proclaimed, "Deutscher Arzt" (i.e. German physician).[66] Dr. Giuseppe Cuneo, who arrived in the 1880s, was the first Italian doctor in Denver.[67] Dr. Rodolfo Albi, who came to Denver in 1902, was described as "popular among both Italians and Americans" and his wife was the first licensed Italian midwife in Denver.[67] In 1906 a dispensary was opened in West Denver " to provide service for indigent Italians;" however, an attempt to found an Italian hospital was unsuccessful.[68] Most of the physicians who cared for Denver's minorities were not, of course, minorities themselves. Dr. Kate Yont, descended from an old New York family, took a special interest in Denver's "Italian colony," teaching women the fundamentals of proper diet and helping families obtain American citizenship.[69]

The most visible minority, perhaps, was the Russian Jews. Following the pogroms of 1905, they immigrated to the United States in great numbers, seeking relief from the Czar's persecution. Many were tuberculous, and nearly all were impoverished, malnourished, and imbued with the prejudices and fears of generations of ghetto survival. An incident that occurred in 1908 is illustrative.[70] That spring, Denver was visited by a famous Italian orthopedic surgeon, Dr. Cesare Ghillini. One morning, as the doctor was walking downtown, he encountered a *Denver Post* newsboy hobbling along on "terribly deformed and misshapen feet." Sympathetic to the boy's plight, he offered young Nathan Siegel's parents the opportunity to have the defects corrected at no cost. The parents, "ignorant and oppressed" Russian Jews, were certain that the surgeon intended to cut off the child's feet. It was only after much persuasion that the procedure was done.

The same fear and ignorance led to misunderstandings regarding sanitation and such public health measures as quarantine. The city's chief milk inspector complained of the impossibility of monitoring the "one cow dairies" in the Jewish district.[71] The editor of the *Denver Medical Times* was sympathetic to "this colony of people who have fled to America as a haven from reputedly terrible oppression in Europe."[72] Nevertheless, he added:

> If they are to be a chronic source of danger to the community which has received them; if they are to be a continuous breeding ground for such diseases as diphtheria and scarlet fever; and if they constantly refuse to obey sanitary laws; one can perhaps understand a part of the reason for their having been considered undesirables in their former place . . .[72]

The doctor pointed out that he was not intolerant and that his words were meant to be in the best interests of the Russian Jews themselves. The Russian Jews learned fast and it wasn't long before their offspring, and those of other minorities, were, themselves, graduating from Colorado's medical schools.

Elsner, Bancroft, and Other Doctors

Denver has always been able to attract good physicians. In the earliest days, the lure was gold and the mystique of the new frontier. Later, they came as part of the post-Civil War migration. In many instances, they or a member of their family had tuberculosis, and they came to regain their health in Colorado's salubrious climate. When the A.M.A. convention was held in Denver in 1898, many of the visiting physicians were impressed with Denver's professional climate as well, and on their return home, they spread the word that Denver was a credible medical community and a good place to live.

There were many outstanding physicians in early Denver.[73] Dr. Richard Buckingham, who arrived by covered wagon, helped create and served as first president of both the Denver and territorial medical societies, helped write the state's constitution, served as Denver's mayor, and participated in the formation of the city's public school system.[74] He was also famous for having delivered his own great-grandchildren. William McClelland, who traded a wagon-load of bacon for a lot in Denver, also helped organize the medical societies. He wrote several early articles which helped to popularize the therapeutic benefits of Denver's climate. Arnold Stedman helped found Denver's first medical school and built its first professional building. William R. Whitehead, who had the unusual distinction of serving as a physician in both the Crimean War (with the Russians) and the Civil War (with the Confederates), was a well known surgeon and professor of anatomy. There were many others, some of them cited elsewhere in this book. A Denver surgeon described the successful leaders of Denver's medical community:

> They lived in well-appointed homes [and] visited their patients in excellent carriages drawn by beautiful horses. Not a few accumulated considerable wealth [and] all of the genuine pleasures of life were theirs . . .[75]

Two of Denver's early physicians were especially outstanding and, in many ways representative of their contemporaries. In many respects, Dr. John Elsner and Dr. Frederick J. Bancroft were similar; in others they were very different.[76] Both came to Denver from the Northeast, arriving within a month of each other in 1866, and both had served the Union in the Civil War. Elsner came with a wagon train, Bancroft in an overland coach. Their offices faced each other above the First National Bank at 15th and Blake. Later, both married and established combination office-homes in downtown Denver. As city physician, Bancroft urged the establishment of a county hospital in 1866; as county physician, Elsner established the hospital a few years later. Both helped found the Denver and territorial (later state) medical societies, both had large private practices, and each helped to start a medical school in Denver. Bancroft was one of the founders of St. Luke's Hospital and Elsner

helped establish the National Jewish Hospital. Both were active in their respective religious organizations, but neither appears to have been "religious" in the orthodox sense.

The two doctors were also, in many ways, very different from each other. Bancroft was a huge, muscular man famed for his large black beard and his enormous appetite. He was also well known for his sense of humor, documented in a number of anecdotes which have survived. His background was conservative and rural New England and his ancestors were farmers and country teachers. He lived in Denver, but he had a farm, pioneered in agricultural irrigation, enjoyed hunting and fishing, and liked dogs and horses. He was not interested in mining or mining speculations. As chief surgeon to the Denver and Rio Grande, Bancroft had free access to the railroad, but he did little traveling around the state and there is no record of his ever visiting any of the mining camps. He and Mrs. Bancroft were Episcopalians and members of Denver society. Mrs. Bancroft belonged to the right organizations and attended the right social affairs. Dr. Bancroft's friends included governors, bankers, judges, and publishers. He was the first president of Denver's school board and the first president of the State Historical Society, but he was not an intellectual. According to his granddaughter, Caroline, he fell asleep at operas and concerts, and he may have never have read a non-medical book.

Elsner appears to have been a small man, beardless, and although he may have had a sense of humor, there are no anecdotes extant to docu-

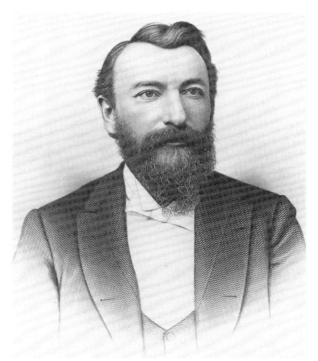

7.7 Dr. John Elsner.

ment it. His background was Eastern European—Austrian, Jewish, urban, intellectual, and liberal. His father had participated in the revolutionary events of 1848, and as a result, the family had to make a hasty move to the U.S. Elsner's brothers were both physicians, and he graduated from Bellevue Hospital Medical School in New York City. Elsner was an amateur geologist and it was a mining investment that brought him to Colorado. Unlike Bancroft, he enjoyed using his railroad pass. Over the years he visited many of the mining camps, leaving in his wake the foreskins of more than a hundred Jewish males whom he circumcised in those isolated communities.[77] Elsner was a prominent and successful physician, but, as Jews, he and Mrs. Elsner were definitely not a part of Denver society. Bancroft and Elsner both helped to found medical schools. Bancroft's school was part of the Methodist's University of Denver, with its select and socially prominent faculty. Elsner was one of those who had not been invited to serve on D.U.'s faculty. This equally talented group organized their own school, the Gross College of Medicine. Bancroft and Elsner started out as general practitioners. Eventually, Elsner became the equivalent of today's internist, while Bancroft specialized in surgery.

Elsner, the sophisticated urbanite, did not especially enjoy farming or outdoors activities. At their home, the Denver equivalent of a Parisian salon, the Elsners entertained famous actors, opera stars, and writers. The apogee of early Rocky Mountain culture, Oscar Wilde's visit to Colorado, included a dinner at the Elsner's. Dr. Elsner was said to have the largest private library in Denver, "all classical [including] rare volumes, vellum bound, with brazen clasps and corners which would make the mouth of a virtuoso water."[78] In addition, the doctor had an extensive collection of minerals, and in all, the house was said to be "so full of modern paintings, old Sevres, curios and antiques, that it was almost impossible to move around."[79]

With the approach of the twentieth century, the two Denver medical pioneers, both of whom had been educated before the Civil War, had become professionally outdated, their leadership roles supplanted by their younger and more modern colleagues. Bancroft died in 1903 and Elsner, who was ten years younger, in 1922.

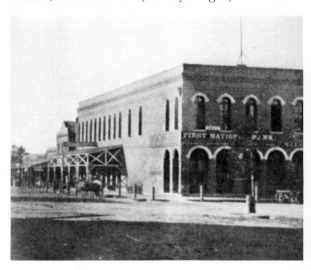

St. Joseph's Hospital

Although Central City had been Bishop Machebeuf's choice as the site for the Catholic Church's first hospital in Colorado, Denver was where it was eventually located. Financed by a grand raffle, the hospital was to be an impressive structure. Unfortunately, the treasurer absconded with the building fund and a small rented house had to suffice. The hospital's original name, St. Vincent's Home, was changed to St. Joseph's. Finally, it was to be organized, administered, and staffed by the Sisters of Charity of Leavenworth. Fortunately, the last of these original plans held fast, for it was the tireless efforts of the sisters that saw Denver's first private hospital through difficult times.[80]

In its first year, the "hospital" was moved from its original site to a building which had the advantage of being larger and the disadvantage of being in Denver's red light district. Next it was moved to a site which had served as one of Denver's pioneer hotels. The $80 a month rent absorbed just about all of the hospital's income, and the sisters spent the next three years campaigning for a building of their own. In 1876 a new brick, three-story, eighty-bed hospital was

7.9 Drs. Elsner and Bancroft arrived in Denver in 1866 and opened their offices in the First National Bank building.

7.8 Dr. Frederick J. Bancroft.

dedicated at 18th Avenue and Humboldt Street. The decade between 1890 and 1900 saw another major building effort result in the 150-bed, twin-towered hospital which served, with various additions and modifications, until recent times. Ten thousand dollars was generated by a "gigantic city-wide bazaar" and a "monster euchre party" presided over by Mrs. J. J. ("Unsinkable Molly") Brown.[81]

St. Joseph's admissions books offer a fascinating catalogue of hospital medicine in early Denver. The first patient, appropriately enough, was an Irishman named Dennis O'Morrow. Dennis's illness was one of the more common causes of hospitalization in early Denver, typhoid. He died a month later, at the age of twenty-six. Eleven of the first month's thirty admissions had typhoid, and seven patients died. The admissions books tersely listed, over the first two decades, the usual litany of nineteenth century diagnoses—consumption, erysipelas, insanity, rheumatism, mountain fever, nervous debility, diphtheria, dropsy, dyspepsia, and so on. In 1894 the diagnoses became more descriptive. The hospital contracted to serve various businesses and factories, as well as the Denver Tramway Company and the Union Pacific Railroad, and many trauma cases were admitted. From the admissions books:

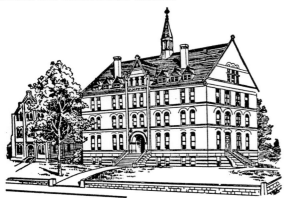

Injured at Brown Palace by barrel of brandy falling on his right leg.

Right arm broken by a horse falling on him whilst leaving barn.

Run down by tramway—both legs broken (11 years old).

Was shot!! In drunken row!! Patient died.

In addition to many miners, railroad men, and laborers, St. Joseph's patients included one or more of the following: "Capitalist . . . health seeker . . . gambler . . . cow man . . . speculator . . . popcorn seller . . . and lady of leisure." It was estimated that twenty percent of the patients were indigent. In 1905 the maximum weekly charge for a private room was $25, while a ward bed could be had for $7.82 There were more than 1,600 admissions that year, and among those patients stating their religion, more than half were Protestant, more than five percent were Jewish, and there were three Christian Scientists.

St. Luke's Hospital

By 1874 Denver's poor had the County Hospital, and its working classes and Catholics had St. Joseph's. But, when the wife of the new Episcopal bishop was asked whether there was a "Church" (i.e. Protestant) hospital in Denver, she had to respond, "No." This was unacceptable to Mrs. John Franklin Spalding, and, as a result, St. Luke's Hospital was opened seven years later.[83] The Episcopalians represented a considerable segment of Denver's largely Protestant social and economic elite, and St. Luke's was identified as Denver's "establishment" hospital. Funds for St. Luke's were not raised by nuns walking the mining camps in sensible shoes and asking for a few pennies from shame-faced miners in saloons, or from the efforts of wealthy but socially "outre" types like Molly Brown. St. Luke's Cathedral Ladies' Hospital Aid Society was composed of well-shod young ladies and matrons with such establishment names as Kountze, Buchtel, Adams, and Bancroft. Mrs. Bishop Spalding was elected president and remained in that office for half a century.

The first St. Luke's Hospital was a converted hotel, two stories, wooden, and containing twenty-one rooms and three wards. Situated on suburban Federal Boulevard, the hospital's *Announcement* proclaimed it's view "the most varied and beautiful that can be found in the whole State of Colorado."[84] The medical staff included some of Denver's most prominent physicians.[85] The *Announcement* also pointed out that "The Hospital is not intended for that class of patients who would be received at the County Hospital" and that the charge was $7 a week or more, "according to accommodations required." A charity bed, named the "Easter Free Bed," was endowed, and soon followed by a second, "The Christian's Cot."[86] The first annual Charity Ball was held at the elegant Windsor Hotel the following year; tickets were ten dollars a couple and the ladies' gowns were described, in great detail, in the society columns. Funds were also raised from lifetime memberships (railroad and banking magnate David Moffat, was a member) and by solicitations from the ladies' wealthy friends back east.

7.10 St. Joseph's Hospital, founded in 1873, is the oldest continuously operated private hospital in Colorado.

Although the *Rocky Mountain News* reported that the hospital had been enlarged to forty beds and "thoroughly refitted and refurnished . . . with a telephone connection with the city and an ambulance to convey patients," its suburban location had proven inconvenient.[87] In addition, many of the the doctors found it dangerous to drive through the "bottoms" of the city at night. Land was purchased near Denver's elegant Capitol Hill, and a former chief justice of Colorado's supreme court, Moses Hallett, served as fund raiser. In 1891, the new hospital was opened on the site of its present location.[88]

Other Hospitals

As the city continued to grow, additional hospitals were added to the original three. St. Anthony's Hospital was built in 1893. Administered by the Sisters of St. Francis, the four-story brick building was described in 1901 as having 211 beds and a staff of thirty-six physicians, two "resident interns," and forty sisters.[89] St. Anthony's was proud of the fact that it was far enough away from downtown "to escape the noise and smoke, yet directly connected with the city by electric car line."

Mercy Hospital was opened in 1902 by the Sisters of Mercy, the same order which had previously founded hospitals in the mining camps of Cripple Creek and Ouray.[90] With accommodations for about forty patients, it advertised its proximity to City Park, where "convalescents [could] seek moderate exercise and fresh air as a diversion from the tedium of long illness."

Several hospitals were for women and/or children. Mother's and Children's Home was opened in 1899. With two wards and private rooms "for ladies who desire their own physician and special care." The hospital provided "trained nurses . . . good food . . . and beds as comfortable as woven wire springs and sanitary mattresses can make them."[91] The Maternity Hospital opened in 1901 and the Denver Maternity and Woman's Hospital in 1902.[92] The latter's eighteen beds included "two endowed for free patients" and the hospital's policy was "to care for as many indigent and deserving women as means and equipment will allow." In 1910 the house which had been the Denver Maternity and Woman's Hospital became the original site of today's Children's Hospital.[93] In 1917 Children's Hospital was moved to a new 135-bed hospital at its present location in central Denver. In addition to its hospitals, Denver had numerous facilities for lying-in, convalescent, and tuberculous patients in private residences around the city. Eventually, a number of large, well equipped tuberculosis sanitaria were built, several of which evolved into major hospitals, including Lutheran, Swedish, and Porter Hospitals (Chapter 15). In 1918 the army opened General Hospital No. 21 in Aurora.[94] In 1920 its name was changed to Fitzsimons General Hospital; it included seventy-three buildings and was, at that time, the largest army hospital in the country. It had about 2,500 beds, and although a general hospital, the emphasis was on tuberculosis, as indicated in an article about the hospital entitled, "How Uncle Sam Treats Boys of T.B. Brigade."[95] Presbyterian Hospital was opened in 1923, completing Denver's "hospital row" east of downtown. Beth Israel Hospital and the University of Colorado's Colorado General Hospital (now University Hospital) completed the panoply.

Later Days

In his role as city physician in 1873, Dr. Bancroft compiled Denver's first mortality report.[97] That year in Denver there were approximately thirteen deaths for every thousand members of the population. The leading cause of death (nearly one out of four) was pulmonary tuberculosis, followed by typhoid, pneumonia, and infantile gastroenteritis. Nearly ten percent of deaths were due to accidents, suicide, or homicide—including five drug overdoses.

In succeeding years, Denver's mortality rate fluctuated above and below that of 1873.[98] In 1914, with the population grown from 14,000 to 245,000, it was still about 1.3%. This was slightly less than that of Chicago and New York City. Interestingly, over this thirty year span, there had been little change, not only in the mortality rate, but in the causes of death. Tuberculosis was still first, and infectious diseases, now including diphtheria and scarlet fever, formed the largest single category.[99] The intervening years had seen improvements in public health measures, diagnosis and treatment, medical education and knowledge, and hospitals and technology. On the other hand, Denver had acquired a number of big city problems. Its population had become more dense, and a large segment were poorly housed, clothed, and fed. Many had come with terminal tuberculosis, and although physicians had become more adept at diagnosing and controlling infectious diseases, they still lacked specific therapies such as antibiotics. By the beginning of World War I, Denver, the onetime frontier town, was not very much different, medically, from other American cities of its size.

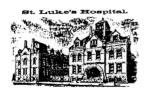

7.11 St. Luke's Hospital was founded in 1881.

8 Colorado—North, South, East, West

If there is any place in the world where a physician should be an all-around man it is in the country . . . Any man who has spent ten years in country practice has a great many amusing, as well as instructive incidents, to remember.

M.S. Chenoweth, M.D. (Elbert County), 1898[1]

THUS FAR, WE HAVE DISCUSSED medicine in early Colorado in the mining camps and in Denver. The remaining half of the state comprises Colorado's eastern, western, northern, and southern periphery—the high plains of the east, the Great Basin and canyons of the west, the parks and river valleys of the north, and the San Luis Valley and coal mining camps of the south. Here, on farms and ranches and in small towns, medicine was not terribly different from rural areas in Pennsylvania, Georgia, or Ohio. The topography did tend to make living conditions somewhat harsher. Water was generally scarce, trees were sparse, and the countryside ranged from open grassland to brown and barren mesas and canyons. Temperatures varied over a wide spectrum and the weather was erratic. Towns were small and far between, distances were great, and many "roads" were really trails made periodically impassable by wash-outs and snowdrifts.

The classic early-day Colorado farm or ranch house was a sixteen by twenty-four foot frame structure, one, or sometimes two, stories high. Under its pitched roof there were two to four rooms, and as the family grew, an "L" might be added later. The whole thing rested on blocks, and the bottom edge was banked with dried manure to help keep out the cold. The cookstove was the only source of heat and the "plumbing," a well and a privy, was outdoors. In forested areas, log cabins were common. On the prairies,

less privileged homesteaders often made do with a sod house. The typical "soddy" was built of foot-wide bricks of prairie sod with an earthen floor and a roof of thatch and prairie grass laid over branches and tree limbs. The walls and roof were chinked with mud. Although ugly to look at, soddies were probably better insulated than the more attractive frame houses, but their furnishings were even more sparse. Together with a few sheds and a wagon, an early homestead provided a stark silouette, barely relieved perhaps by a single tree, against a background of surrounding plains, high plateaus, or canyonlands.[2]

Life on the early-day farm or ranch was often as stark as the environment. The workday was long and tedious, unrelieved by amusements or, in the more isolated areas, even a neighbor's visit. Diets were often nutritionally unbalanced, especially in the winter, and there was no means of refrigeration in the summer. More fortunate families had a cow or goat to provide fresh, though unpasteurized, milk. Ventilation was poor and windows were few, but flies were common, often attracted by nearby farm animals. With water scarce and hot water even scarcer, bathing was a luxury. Clothing was worn in layers in the winter and infrequently changed and laundered. Vermin were common. An early visitor commented: "Bugs are a great pest in Colorado . . . Many careful housewives take their beds to pieces every week and put carbolic acid on them."[3]

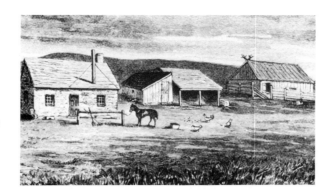

8.1 Idyllic as it now seems, the farm or ranch was the source of as much disease as the ugliest big-city slum.

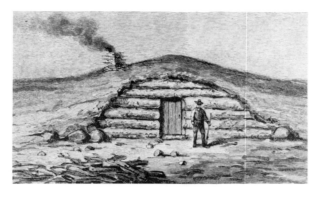

8.2 The sod house provided warmth and shelter—and little else.

structions in the *Colorado Medical Journal* for the construction of sanitary outhouses—complete with brick vault, trap doors, and compartments for dry ash and slaked lime.

Just as certain ailments were popularly associated with the cities or the mining camps, others tended to be viewed, correctly or incorrectly, as characteristic of rural areas. In both the southwestern and northwestern parts of the state, goiter was common, presumably due to a local deficiency of dietary iodine.[5] Less dramatic, but irritatingly frequent, was prairie itch, a dermatitis which may have actually been scabies. Prairie itch (often accompanied by lice) was the particular bane of the cowboy. If nineteenth century advertisements had featured cowboys, they might have shown him scratching rather than smoking. Pueblo's Dr. Will Davis published one cowboy's cure for prairie itch—sponging the skin with bichloride of mercury in alcohol.[6]

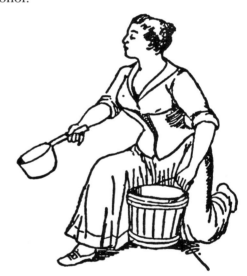

Even though drinking water was usually supplied from wells, Dr. J. T. Melvin, an early Colorado country doctor, pointed out that "the pollution of our rural water supply presents a problem no less vital than that which confronts urban communities."[4] He noted that, "examination of the water from village wells, and even from those of isolated ranches, often shows a surprising amount of unsuspected pollution." Although country water might taste and look pure, it's bacterial contamination is not surprising. The homestead's well was typically located "a few feet from the stable yard, and but a short distance from the outhouse, with the kitchen drain in close proximity." Under those circumstances, Dr. Melvin asked, "How can it fail to become contaminated?" The family's drinking water was usually kept in a wooden bucket in the house and drunk from a common ladle or cup. Dr. Melvin's major sanitary concern, however, was the outhouse:

8.3 An improperly located well and the drinking bucket provided sources of contamination and disease.

> Chief among all the offenders against public health . . . is the universal country outhouse . . . This I believe to be responsible for more ill health in the country than any other one cause. Usually unprotected, exposed and dilapidated . . . , with nothing but a shallow hole dug in the porous soil, it poisons air and water in every direction.

Outhouses, said the doctor, require a "certain amount of intelligent attention and care . . . a thing which the average American man or woman will not give to any contrivance of this nature." Nevertheless, Dr. Melvin provided in-

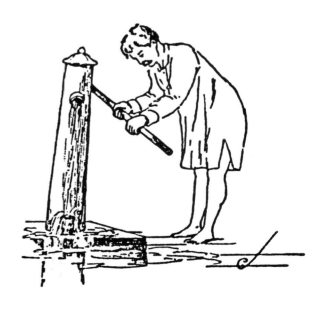

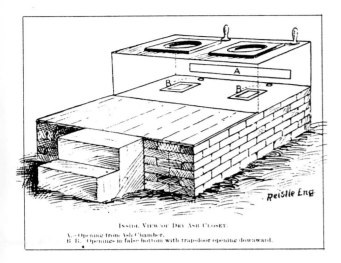

INSIDE VIEW OF DRY ASH CLOSET.
A.—Opening from Ash Chamber.
B B.—Openings in false bottom with trapdoor opening downward.

head of the State Board of Health, Dr. Sherman Williams. Dr. Williams recalled, years later, that the dried rabbit spinal cords used in preparing the vaccine were both "expensive and scarce." Nevertheless, none of his nine patients died.

Traumatic injuries were common in rural areas, but there is little mention of lightning or frostbite injuries in Colorado's early medical literature, and heatstroke is only commented on for its rarity in Colorado. Although the remarkable heat and dryness of the climate were said to cause "hams to lose from 6 to 10 percent of their weight in a compatively short time [and] furniture to shrink and . . . fall to pieces," and although "the sun pours his rays down through a clear atmosphere with unrelenting vigor," Dr. H. A. Lemen could find "no well authenticated case of sunstroke . . . in Colorado."[12]

8.4 Dr. Melvin provided the homesteader with detailed plans for a sanitary outhouse. This is his two-seater version.

Rattlesnakes were another environmental hazard. In some areas on the eastern plains, rattlers were said to be so common that some folks carried a small bottle of turpentine. The turpentine was applied to the bite after first sucking the wound, incising it, and using a tourniquet to promote bleeding.[13] Dr. John Chase recalled that once, while bicycling near Sedalia, a rattler became entangled in the spokes of his front wheel. While it was possible that "since wheels were invented, some man may have dismounted more gracefully than I did," he chuckled, "no one on earth ever got off quicker."[14] Most physicians cauterized rattlesnake bites with silver nitrate, supplementing this treatment with spirits of ammonia and liberal doses of whiskey.

Tetanus was a much more serious "country" disease. Although by no means limited to the country, this frequently fatal infection was due to the contamination of lacerations and wounds such as those due to splinters or the perennial rusty nail. Country people were fearful of tetanus and one doctor recalled an emergency call— "Mama has the lockjaw"—which turned out, after a hurried housecall, to be a dislocated jaw.[7] Occasional bona fide cases did occur. In 1889, for example, a sixteen-year-old boy in Morrison was reported as having tetanus, with "paroxysms so violent that extension of the arm would throw a heavy man forcibly from him."[9]

Botulism was another "country" disease. Like tetanus, it is also due to a powerful bacterial toxin and was often fatal. Unlike tetanus, the toxin is ingested, typically in improperly canned and preserved foods. Since home canning was a way of life on the farm and ranch, outbreaks of botulism occurred periodically. Typical were reports of five deaths on a farm near Sterling due to home canned beans, a death in the Swenson family in Longmont due to home canned corn, and two deaths in Calcite due to home canned tomatoes.[9]

Nothing spread more fear among country people, however, than word of a mad dog and rabies. Colorado's first reported case was in 1899, in an eight-year-old boy who was bitten on the upper lip by a stray dog.[10] The child died, "in great fear and agony," after five days of illness. The following year an outbreak of rabies in animals was reported in Douglas County and there were two more fatal cases in humans.[11] In 1917 nine passengers on the Denver—Longmont train were bitten by a stray dog. The victims were brought to Denver, where they were treated over the next three weeks with daily injections of a vaccine prepared by the

Injuries of all kinds were common on the farm and ranch and the most serious ones were usually due to farm machinery. While working on a ranch, visiting Englishman Richard B. Townshend, author of the classic *Tenderfoot in Colorado*, fell into a mower and suffered severe lacerations to his leg.[15] He recalled that, although ranchmen had "a rough skill in surgery in those days, more than that was wanted for my hurts." He was taken in a hay wagon sixty-five miles to Denver and sewn up by a surgeon. Back on the ranch, and after a prolonged recuperation, Townshend soon suffered another injury common on farms and ranches, a broken bone. Once again he was carted off to Denver, this time to have his fractured leg set.

Riding accidents were also common. In his large rural practice in Sterling, Dr. Hall treated forty-four accidents in horseback riders, "very largely among the cowboys of the region."[16] There were six head injuries, the most serious in a young man who had been dragged for a mile and who had "not been entirely sound of mind since." Hall recorded numerous fractures (only one of which was compound), dislocations, and sprains, as well as lacerations and abrasions—but no deaths.

Home Remedies

In the country, the doctor was often called only as a last resort. Money was not readily available, and many farm and ranch people did not feel it was right to call a doctor unless they could pay him. In some areas, the distances were simply too great, the homestead too remote, and a doctor's services simply unavailable.

Mother, or a neighbor woman, often took care of the family's medical needs. One chronicler recalled that when a cowboy was run into a fence by a wild bronc on a northwestern Colorado ranch, it was the rancher's wife, assisted by another lady, who put five stitches into his lacerated leg.[17] Table salt was used as an antiseptic and herbs to staunch the flow of blood. That cowboy recovered sufficiently to become a famous bronco rider in Buffalo Bill's troupe. On the range, "cookie" often served as the cowboy's physician and surgeon. As cowboy folklorist Ramon Adams put it, the cook "was called upon to create a dosage good for any ailment . . . from

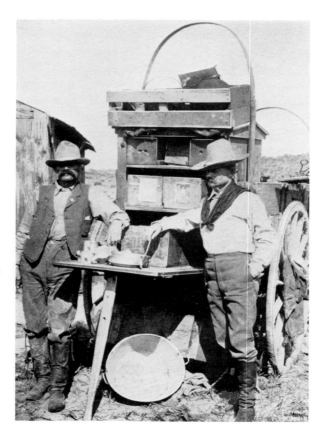

8.5 The ranch cook often provided more than meals to the cowboys. Far from any professional medical care, he often served as the ranch's "doc."

bellyache to boils, from bruises to broken bones."[18] Sometimes it was his fellow cowboys who provided medical care. When one boistrous cowboy who had come to town "got a hole bored in him," his buddies laid him on the saloon's bar and found "an ominous bluish hole just over the hip."[19] One of the cowboys was afraid he was "gut-shot," a sure death sentence, but just then the wounded man woke up and opined, "It don't feel like I was gut-shot . . . Is there any of my insides sticking out?" One of the cooler heads felt around the wound and discovered the bullet just under the skin. It had apparently ricocheted off the bone and traveled subcutaneously around the pelvis. Fortified, perhaps, by a glass or two added to his previous intake, the patient urged his buddy to "carve away." A razor was found and the cowboy-surgeon extracted the bullet and dressed the wound. The patient was put to sleep in a room "well away from the bar."

In town, the local druggist often played the role of physician, making diagnoses, providing medicines, and even performing minor procedures. Occasionally, even the town's school teacher had to act as doctor. When an Ault, Colorado, schoolgirl who went down a rough wooden slide wound up with a "huge sliver of dirty wood sinking fast into her fat little bottom," her teacher provided emergency medical care.[20] Unable to grasp the deeply embedded sliver with her fingers, the schoolmarm clamped down on it with her teeth and pulled it out—to the accompaniment of the patient's younger sister's cries of: " The teacher's biting Sally's ass . . ."

Some farm and ranch women attained reputations as midwives and "nurses" and were the sole sources of medical care. In one remote region in southern Colorado, a doctor made rounds once a year; at all other times, Rebecca Lopez attended to the inhabitants' medical needs.[21] It was impossible, it was said, to enumerate her many accomplishments as combined nurse, midwife, and "even as doctor." At times, such non-professional medical care was less effective. One Colorado pioneer recalled having cut her foot as a little girl. Instead of calling for a doctor to stitch it, her father sent for the local "nurse."[22] She sealed the wound with pitch. The next morning, the child was in such pain that her mother had to remove the pitch with lard and warm water. The wound took months to heal and left a large scar. On the other hand, some lay nurses brought more than medical attention to their patients. Mrs. Laura Wright, the "Angel of Bob Creek," often carried food and blankets to poor families throughout two counties in

W. P. DOOLEY, M. D.
PHYSICIAN & SURGEON

Office Phone Eaton 191
Residence Phone, Eaton 192

Office in First National Bank Building
Eaton, Colorado

R

Protargol 5% sol. ℥iv
Sig. as directed
Dooley

If this prescription is taken to *Gayman's Pharmacy* it will be properly filled
EATON, COLO.

southeastern Colorado.[23] A few of the "prairie nightingales" were professionally trained nurses. Alice and Sadie Mosser were two such nurses who, from their sod house homes, cared for many homesteader families on the northeastern Colorado plains.[23]

Innumerable time-honored remedies were available to country families, handed down through generations, recommended by neighbors, or published in the many home medical references, recipe books, and other popular sources. A homestead mother's remedies might have included turpentine and lard salve for a sore throat, alum mixed with sugar or dissolved in molasses for croup, raw bacon or salt pork laid on a rash or a burn, a mustard and flour plaster for severe cough or pneumonia, onion and sugar syrup for colds, and vinegar and honey, or sulfur and molasses, as a general "pick-me-up" or tonic. Other favorites included arnica, powdered rhubarb, castor oil, camphor, horehound, sassafras bark, wild sage and chokecherry teas, oil of wintergreen, baking soda and Epsom salts. Dr. Ralph Danielson recalled that, as a child in the railroad town of Basalt, a little bag of asafetida was hung around his neck to ward off various illnesses. The pungent odor tended to keep people at a distance, perhaps accounting for any effect the asafetida might have had in in preventing contagious disease.[24]

Almanacs and cookbooks often contained medical advice. The *Denver Quaker Cook Book* provided a number of interesting remedies.[25]

Diarrhea: Tinctures of capsicum, opium, and rhubarb, essence of peppermint, and spirits of camphor—all in equal parts. Take 15 - 20 drops every fifteen minutes. 'This alone is well worth the price of the book.'

Ringworm: Smoke a fine Cuban cigar and take one-half inch of ash. Wet the skin with saliva and rub the ashes in thoroughly; 'do this three times each day and in a week all will be smooth and well.'

Nervous prostration: 'Onions . . . are almost the best nervine known [and] there is nothing else that will so quickly relieve and tone up a worn-out system.'

Country Doctors

Colorado's early doctors came for health reasons, or to mine gold and silver, or to practice in the city, and they settled in the mountains, or in Denver or Colorado Springs. They and their wives saw little reason to live in the remote little towns of the countryside. Those who did settle in rural areas found themselves, like Sterling's Dr. Hall,

isolated as if upon an island in mid-ocean . . . My territory was 8,000 square miles. The nearest doctor to the west was at Evans, one hundred miles away, and east was at North Platte, Nebraska, one hundred and forty miles away . . . and I have been six months without seeing another doctor. There was no hospital or nurse . . . In our first winter, the housekeeper and I ate buffalo meat every day for three months.[26]

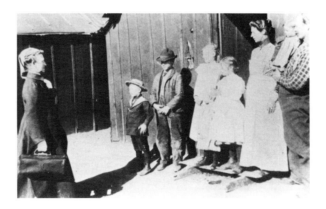

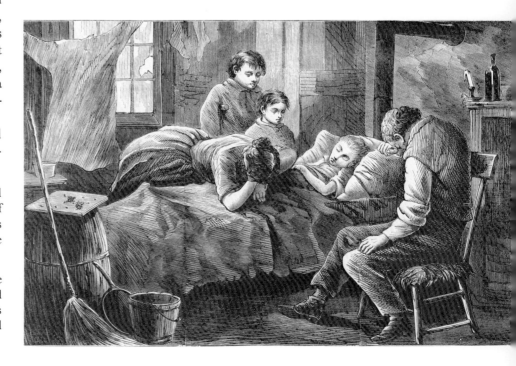

8.6 In rural areas, the local druggist often provided the doctor with his prescription blanks. In the absence of a doctor, he often provided medical care as well.

8.7 Some rural families depended on a neighbor or themselves for medical care. If they were fortunate, like this Weld county family, a visiting nurse might come by every once in a while.

8.8 Too poor and too proud to call a doctor to their isolated homestead, some rural families depended on home remedies, medical guidebooks, and fate.

74

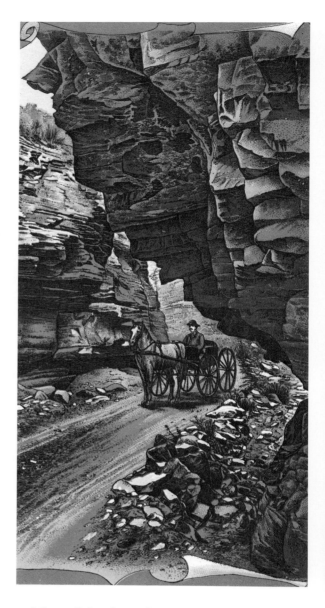

Hall, a New Englander, had impeccable credentials. He was a graduate of Amherst College and Harvard Medical School and had interned at Boston City Hospital. After completing his training, he immediately went west, and in 1883, the twenty-three-year-old doctor settled in Sterling, a town of 250 souls on the plains of northeastern Colorado. It was a world away from Boston and the lush New England countryside.[27]

Hall found that his patients comprised "an average American farming population," and as the only doctor in the area, he had to be prepared for virtually any medical problem. Hall catalogued his first thousand cases, and they provide us with a breakdown of a country doctor's practice.[28] Of his thousand patients, 55% were medical—two-thirds adult and one-third pediatric. In addition, 9% were surgical, 8% obstetric, 6% gynecologic, and 3 - 4% each were orthopedic, ophthalmologic, otolaryngologic, urologic, dermatologic, or suffered from "nervous diseases."

As another pioneer, Dr. G. Law of Greeley, put it, "the country doctor in Colorado . . . had to become as good an all-around man as he could make himself."[29] When he was still the only doctor in the area, his patients expected him to be available seven days a week, twenty-four hours a day. Some doctors circuit rode across large domains, advertising their expected arrivals on handbills or in the local newspapers. One northern Colorado newspaper contained the announcement, for example, that "Dr. --- will be in Julesburg, Sunday, to look after his practice in that locality."[30]

Sometimes patients traveled long distances to the doctor. Dr. Hall recalled a cowboy who had dislocated his shoulder when his horse stepped into a badger hole. With his arm in a sling, the cowboy spent three hours riding the thirty miles to Snyder, where he then caught the train to Sterling.[31]

Others sought medical advice through the mail. W. A. Hopkins, a rancher near Nucla, a town with no doctor or druggist, and forty miles away from the railroad, wrote to Cripple Creek's Dr. W.E. Driscoll.[32] The letter which began with the chief complaint of "I am bothered with what I call catarrh of the stomach . . . ," provided the doctor with a reasonable summary of Mr. Hopkins' medical status. In addition, the rancher described some of his wife's complaints, including "a womb which is tipped or fallen," constipation, and what sounds like attacks of migraine headaches. He asked the doctor for "liquid medicine" which, he noted, could be sent to Nucla by stage.

8.10 The country doctor, especially in Colorado, faced some major challenges on his more distant housecalls—even when the weather was decent.

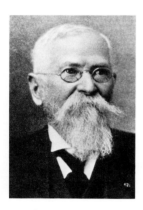

8.9 Greeley's Dr. G. Law stated the credo of the country doctor: " . . . to become as good an all-around man as he could make himself."

Most of the time, the country doctor traveled to his patient, especially in emergency situations. Some of these "housecalls" involved long distances and major hardships. Dr. Law, for example, traveled sixty-five miles one winter night, "to set a broken leg" and Grand Junction's Dr. A. B. Hubbard rode his horse 200 miles to attend a surgical case in Rangely.[33] Colorado's winters were not always conducive to such excursions. Limon's Dr. W. H. Rothwell rode thirty miles "through two feet of snow . . . in the face of a blinding blizzard" to attend a couple of frozen sheepherders.[34] Suffering, himself, from frostbitten hands and feet, the doctor, "after working for several hours . . . brought the sheepherders back to consciousness." Dr. C. E. Tennant was better prepared when called across the border to Wyoming late one January; he travelled the fifty miles by "bobsled."[35] By 1916 transportation had become faster, though not necessarily safer, for the country doctor. That year, Dr. F. G. Dryden was killed in an auto accident near Wootten and Dr. John Solandt, Hayden's "most popular citizen," was killed in an auto accident while making a house call.[36]

Once having arrived at his destination, the doctor might encounter anything. Dr. Law rode twenty miles from Greeley to find a woman "who had been in labor a great many hours, her child's arm hanging in the vagina and its shoulder tightly wedged into the pelvis."[37] Dr. Chenoweth found a woman whose "abdominal cavity was as full of fluid as it was possible to be without rupturing ... Aspiration revealed viscid, foul-smelling pus."[38] Dr. Melvin rode twenty miles from Saguache to attend a cowboy who was said to "have some kind of stomach ache." The doctor's report was succinct:

> I found him in collapse [and] suspected a ruptured [abdominal] abscess ... With the assistance of another cowboy he was placed under chloroform and the abdomen opened. A teacupful of pus escaped. The appendix was perforated in two places and was removed. The [abdominal] cavity was flushed with boiled saline solution. Closed the wound with two layers of sutures.[39]

All three of these patients survived. Dr. Melvin noted that his cowboy with appendicitis recovered "without special interest" and that he "drove to my office in twenty days."

Sometimes the doctor arrived to non-medical surprises. Dr. Charles Gardiner, having ridden all the way from Meeker to a distant ranch, found himself in the middle of a family feud, dodging bullets.[40] Dr. Frederick Bancroft traveled from Denver to Deertrail to care for a cowboy with a severe gunshot wound of his leg.[41] Just as he was about to amputate, the cowboy's drunken brother warned him that if his brother died, so would the doctor. Bancroft, armed with his own six-shooter, later told why the cowboy's threat hadn't worried him—he would know, well before the brother, if his patient was about to die.

In the latter half of the 1880s, Colorado's rural communities were deluged by physicians. By 1886 Longmont (in Boulder County) had a physician-to-population ratio of 1:160, Loveland (in Larimer County) a ratio of 1:100, Florence (in Fremont County) a ratio of 1:20, and tiny Hotchkiss (in Delta County) had two physicians for its thirty inhabitants.[42] For some, like Dr. Hall, country practice lasted only a few years and led to specialized practices in bigger cities. Some country doctors moved from one small town to another, until they found a suitable locale. Dr. Charles W. Williams came to tiny Minneapolis, Colorado, in 1887, then moved,

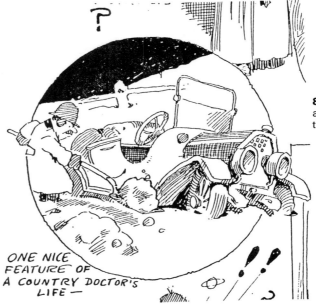

8.11 Even with the advent of the automobile there were problems.

ONE NICE FEATURE OF A COUNTRY DOCTOR'S LIFE —

successively, to Elizabeth, Pueblo, Overton, and finally to Manzanola.[43] Dr. O. E. Sperry moved from La Porte to the Hardscrabble district and then to Rosita, Westcliffe, and finally, to Querida.[44] Dr. F.M. Means, on the other hand, came to Holyoke and remained there to practice for fifty-five years, delivering more than 5,000 babies.[45] Dr. J. R. Trotter practiced for nearly fifty years in Mancos, Dr. G. E. Van Der Schouw for forty-five years in Fowler, and Dr. Robert Denney for sixty years in Elbert County.[46]

As physicians continued to pour into Colorado, the competition for patients became more intense. In the smaller communities, in particu-

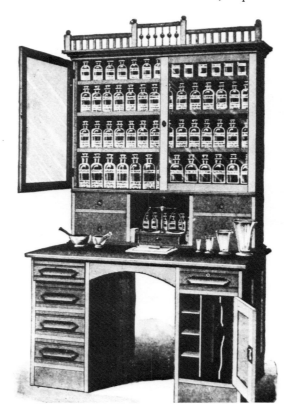

8.12 The "dispensing doctor" kept his medicine cabinet well stocked.

lar, this sometimes led to hard feelings among the doctors. Many rural doctors operated their own drugstores or were "dispensing" physicians, i.e. sold medications directly to their patients. The medical societies considered this practice to be unethical, or at least borderline, but there was little they could do about it, especially in communities which were not large enough to support a druggist. Greeley's Dr. W. W. Harmer probably spoke for many of his fellows when he announced, at the annual meeting of the State Medical Society, that he was proud to be a country physician and a "dispenser." He dispensed drugs, he said, because he thought it to be medically beneficial to his patients and financially beneficial to his family. Furthermore, he felt "no obligation to look out for the welfare of the druggist."[47] As the financial pressures of competition grew, some physicians took on non-medical occupations. Manzanola's Dr. Williams, for example, in addition to practicing medicine and running a drug store, was the town's postmaster and ran an eighty acre spread. It was noted, however, that "he has not neglected his practice, but employs a clerk to attend to the post office and drug store during his absence on professional business."[48] Canon City's Dr. Thomas Craven owned a drug store, worked for the railroad, and ran a gold mining company.[48]

Many physicians also participated in local civic activities. Many served on school boards or were elected to various municipal and county offices. Dr. Craven served as president of his local school board, treasurer of Fremont County, and mayor of Canon City.[49] Dr. Hall served as mayor of Sterling and Dr. W. Cummings was the first mayor of Montrose.[50] Dr. W. A. E. DeBecque founded the town which bears his name.[51]

Dr. Michael Beshoar was one of the most versatile and colorful of Colorado's early country doctors.[52] Coming to Pueblo after serving both the Confederacy and, after his capture, the Union as a surgeon, Beshoar moved to Trinidad in 1867. He established a wide-ranging medical practice, opened the first drugstore between Denver and Santa Fe, founded both city's newspapers, was elected to various territorial, state, county, and municipal offices (including that of school superintendent), had many friends and enemies, and for many years was one of southern Colorado's leading political, journalistic, medical, social, commercial, and educational forces. Also, and this was unusual among Colorado's physicians, he was a Democrat.[53]

Hospitals and Medical Societies

The continually expanding population of Colorado's countryside led to a need for local hospitals. Some of the earliest rural hospitals were built by doctors. That was literally the case in Meeker, a tiny ranching town in northwestern Colorado. The town's lone physician, Dr. Gardiner, begged some lumber from the nearby sawmill, and together with some of the "boys," used the unpainted pine to build his 15 x 15 foot "hospital" on the town's only thoroughfare.[54] There were two bunks for patients, drinking water was stored in a whisky barrel, a cookstove provided heat, and the healthier of the two patients was expected to do the cooking. Dr. Gardiner served as "surgeon in chief, superintendent, and general nurse." One night, some mischievous cowboys painted the words, "The shortest road to hell," in foot-high black letters across the front of the hospital. Nevertheless, the two beds were soon filled. One patient was an older Mormon gentleman who had been shot in the abdomen and who was described as "mean, surly, fanatical . . . and all beard." The other was a young cowboy who had broken his leg. He was described as "careless, happy-go-lucky . . . with a mop of golden hair, and a smiling face." The cowboy did the cooking.

In Mancos Dr. Trotter bought a large old house and converted nine of its rooms for inpatients.[55] In Loveland, Dr. W. B. Sutherland used the upper floor of his home as a "hospital."[56] In the larger towns, private homes did not suffice. In Fort Collins, six physicians formed a hospital association, borrowed the necessary capital, and built a twenty-five bed hospital.[57] In La Junta some $25,000 in subscriptions was raised to construct a twenty-five bed hospital.[58] In some of Colorado's towns, hospital names,

8.13 Rural communities had hospitals ranging from a few rooms in the doctor's office-home, to more impressive structures. Canon City's Graves' Hospital was built by Dr. Charles Graves in the early 1900s. It had twenty-five beds.

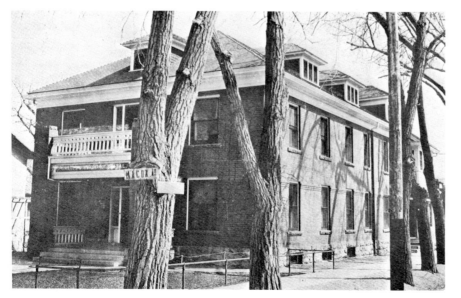

owners, and locations changed over the years, and it is difficult to trace some of their histories. Lamar, for example, had its Great Plains Sanitarium, Cherry Tree Hospital, Friend Sanitorium, Mrs. Everett's "lying-in house," a pesthouse, a "hospital" over the Ben Mar Hotel Annex, and Lamar General, Southeast, and Maxwell hospitals.[59]

Isolated in small communities, without the stimulation of colleagues, libraries, or medical society meetings, most of the early country doctors, Dr. Law recalled

> were subscribers to the best medical journals . . . and kept buying new books and reading them. Even now, we 'old fellows' do not feel very lonesome in the presence of the newest [medical school] graduate, even if he does look down with pity and scorn on our old buggy cases.[60]

In later years, county medical societies were organized. One of their purposes was to provide continuing medical education for their members. At Morgan County Medical Society meetings, each member was required to present an interesting case when his name was called.[61] In 1909 examples of "myelogenous anemia, hydatid mole, cervical abscess, and postpartum dementia" were presented by Morgan County physicians to their colleagues. Sometimes guest lecturers presented "very advanced" topics. In 1915, a Chicago physician was invited to present his experience with human organ transplantation to the Weld County Medical Society.[62] That night's meeting was notable for its unusually large turnout. The attendees were especially impressed by the visiting doctor's success with testis transplants, especially when he cited the addition of a testis to his own "armamentarium." In his official report (and with tongue in cheek), the society's reporter noted:

> The long sought for elixir vitae seems to have arrived . . . The satisfying sentiments which diffused the countenances of the members as they realized how close they were to the desired haven cannot be adequately expressed by the feeble adjectives of the English language.[62]

Hispanics

Hispanics were the major minority group in rural Colorado. The first permanent Hispanic residents arrived before the Anglos, in the early 1850s. Land grant settlers from northern New Mexico, they migrated to the southern San Luis Valley, built adobe houses and churches, plazas and irrigation ditches, and founded such communities as San Luis, Guadelupe, and Conejos.

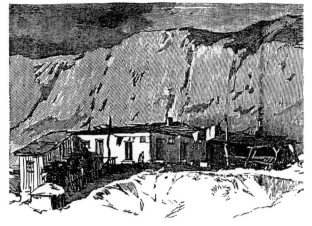

8.14 Southern Colorado's Hispanics depended for the most part on their own folk doctors and medicines. They were generally poor and socially, economically, and medically isolated from their Anglo neighbors.

Many were descended from Spanish ancestors who, often admixed with Mexican, Pueblo, Navajo, and other Indians, had come to New Mexico from old Mexico in the 1600s. Even after the Gold Rush, many of Colorado's Hispanic communities remained essentially isolated from the mainstream, with only a few Anglo merchants and Mormon towns to disturb the otherwise homogeneous Spanish-Mexican environment. Many of the people spoke only Spanish, the Catholic church and the mystical traditions of the Penitentes were dominant, and the economy was agricultural and predominantly poor. Families were large, closely knit, and often housed under the same or nearby roofs. Illiteracy and infant mortality rates were high.

The Hispanic concept of disease was based on several precepts. Some diseases, as in classic European medicine, were believed to be due to internal imbalances, especially of heat and cold. Other diseases were attributed to the structural dislocation of bones and organs. In the condition known as *suspendida*, the abdominal organs were believed to be pulled up tightly against the diaphragm. Displacement of the bones of the cranial vault (*mollera caida*) was responsible for certain infantile disorders. Emotional problems such as anger (*bilis*, or bile) and fright (*sustus*) could lead to illness. Finally, witchcraft (*brujeria*) could result in injury or disease through such means as the evil eye (*mal ojo*). Dr. Beshoar described two traditional illnesses, both of which had sexual connotations.[63] One was *empapelada*, a fatal illness which a wronged husband introduced into the vagina of his faithless wife by placing a piece of paper on his penis. The other was *oxalate* (or *salamander*), caused by a "lecherous reptile" which entered a woman's vagina and "once inside . . . luxuriates on the flesh of the woman until she dies." Beshoar equated *empapelada* with vaginitis and *oxalote* with chronic endometritis and other endometrial disorders. The psychological effects of *oxalote*, in particular,

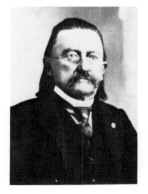

8.15 Trinidad's Dr. Michael Beshoar was one of the few M.D.s who provided medical care to Hispanics.

were devastating, and Beshoar had to resort to various tricks to pursuade its victims that he had been able to extract the pathogenic intruder.

Colorado's early Hispanics generally regarded illness with a mixture of faith and fear, fatalism and stoicism. Nevertheless, they did have a complex system of medical treatment which combined Old World and Indian remedies with religious, mystical, and traditional beliefs and values. Men, and more often, women *curanderas* and *medicas* (folk doctors), *yerbalistas* (herbalists), *sobandos* (masseurs), *parteras* (midwives), and *arbolarios* (witchdoctors) were available to provide their services. In fact, most healers combined one or all of these specialties into their practices.

Medical treatment included massages and manipulations, taboos, the use of medallions and fetishes, prayers and incantations, cupping and lancing, and all sorts of maneuvers and magical procedures. Some of the more picturesque remedies included such items as newborn pigs, cat's blood, black hens, and human umbilical cord.[64] The most extensive therapeutic system, however, was based on herbal medicine, some of it derived from old Spanish lore, some from Indian remedies, and some using the leaves, roots, barks, resins, seeds, and flowers obtained from the grasses, bushes, weeds, trees, and other flora of New Mexico and Colorado. The long list of Hispanic botanicals included the Spanish remedies *alhucema* (lavender) for colic and *manzanilla* (chamomile) for dyspepsia, colds, fevers, and menstrual cramps. The Indian remedies *inmortal* (antelope horns) were used to facilitate labor and *osha* for virtually any illness.[65] *Cachana* (or "blazing star") root was said to be effective in counteracting the evil eye, wild tobacco leaves were made into a poultice for rheumatism and muscle pains, and *yerba del buey* (gumweed) was the treatment of choice for gonorrhea. Cottonwood bark was burned and mixed with blue corn meal and water to make an unguent for skin infections.[66] Pleurisy was treated by drinking various teas, inhaling the fumes formed by steaming cedar twigs under a blanket "tent," and rubbing a mixture of aromatic herbs and prickly pear pulp on the chest.

As time went on, some Hispanics began to turn to Anglo physicians such as Del Norte's Dr. Jonathan McFadzean. In 1907 McFadzean was asked to present a paper to the San Luis Valley Medical Association on "the Mexican from the viewpoint of the medical practitioner."[67] The result was a remarkable mixture of social and medical observation, colored by both prejudice and sensitivity. Although uncertain as to why he had been assigned this topic, the doctor thought that the occasion did provide an opportunity "to direct attention to the better side of this unfortunate and inferior race and to render some small measure of justice to [a people] berated by fully ninety-nine per cent of Americans." McFadzean began by pointing out the closeness of "Mexican" families ("They share in a remarkable degree each other's joys and sorrows") and their solicitude for the aged, indigent, infirm, and orphans. They cared for each other, "no matter how small the house or . . . poor the breadwinner." Although "their honesty is impugned by all classes of our citizens," the doctor had encountered a few "deadbeats" and had "seen Mexicans suffer long and intensely rather than employ a physician" when they knew they could not pay his bill.

McFadzean ascribed the fact that the "Mexicans" were "small, withered and stunted" to the effects of inadequate diet, overcrowding, poor ventilation, and early marriage. Infant mortality was high and tuberculosis and "dyspepsia" were common. Syphilis was better "tolerated [than in] whites," but "gonorrhea shows [them] no special favor." The rarity of postpartum or puerperal fever was remarkable, Dr. McFadzean noted, especially "when one considers the . . . filthy sheep skins on which they are confined, pole and dirt ceilings, mud floors with the accumulated filth and expectoration of generations, and the absence . . . of even soap and hot water."

The doctor found his Hispanic patients to be stoic and to "bear minor surgical operations . . . without anaesthesia, also the most difficult cases of labor." Their attitude was fatalistic, and a death was often followed by the comment, "The doctor did well, but God, the Great Physician, willed otherwise." There were few illegitimate births and McFadzean recalled that he had never been approached by Hispanics "to perform the atrocious crime of abortion."

Finally, the doctor reminded his medical colleagues: "You are in a position by counsel and admonition to do much toward ameliorating their miseries and bettering their condition."[67]

Although many still adhered to traditional Hispanic medicine and healers, there was evidence of increasing acceptance of Anglo medicine. With regard to smallpox, for example, the traditional opinion was that the disease was ordained by the will of God and that "infection will afford them [Hispanics] a better chance of salvation."[68] In 1902 Trinidad's Dr. T. J. Forhan observed:

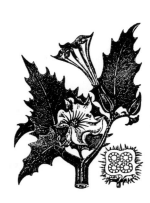

8.16 The Hispanics of the Southwest had an extensive number of botanical remedies. Stramonium was used as a salve to relieve the pain of arthritis.

These old-time prejudices are fast disappearing. Many Mexicans ... now seek vaccination and make no objection when house calls are made for this purpose.[68]

Coal Camps and Minnequa Hospital

Colorado's huge coal reserves were tapped early in its history, and coal mining grew with the state, providing energy to heat its homes and to fire its railroads and its steel and other industries. By 1910 there were 15,000 coal miners in the state, accounting, with coke and other coal industry workers and their families, for more than five percent of the population.[69] The majority lived in coal camps in the southern part of the state, distributed along a fifty mile belt between Trinidad and Walsenburg. The remainder were scattered elsewhere—in Boulder County north of Denver, parts of the Western Slope, the area west of Pueblo, and other sites. Working in a hazardous occupation and mainly foreign-born, illiterate, and poor, the coal miners and their families were sequestered in company camps and towns near the mines, living under a semi-feudal socio-economic system. The medical aspects of coal mining and of life in the coal camps are an interesting and unique aspect of early Colorado's medical history.

In addition to the miners, who earned between $2.50 and $4.00 a day, the mines employed trimmers, dumpers, trackmen, loaders, mule drivers, and other workers.[70] Boys as young as ten years of age were employed to do some of the lighter work; they were paid a dollar a day. Most of the mining was done by men swinging picks. A vein's face was undermined by pick, an explosive charge was fired, the loosened chunks of coal were broken up and loaded onto mule cars, hauled to the surface, sorted and processed, and the coal hauled off by train. Some of it was converted in huge ovens to coke for the steel industry. Each mine was administered by a superintendent, while foremen supervised the actual work in the mines. Coal mining in Colorado was dominated by the huge Colorado Fuel and Iron Company (CF & I) and several smaller companies.

The mines were unhealthy places in which to work. Ventilation was poor and clouds of coal dust were inhaled by the miners and other workers. In a few years, a miner's lungs were as black as the coal he mined. Dr. H. A. Lemen presented a patient with "black lung," or "phthisis pulmonalis nigra," to the State Medical Society in 1881—a 49 year old miner he had admitted to Arapahoe County Hospital:

> He was expectorating daily large quantities of the fluid a specimen of which I exhibit to you in this bottle. He not infrequently expectorated ... two pints in 24 hours ... As you see, the fluid is quite black. The sentence that I am now reading was written with this fluid ... The pen used has never been in ink![71]

Lemen described how carbon particles were carried to the lungs, "lodged upon the respiratory surfaces [and] mechanically, or by leucocytotic diapedesis, make their way to the alveolar walls, lymph spaces and vessels, and peribronchial tissues."

Although the pathogenetic role of carbon particles has been somewhat controversial, and the issue has been charged with political and economic considerations, there is little doubt that coal mining is associated with chronic lung disease. This has been recently termed "coal worker's pneumoconiosis" and is distinct from the hard rock miner's silicosis, although the two many occur in combination.[72] The effects of this pulmonary disease are insidious and generally inapparent until many years of mining have elapsed. During their active working years, the miners were more concerned with other medical problems such as bronchitis and pneumonia, the "rheumatism" which they associated with dampness, and headaches due to breathing gases generated by blasting. Such gases, or "after-damp," often contained high concentrations of carbon monoxide. Canaries were used to detect the lethal gas.[73] When the canary died, the miners knew it was time to leave.

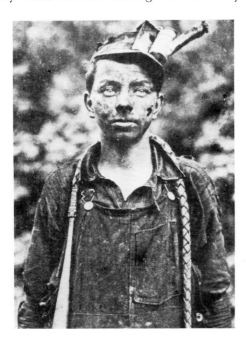

8.17 Even children worked in the coal mines. They were subject to the same dangers and illnesses as adults.

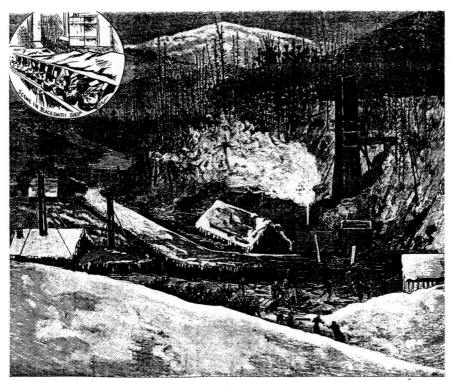

8.18 In 1884 a coal mine explosion near Crested Butte killed sixty miners. There were virtually no safety precautions in those days.

8.19 A few efforts were made to teach mine supervisors and foremen some first aid, and contests were held at county fairs.

Of even greater concern, however, were the injuries associated with mining accidents—cave-ins, floods, falls, the hazards of machinery—all occurring in semi-darkness and close confines, sometimes miles inside the earth. Most dreaded, however, by even the most hardened miners, were the massive explosions which might, at any time and without warning, suddenly roar through a mine—blowing some men to bits, asphyxiating others with noxious gases, and trapping still others beyond the reach of rescuers. Such explosions were the result of the accumulation, over the ages, of the gaseous and inflammable byproducts of coal formation. It was said that "if you wish to hear gruesome and blood chilling stories, listen to veteran coal miners who have gone through mine explosions . . ."[74] Explosive gases were especially frequent in Colorado's mines, a fact which led to the retention of pick-mining in Colorado while mechanical, but spark-generating, methods were being introduced elsewhere. Nevertheless, the list of disastrous mine explosions in Colorado is a long one. In 1910, 16,000 feet into the mine at Starkville, an explosion killed twenty-seven Austrians, thirteen Italians, four Russians, five Mexicans, "six white Americans and one colored American."[75] The same year, many more were killed in the mines at Delagua and Primero. Each successive year saw its disasters and in 1917, 121 miners died in an explosion at the Hastings mine.

In the two decades prior to 1908, there were, in the United States, more than 29,000 fatalities due to accidents in the coal mining industry. The rate of fatal accidents was higher than that of the other twelve major coal producing nations, more than twice that of Great Britain and higher, even, than primitive Russia.[76] Furthermore, the rate of fatalities in the United States was increasing rather than, as in other nations, decreasing. The major causes of accidental death in the coal mines, in order of frequency, were cave-ins (forty-seven percent), explosions (twenty-five percent), and "mine cars, mules, and other transportation (fifteen percent)."[77] During the five year period from 1913 through 1917, there were 481 accidental coal mining deaths in Colorado, an average of 7.5 deaths per 1,000 workers.[78] At that rate, over a workspan of thirty years, a coal mine worker had a nearly one-in-twenty chance of being killed in a mining accident. Non-fatal accidents were, of course, much more common, many of them serious and involving the loss of fingers, limbs, or eyes.

Depending on who was asked, blame for the high rate of coal mining accidents was placed on the carelessness of the miners, the greed of the companies, the indifference of the government, or the inevitability of fate. Little appears to have been done to educate the miners in accident prevention or emergency medicine; however, much was made of the first aid contests held at the annual Trinidad-Las Animas County Fairs. That of 1912 was said to have generated "an unusual amount of interest throughout the southern coal district [and was] attended by several thousand persons."[79] The events of "these friendly tournaments . . . were made to conform absolutely with those experienced in time of fire, explosion, fall of rock or other emergency" and were judged by several military surgeons. The team from the Maitland mine was awarded first prize, a silver loving cup.[80]

At least one physician was concerned enough to devise a miner's first aid kit. The inventor, Primero's Dr. W. W. Gage, noted that the kit

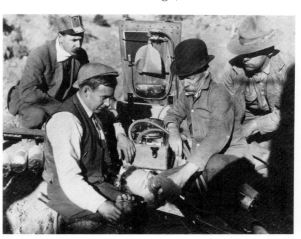

was designed to be attached to the miner's dinner pail, "the one article that always goes [into the mine] with its owner."[81] This neat little packet contained bandages, gauze, splints, tape, and spirits of ammonia. One has the feeling, however, that many miners found a way to remember their lunch and forget their kit.

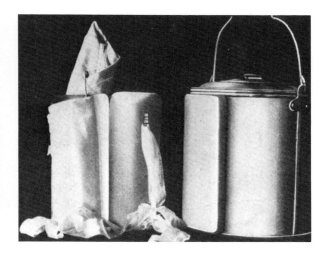

The coal camps were a remarkable institution. They were company towns, with rows of small frame houses for the miners and their families, and a church, school, general store, and saloon owned or controlled by the company. Virtually everything was provided by the company—food, water, housing, entertainment, medical care— all for a charge. The inhabitants were "encouraged" to make their purchases at the company store. Laws were enforced by company-controlled sheriffs and judges. The workers and their families represented dozens of nationalities and languages—Slavic, Italian, German, Hispanic, Oriental, Greek, Scandanavian, and so on—and many spoke no English. It was said that the companies preferred it that way; non-English speaking workers were easier to control and less likely to be influenced by the unions.

Some of the camps were said to be models of benevolent corporate paternalism. The company physician at Sopris, Dr. T. J. Forhan, described the good and bad features of his camp.[82] In general, he found that houses which belonged to the company were "kept in good repair [although built] in a very hurried way and not as substantial as they might be . . . fairly cold in winter, but otherwise fairly comfortable." On the other hand, he noted, a number of "shacks" which had been built by previous workers on company property were still in use:

There are about 54 houses up the canyon . . . of which 8 are habitable and 46 simply awful . . . Old dry goods boxes, soap boxes, old pieces of corrugated iron, powder cans, barrel staves and

every available thing that would stop a hole were used in construction . . . I have had to remove a mother in labor [during a rainstorm] to keep her dry . . . In the canyon there may be half dozen [water closets] . . . Many of them are a few boards thrown together with a hole in the ground not 2 feet deep . . . Some are constructed of gunny sacks . . . The children adopt the primitive plan of squatting beside the house and turning loose.[82]

Dr. Beshoar found that the amount of drinking water supplied to the camp at Hastings was inadequate, and as a result, the "ignorant families" sank their own inadequately constructed wells. The result was periodic outbreaks of typhoid, and he noted, the same conditions prevailed in the camps at Berwind and Starkville.[83] At Sopris, Dr. Forhan found that water from the Purgatoire River was pumped into a reservoir near the mine, and from there piped to the town, where it arrived brown with mud and black with coal dust.[84] A family would fill their barrel with water and toss in some powdered alum; then the barrel would "broil" in the sun for a week or so. Not unexpectedly, the insides of these water barrels became "covered with a thick, slimy, green deposit," yet, each week, the process was repeated, usually without even bothering to wash the barrel.

Each month, one dollar was deducted from the worker's pay check, entitling him and his family to free health care at the camp. The larger camps had a dispensary and a doctor on the premises. The doctor was paid a salary, usually one hundred dollars a month, and provided with a house and (of course) free coal.[85] In return, he was to provide "gratuitous service for all cases except those of confinement, venereal diseases and fight bruises." Some of the coal camp doctors left and became prominent physicians and civic leaders. Dr. T. D. Baird, the camp doctor in Pictou, was mayor of Walsenburg, a member of the State Medical Board, and the Board of Regents.[86] For others, the coal camp provided a convenient refuge from the competition of private practice.

Practice in the camps must have been gratifying in some ways and terribly frustrating in others. Many of the camps' inhabitants spoke no English and retained their Old World ways. Dr. A. W. Scarlet was called to see the three year old son of an Austrian miner at the Spring Gulch camp. The boy was in severe pain and the doctor diagnosed an intussusception.[87] He treated the boy successfully and left medication with orders that it be administered regularly. When he returned, the condition had recurred, and the boy was terminal. When Dr. Scarlet

8.20 Dr. W.W. Gage's miner's emergency kit was attached to the miner's lunch pail in the hope that this would ensure its actually being taken into the mine.

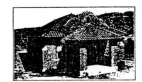

8.21 This neat little CF & I dispensary was located in one of the coal camps and probably manned by a company doctor.

asked the father whether he had given the boy his medicine, the father replied that

> They were afraid he would not wake up if they gave him any more medicine, so they had given him instead some 'Old Country' remedies which a neighbor woman had brought in. As the child was beyond aid, I made no comment. I requested a post-mortem but was refused. This case illustrates the embarrassments often met with . . .[87]

The camp doctors also had to deal with company rules. Each doctor received an allowance of three cents per capita for medicines:

> In one camp the doctor's monthly bill for drugs was $25 or more, and he was receiving about $12 from the company. That would put him nearly $150 in the hole at the end of the year.[88]

The doctors also found themselves at odds with mine superintendents who were not always sensitive to medical considerations, especially when company money was involved:

> The insanitary plight [of the camps] is due very largely to the fact that the hands of the camp physician are tied by the superintendent. For a man who has made hygienic science a special study, to have his recommendations thwarted by a block-headed super . . . is little less than a crime . . .[89]

When one doctor reported that his camp was unsanitary and needed to be cleaned up, the superintendent told him to do it himself. Another, taking measures to deal with a typhoid outbreak, was advised "to be careful, or you will step on someone's toes." The physicians of Huerfano county, company and non-company alike, were said to be in fear of the county's political boss, Sheriff Jeff Farr. A Walsenburg physician who had the temerity to oppose the sheriff was promptly arrested on a charge of "immoral practice" and held in jail for weeks without a trial.[90]

Camp doctors were not equipped to deal with the more serious and complicated cases. Colorado Fuel and Iron employees were transported to the company's hospital in Pueblo, Victor-American workers went to Mount San Raphael

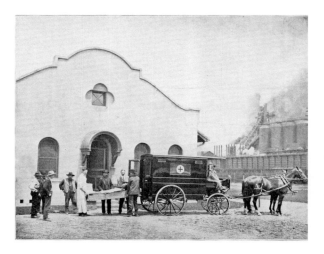

8.23 Seriously ill or injured patients from Pueblo's steel mills or from distant CF & I coal and coke camps in Colorado and Wyoming were transported to Minnequa Hospital.

Hospital in Trinidad, and other companies had arrangements with hospitals in Denver and other cities. The CF & I's Minnequa Hospital was a remarkable institution, the center of a huge and far-flung medical-industrial complex which was a model of turn-of-the-century industrial medicine.[91] Its beginnings were humble enough. In 1881 Dr. Richard W. Corwin, twenty-eight years old and just out of his residency, was put in charge of the company's medical facility in Pueblo, a six room house on Furnace Street across from the company's new steelworks. The following year, a thirty bed hospital was built, and over the years, both the company and the hospital continued to expand.[92] By 1900 CF & I was providing medical care for 60,000 workers and their families, not only for Pueblo's steelworkers but for the miners and other workers at the coal camps and other company operations around Colorado and other Western states.

In 1902 the CF & I's new Minnequa Hospital was opened. Largely the creation of Corwin, it was a breathtaking facility, thirteen Spanish mission style buildings with ironwork balconies and red tile roofs and a mountain view from its twenty landscaped acres on Lake Minnequa. Virtually every modern convenience was provided, including a lead-lined operating room, the newest sanitary, lighting, and plumbing technologies (including showers instead of tubs), and inclined runways to accommodate the handicapped. In addition to the 200 bed hospital (expandable to nearly 400 beds), the complex included "a smoking and game room for convalescents," a pathology laboratory, and physicians' and nurses' residences.[93] The ambulance team was "swift and safe" and was been equipped with a new horse-drawn "rubber-tired, spring, sling stretcher ambulance." Dr. Corwin insisted that no expense be spared, and the company had spent what was then the as-

8.22 The CF & I's Minnequa Hospital in Pueblo was an imposing facility.

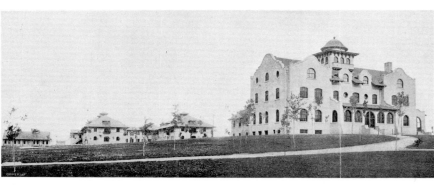

tounding sum of $300,000 in acceding to his wishes. In addition to Corwin as chief surgeon, the hospital was staffed by nine other physicians, five interns and a large number of consultants.

The need for an expanded facility had not been overestimated. By 1911 CF & I's population had increased to 80,000, and the steel mill and the coal camps were sending in thousands of patients each year. Many of these were injuries related to the hazards of the mines, coke ovens, and steel mills. After thirty years with the company, Dr. Corwin was able to survey more than 11,000 fractures—including about 1,000 amputations.[94] In addition, there had been innumerable abrasions, contusions, crushings, lacerations, burns, sprains, strains, dislocations, and other injuries.

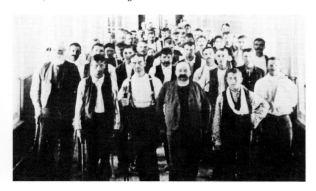

Dr. Corwin had become not only a nationally recognized expert in trauma surgery, hospital administration, and industrial medicine, but a leader in what was becoming known as "social medicine." Realizing that "physical, mental, and moral development go hand in hand," and dealing with a largely uneducated foreign-born population, "a task made none the easier by their speaking forty-seven languages . . . ," Corwin pursuaded the company "to establish a sociological department for the purpose of improving the condition of the men and families".[95] After nearly a half century in charge of the CF & I medical system, Corwin died in 1929. Shortly after his death, Minnequa Hospital was renamed Corwin Hospital.[96]

Despite the new hospital and the CF & I's "sociological department," the semi-feudal system of the mining camps had become increasingly unacceptable to its employees. In 1913, the coal workers began a strike which, in the next year or so, would be unsurpassed in bitterness, hardship, and violence. The confrontation has been portrayed many times as an epic encounter. On one side were the the companies and their representatives—greedy owners, corrupt officials, sadistic sheriffs, heartless militia, and hired thugs and scabs—and on the other,

the miners and their families and friends—courageous union organizers, idealistic reformers, outspoken journalists, and the beatific alter ego of the labor movement, Mother Jones. It was a show-down between John D. Rockefeller, Jr., WASP super-millionaire, and Louis Tikas, a Greek-born miner and union man. Not surprisingly, Rockefeller survived, though not untarnished, and Tikas died, a martyr and a hero.

The doctors found themselves in, or sometimes between, the two hostile camps. On the one side, there was Dr. John Chase, prominent Denver ophthalmologist, mine investor, and adjutant general of the Colorado National Guard. Chase had established his anti-union reputation in the Cripple Creek strike of 1904. Now, as the guard's commander in the 1913-14 strike, he had incarcerated Mother Jones in Mount San Raphael Hospital and led a mounted saber-charge against marching women protestors in Trinidad.[97] Ultimately, Chase was accused of brutality, incompetence, and corruption and was forced to resign in 1916.

On the other side, there was Dr. Benjamin Beshoar, the son of Trinidad's pioneer Dr. Michael, who, it was said, had taught his children "compassion for the poor and the minorities."[98] Ben was the union doctor, and, as such, was subject to the same abuse and dangers as the striking miners. When the miners continued to refuse to capitulate, they and their families were forced out of the camps. They set up tent colonies nearby, literally under the guns of the guard. The tents were cold and drafty, food was inadequate, sanitation was primitive, and Dr. Beshoar was kept busy caring for the men, women and children of the colonies. When it came time for a miner's wife, Emma Zanatell, to deliver her twins, the camp doctor refused to come. After a long delay, Dr. Beshoar finally arrived from Trinidad, soaking wet. The sheriff's deputies had fired at his car, and he had crawled the rest of the way up a gully.[99] The twins were stillborn. The next day, as her babies were being buried, guardsmen raided the camp and threatened to burn down Emma's tent.

Violence had been used by both sides, and dozens had already died when, on April 20, 1914, the guard raided the tent colony at Ludlow. The scene was chaotic and brutal and the victims were mainly women and children. It was said that the guard's officers refused to allow doctors or Red Cross nurses "to minister to the wounded . . . Physicians who went there under flags of truce were driven back by bullets."[100] A company physician was said to have accom-

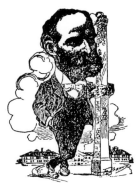

8.24 The workers represented a remarkable diversity of nationalities and languages, providing some interesting challenges to the CF & I's medical staff.

8.25 Dr. Richard Corwin was one of the nation's pioneers in industrial and social medicine.

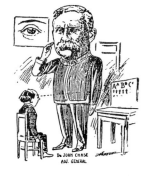

8.26 A Denver ophthalmologist, Dr. John Chase, commanded the Colorado Guard during the coal strike of 1913-1914.

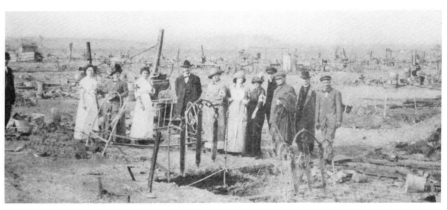

8.27 Medical workers after the disaster at Ludlow.

panied the troops, but it is not known whether he rendered any medical assistance.[101] Mrs. Jolly, a miner's wife and former nurse at Minnequa Hospital, pinned red crosses on her white dress, but the soldiers fired at her anyway.[102] Dr. Aca Harvey drove his buggy out from Aguilar, but he was trapped by gunfire and was unable to reach the colony. His white flag was filled with bullet holes. He did manage to treat several strikers who had been shot nearby.[103]

When rescuers were finally allowed to enter the colony, they found a scene of utter devastation. Many of the tents had caught fire. Under Alcarita Pedregon's burnt out tent, in a tiny pit in which they had sought shelter from the soldiers, were the bodies of thirteen women and children. Dr. Perry Jaffa, the county physician, later testified that the victims had died of asphyxia rather than from burns. He described the pit as "six feet in diameter . . . They were all jammed in so small a place."[104] The guard's officers testified that they had probably died before the fire, perhaps having accidentally trapped themselves in the pit. Shortly afterward, union organizer Louis Tikas was arrested, beaten and shot. His body was examined by Drs. Jaffa and Beshoar and an autopsy was done.[105] Dr. Jaffa described the wounds in detail, and both doctors testified that he had been shot in the back.

The following week, *Colorado Medicine* reported that a National Guard physician, Major Pliny Lester of Walsenburg, "was treacherously shot in the back by striking miners while in the line of duty at Ludlow."[106] Many of the state's physicians, generally conservative politically, sided with the mine owners. Six months after Ludlow, Denver's Dr. H.G. Wetherill was still writing letters to the editor urging a "balanced" view of the situation. In response to the editor's inquiry as to whether the doctor wished to have his letter published anonymously, Wetherill replied:

> If you use my name . . . I shall not hold you responsible if my property is burned, my house dynamited, or my anatomy perforated . . . after the usual methods of argument and retribution employed by the Western Federation of Miners and the United Mine Workers.[107]

The strike had been described as "a civil war, and a bloody one at that."[108] It was followed by Mr. Rockefeller's Industrial Representation Plan of 1915 and, gradually, by a variety of reforms, including improvements in mine safety, living conditions, sanitation, and health care. Employees' representatives were given a voice in the selection of camp physicians, and by the 1920s, a monthly charge of $1.50 entitled the CF & I miner to full medical care and his family to partial coverage. The president of the company himself came to a worker's meeting in Sopris, to explain the new health plan. A visitor inspecting the status of the coal camps reported that "in all the camps we found employees well satisfied with the medical service."[108] The ultimate praise, however, came from a union man, a "motor driver in one of the mines," who stated his opinion of the company's hospital: "It is a good place. I have been there and I don't mind giving my money to it."[108]

9 DOCTORS

The doctor must be bold as a lion with one patient, as patient as Job with another, and as gentle as a lamb with the next . . . While others are resting or refreshed with sleep, he must go no matter whether he be drowned by the rains or choked by the dust. At noon or at midnight, he is supposed to answer every call. He is expected to have an eye like an eagle, a heart like a lion, and a hand like a lady.

Gross Medical College Bulletin
Denver, 1895[1]

THE FIRST DOCTOR'S offices in Colorado were in tents or log cabins. The doctor's equipment consisted of whatever he had packed into his black bag before coming overland—perhaps a few knives, probes, and catheters, an amputation saw, some needles and suture, and, if he adhered to the old ways, lancets and a set of cups. He had also brought his own medicines, including calomel, jalap, quinine, laudanum, various salves, and some personal favorites. Bandages, dressings, and splints were likely to be improvised. This was probably what Dr. Levi Russell's "office" contained at the Cherry Creek diggings in 1859. Even in later years, in some of the more primitive locales, the doctor's office might not have changed very much.

In most of Colorado's towns, and certainly in the cities, doctor's offices began to resemble those of their colleagues in towns and cities back east. In smaller communities or in poorer neighborhoods, the doctor's office might be located behind a storefront. In larger towns and cities, it might be above a bank, or in a small professional building downtown. Married physicians often combined their homes and offices. In his classic book of advice to the new physician, Dr. D. W. Cathell recommended that, if the town was large enough, the doctor should locate his office-home in a "genteel" neighborhood, prefer-ably on a corner lot, so that patients could be admitted through a separate entrance on the side street.[2] Dr. Cathell advised the doctor that his office should suggest its "occupant's good taste and gentility, as well as his learning and skill . . . the office of a live, earnest-working, scientific physician, who has a library, takes the journals and makes use of the various instruments science has devised for him." It was not considered unprofessional to tastefully display one's microscope and stethoscope, or to hang up diplomas, certificates, "academic prizes,"

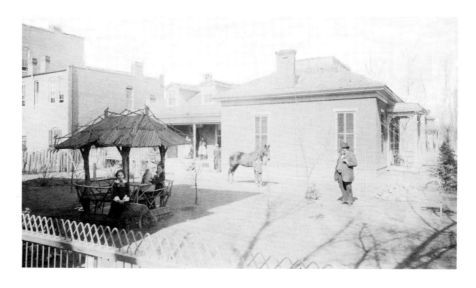

9.1 In 1879 Dr. F. J. Bancroft's combined home and office occupied a corner lot, thereby allowing a separate entrance for his patients. It was located at 16th and Stout streets, in the heart of what is now downtown Denver.

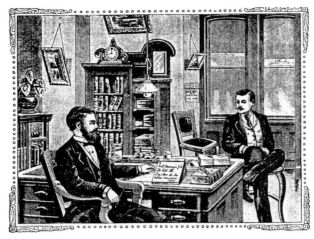

and portraits of "medical celebrities." It would not do, however, to have a

> quackish display of instruments and tools. Keep out of sight such inappropriate or even repulsive objects as catheters, syringes, obstetric forceps, amputating knives, grinning skulls [or] jars of tumors . . . Also, avoid keeping human bones on your desk for use as paperweights.[3]

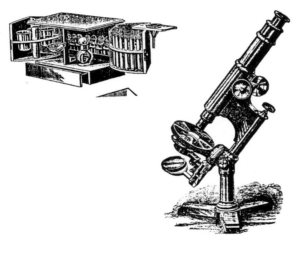

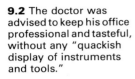

The doctor's office was variously furnished and equipped, depending on whether he was a recent graduate with little capital or a well-established practitioner whose waiting room was filled with paying patients. A modestly furnished office might include a desk and a bookcase, a table or two, an instrument case and a medicine cabinet, and perhaps a simple operating table. After a few years of successful practice, the doctor might invest in a fancy patient's chair-operating table which could be used for both deliveries and minor surgery. One favorite, the "Harvard" chair, had so many adjustments that the patient could be placed in virtually any imaginable position. The Harvard Company located in Canton, Ohio, and not affiliated with the university, advertised a regular model (iron frame and imitation leather) for $48 and a deluxe model (cherry, walnut, or antique oak frame and upholstered with embossed leather or crimson mohair plush) for $75. The Harvard chair's major competitor was, perhaps not coincidentally, manufactured by the Yale Company (also non-university affiliated). It was a little more expensive than the Harvard product. The successful doctor might add all sorts of additional furniture and instruments to his office. An attractive "physician's cabinet"—five feet high, solid oak or walnut with brass mountings, a desk top, five drawers, and four revolving instrument shelves, was available for $25. A solid brass microscope could be purchased for as little as $30 and a Fehlings Urine Test Set, an impressive array of test tubes, funnels, reagent bottles, and other assorted glassware, all in a wooden stand, for $9.

The choice of an office sign was an important matter. Cathell recommended that the ethical doctor not use an office sign as an advertisement, but

> simply to show his office to those looking for him. The signs should be neither too large nor too numerous . . . One of black smalt with gold letters is the neatest and most attractive of all; one such sign on the front wall for day-time, and a glass one with black letters in the window, to be seen at night when your office is lighted . . .[4]

The doctor was urged to be specific and consistent in his office hours:

> Establish regular office hours early in your career, and post them conspicuously in your office. For patients to come strolling in . . . for advice at odd or unreasonable hours . . . amounts almost to persecution.[4]

The doctor had chloroform or ether available for general anaesthesia, cocaine for topical anaesthesia, and carbolic acid or corrosive sublimate for antisepsis. In addition, he was expected to have an array of medicines available in his office. These included cathartics, quinine and other antifebriles, morphine, bromides, belladonna, ergot, and other standards. In addition, he had various tonics, salves, unguents, some of which he concocted himself, and perhaps, a personal remedy or two.

Practice

In 1897 Denver's Dr. George Stover opened his new office.[5] Perhaps he followed the *Denver Medical Times'* advice to "make your office a place of comfort and cheerfulness [and] clean . . . so your patients may enter it . . . with actual eleva-

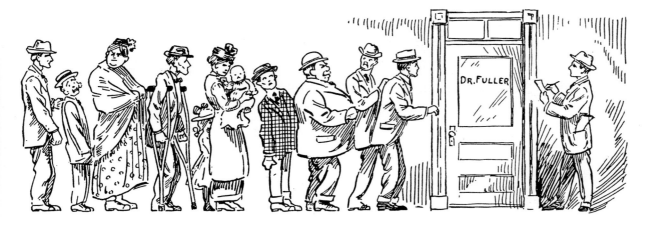

9.5 The new doctor had to be patient—it might be quite some time before he had a waiting room filled with patients.

tion of heart."[5] At any rate, his office newly furnished, "stationery printed, and everything in readiness," the doctor entered his waiting room promptly at the opening of office hours. It was empty. He recalled the day vividly:

> No patients today? Ah! but here comes a vistor; observe the affability with which he is greeted and conducted to the private office,—where he unfolds the benefits of his particular life and accident policy! The next caller leaves me some prescription blanks on the corner drug store. The next is a lady, and now I am sure of a patient, but no - "Will I buy a chance in the raffle for a crazy quilt?" [Next] a trained nurse leaves me her address. I wonder if I will ever employ a nurse? The next is a book agent; well, I may as well get some books, I have plenty of time for reading. Then comes a young man [who wants] an abortion [for his wife] and I refuse . . . Then four or five boys and girls want me to subscribe to a daily paper . . . Then a lady looking for another physician . . . I am afforded opportunities to buy all sorts of merchandise, from wire coat hangers to autographed etchings.[5]

Finally—a patient, a woman who came in, allegedly, for treatment of an "acne pimple on her dimpled chin," but who actually had her own wares to sell. Subsequently, the new doctor learned that "others had danced to her pipings, and paid roundly in cash for the privilege." And so it went, day after day. At last, "an occasional bona fide patient dropped in and I began to feel that I had at last broken the barriers. With renewed hope I looked foward to the day when I should be spoken of by the public . . ."

Regardless of his feelings, the new doctor was advised to "be polite and courteous to every one . . . [since] true politeness is a seed that . . . bears good fruit."[6]

> If ladies ask you for a donation to aid the heathen (!!!) or to help buy a carpet for their church, or any other laudable object, give willingly and cheerfully. If the tiny boy or girl comes to sell a concert

or festival ticket, buy it laughingly, for contributions this way not only do good, but have other consequences.[6]

Having, at last, achieved a successful practice, the doctor was likely to be provided with all sorts of opportunities to invest his earnings. To fend off this type of office "pest," one doctor suggested placing a sign on the office door. Beginning with the word "NO!" in huge letters, the sign included the following:

> I don't want to double my money in ninety days!
> I don't want to "get in on the ground floor"!
> I don't want to be a charter member![7]

And, for good measure, he added, "I don't want a ticket to the Masked Ball of the firemen, or the policemen, or the mail carriers, or the elevator pilots, or the janitors, or the Busy Bees, or the Helping Hand . . ."

The drug company salesman or "rep" was another frequent visitor. The physician's response to this category of "pest" was unpredictable. It might depend on the skill and personality of the salesman, on whether the doctor's last patient had paid her bill, or on the time of day. The representative of a reputable company was often regarded as an important source of current pharmaceutical information for the physician, especially those who were too busy to read the medical literature. In addition, the doctor appreciated the free samples that accompanied the "rep's" visit.

The mail was another form of office "pest." A La Junta, Colorado, physician wrote to the *Journal of the American Medical Association* about an unpleasant experience with a soap company that claimed its product would cure "erysipelas, eczema, herpes, hemorrhoids . . . and any morbid exudation [of the skin]."[18] This was only one of thousands of instances, he complained, of physicians being "worked" for testimonials and being tricked or seduced into ad-

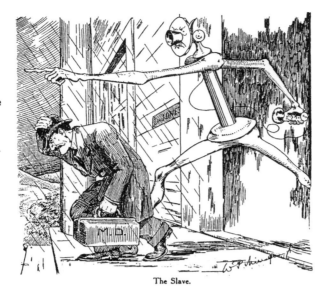

9.6 The telephone made its appearance in Colorado in the late 1870s. It had a major impact on the doctor's daily routine.

The Slave.

vertising such wares to their patients. "Is it not about time," he asked, "that we physicians realized how we are being humbugged and utilized by these proprietary men?"

Another by-product of a successful practice was the proliferation of paper work. Physicians had to fill out insurance data, accident reports, physical examinations for the railroads and mining companies, pension applications, and so on. These were tolerable since they were accompanied by a fee. Birth and death certificates and contagious disease reports were, on the other hand, not reimbursed, and despite what were probably the best of intentions by physicians who realized their importance, these aspects of office paperwork were generally assigned a low priority. Colorado's state registrar reported that many doctors simply did not bother to fill out birth certificates, for example, and those who did, often did so improperly.[9] Busy doctors, faced with mounting stacks of paperwork, became legendary for their inscrutable handwriting. Obviously annoyed by the complaints of his long suffering clerks, the state registrar asked the doctors, " Do you think [they] are specially gifted in the art of deciphering hieroglyphics?"

The successful physician usually wanted to expand his office or perhaps move to a more prestigious location. This meant more plush office furniture, more elaborate equipment, and perhaps even a telephone. Some might point to 1879 as the beginning of modern medical practice in Colorado, that year having seen Dr. Charles Denison and several others become the first physicians in Denver to acquire a telephone.[10] By 1908 there were 600 physicians listed in Denver's telephone directory, and most had two phones.[11] Soon, the telephone was expanded into another physician's love-hate re-

9.7 A reasonable medical library could be put together for about fifty dollars in the 1890s.

lationship, the answering service. In 1915 *Colorado Medicine* reported that

> a rather interesting project is on foot in Denver to establish a physician's . . . telephone exchange through which, when a physician is not at his office or home, patients may be enabled to reach him, or may, at his request, be referred to another physician who is caring for his practice.[12]

By the 1890s, medical advances had become bewildering in their number and complexity. The medical publishing industry was booming and the doctor had to make a major effort if he was to keep up with the rapidly expanding medical literature. The new physician was urged to invest in a personal library. For a total of about $50.00 he could obtain ten to fifteen of the standard textbooks. In 1890 Senn's *Principles of Surgery* cost $4.50 (another dollar for the leather-bound edition). For $20.00, the doctor could add four or five books to his library each year. Most medical journals cost $2.00 or $3.00 for a year's subscription. In addition to one of Colorado's journals, the physician might want to subscribe to one or two national journals. Reprints of journal articles, according to Colorado's Dr. Charles Spivak, were often sent by their authors, unsolicited, to colleagues as a form of advertising.[13] The great majority, Spivak commented, went into the trash, unread.

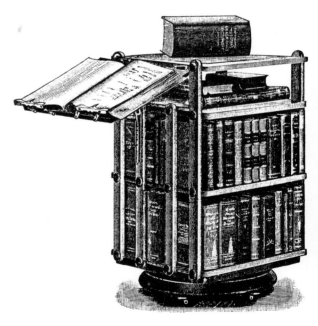

Some doctors were known for their extensive medical libraries.[14] Denver's Dr. J. T. Eskridge subscribed to some forty medical journals from "all corners of the globe." Dr. T. H. Hawkins had "almost every [medical] work of importance published in the English language within the last two decades . . . the ragged back and the luxuriously bound reposing side by side" on the shelves. Those who could afford it, travelled to the major medical centers in the East or in Europe to take postgraduate courses, often by spending some time working with some well-known professor. The "news notes" of Colorado's medical journals contain many reports of Dr. X or Y having returned from New York, Philadelphia, Berlin, or Vienna, after having done some postgraduate work.

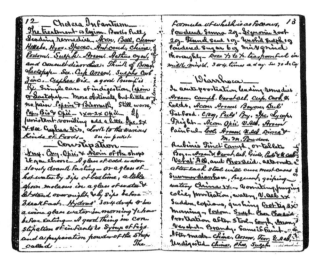

The doctor's office, education, and skills were important in attracting patients and building a successful practice. So, too, was the impression he made upon his potential clientele. Cathell advised the new doctor to "cultivate a professional manner and spirit."[15] In dress, for example,

> keep yourself neat and tidy, and avoid slovenliness and everything approaching carelessness or neglect . . . Do not ignore the fashions of the day [but] do not be a leader in loud or frivolous fashions, appearing as though your starchy foppishness and love of fine clothes had overshadowed everything else.[15]

The doctor's office, he advised, should not to be a "lounging place or smoking-room for horse-jockeys, dog-fanciers, base-ballers, politicians, mimics, chatty blockheads or others whose time hangs heavily on their hands."[15] This was especially important in cultivating a good impression among women, since "females have more sickness than males, and the females of every family have a potent voice in selecting the family physician." With men, caution was to be used when expressing opinions regarding such potentially controversial areas as politics and religion. As for non-medical pursuits, "patients want to think of their physician as interested in medicine and medicine alone." The doctor with a hobby,

for example, was advised to keep under wraps his "miniature museum of . . . impaled butterflies, bugs, miniature ships, snakes, stuffed birds . . . and anything else that will advertise you in any other light than that of a physician."

Housecalls

Patients expected their doctor to make housecalls. In 1895 the cost of a housecall in Denver ranged from two to five dollars. After the first mile, an additional dollar was added for each mile, two dollars at night.[16] Some doctors had a meter-like arrangement attached to a wheel of their buggy in order to measure the mileage. Doctors who made their housecalls on horseback generally preferred an Elliott's or a Western Patent Springs medical saddle bag. Both were made from a single piece of leather, and the twin bags contained inner cases which kept medicines and instruments free from "odious horse smell."[17] When walking or travelling by horse and buggy, the doctor used a hand case or satchel, a trademark of his profession. Of variable size, and usually covered by black pebbled leather and lined with chamois, the doctor's bag typically contained a stethescope, a thermometer, a small surgical kit, bandages, gauze, cotton, a hypodermic syringe kit, alcohol, an antiseptic solution, and a dozen or so medicines. A larger bag, for the doctor who had to be prepared for any emergency, might include splints and plaster, an amputating saw, obstetrical forceps and other larger instruments, and an anaesthetic drop bottle and mask.[18]

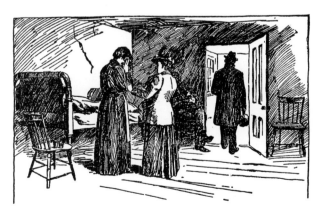

In the city, a housecall usually meant a walk or a short ride to the patient's home. Only occasionally did the city doctor travel across town or into the suburbs: "Dr. T. H. Close made a wild night ride a few days ago to bring a patient with a ruptured appendix to Denver [from the town of Parker] . . "[19] Away from the city, the situation was quite different. Some of the long-

9.8 Many doctors carried their pocket notebook of helpful hints and favorite prescriptions. This notebook was inscribed: "Collated from various authors and personal practice—for *private* use."

9.9 Housecalls were an important part of the doctor's practice. Sometimes he arrived too late.

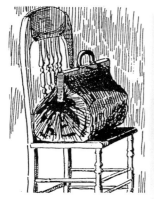

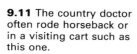

9.10 The doctor's pebbled black leather bag was the symbol of the housecall. In rural areas, it was the medical saddle bag or buggy case. This one combined the features of the two.

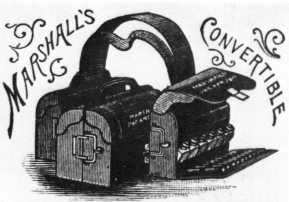

BUGGY-CASE-SADDLE-BAGS

distance "housecalls" made by mining camp and country doctors were mentioned previously. Methods of transportation varied considerably, and sometimes a great deal of ingenuity was required. One doctor on the eastern plains recalled making housecalls on foot, on horseback, by cart, and by sled.[20] In 1914 he purchased his first automobile, a Model T Ford. On one occasion, when the tin lizzie couldn't make it through the snowbanks, the resourceful country doctor commandeered a tractor.

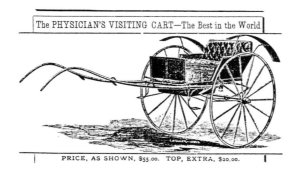

9.11 The country doctor often rode horseback or in a visiting cart such as this one.

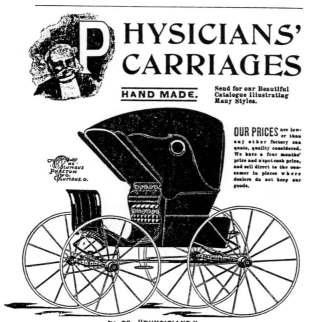

9.12 In the city, the doctor might prefer a more elegant phaeton or brougham.

When the horse was still the usual means of transportation, a doctor generally kept one or two horses in his own barn or in a stable in town. As trails became roads, the horse and buggy became, as one adverstisement proclaimed, "the doctor's best friend." Doctors were as knowledgeable about horses, saddles, harness, and the like as their neighbors. In the city, a bicycle was considered undignified or dangerous, and walking meant that "Dr. Footpace" would have to stop "to parley, and lose valuable time with convalescent patients, old friends, etc."[21] So the city doctor was advised to get a "respectable-looking horse and carriage." The doctor whose practice could not sustain so costly a means of transportation and who was dependent on "a bony horse and a seedy looking . . . buggy," was advised not to "let them stand in front of your office . . . as if to advertise your poverty, lack of taste, or paucity of practice." With a well-appointed carriage, however, it was "proper and ethical [to display] a modest monogram . . ."

Automobiles began to appear in the late 1890s. In rural areas and in the mountains, many Colorado physicians continued to rely on a horse and buggy on dirt roads which were usually deeply rutted or rocky and oftentimes muddy, icy, or snow-packed. Motor cars were unreliable and even dangerous under such circumstances. Colorado's physicians soon adapted to the new means of transportation, however. In the city, with streets congested with pedestrians, bicycles, and horse-drawn vehicles, the speedy new conveyences were not always welcomed. A Denver doctor who drove his automobile down a Denver street at thirty miles an hour in 1914 must have created absolute havoc; he was ticketed and the event was sufficiently newsworthy to appear in print.[22] Like most new drivers, doctors were not fully aware of some of the dangerous features of their contraptions. In 1914 *Colorado Medicine* reported that Craig's Dr. J. E. Downs was knocked unconscious by "the crank handle of his automobile" and that Canon City's Dr. Otis Orendorff received an eye injury while cranking his vehicle.[23] Automobile accidents became common news items in Colorado's medical journals. Again in 1914, another issue of *Colorado Medicine* noted four such accidents: Dr. L. B. Overfelt in a collision with a buggy in Boulder, Dr. C. A. Tennant and his family somersaulting over Willow Creek Pass in northern Colorado, Dr. J. H. Cole in a similar accident near Yampa, and Dr. C. S. Phelan breaking three ribs while attempting to start his car in Salida.[23]

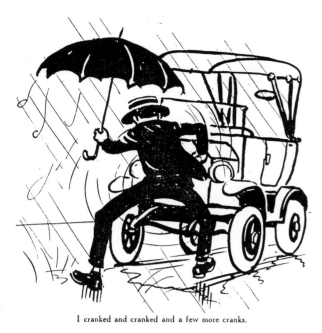

I cranked and cranked and a few more cranks.

Patients

The new doctor, about to begin his practice, was advised:

> In the course of your professional career you will meet humanity in all its aspects and phases . . . A gilt-edged society lady and a hod-carrier, a lawyer, a backwoodsman, a school-miss, a straitlaced old maid, a sailor, and a girlish dude will each use a different kind of language to express the same symptoms . . . Some who are naturally stoical and apathetic will fall into the error of understating their true condition [while] others, of a hysterical or nervous temperament . . . will magnify every detail . . . [24]

Some of his patients made the doctor angry—the malingerer, the hypochondriac, the deadbeat—but probably none more than the patient who sought his advice, only to ignore it. One Colorado physician commented about such patients:

> In the daily drudge of the overworked Doctor . . . when he finds that his advice is disregarded, that his instructions are not carried out, that his medicines are not administered . . . it is enough to drive a sensitive man out of the practice of medicine. [25]

He cited the case of a young tuberculous woman who walked into his office one day. She was carrying a sputum cup filled with blood which she had just coughed up. The doctor gave her a prescription, stressed the seriousness of her condition, and and told her to immediately go home and rest. Three hours later, she was seen carrying a "large bag of vegetables" and running to catch the streetcar. That night, when her hemorrhage recurred, the doctor refused to visit.

Dr. C. A. Hadsell, a general practitioner in the small Western Slope town of Cedaredge, wondered whether some of this "therapeutic infidelity" might be, at least partially, the fault of the doctors themselves:

> Have we not, as a profession, become so deeply interested in microbes, in chemical formulas—in the science of medicine—that we have forgotten and neglected the man? [26]

Hadsell suggested that "faith, without works, in religion, is dead, but we might say work without faith, in the practice of medicine, is dead." The emotional state of the patient—"fear, despair, remorse, etc . . ."—might be just as important in wound healing, for example, as biochemical and physiological phenomena. He asked, in what today might be regarded as a holistic approach, "If the physician can induce suitable emotional states, would it not aid a correct treatment by medication? Is he not justified in using any influence for the betterment of his patient?"

Colleagues

Dr. E.L. Foster was fairly typical of the turn-of-the-century Colorado doctor.[27] Having graduated from a legitimate medical school, and after practicing "back east" for a few years, Foster developed what was probably tuberculosis and came to Colorado for his health. After living the outdoor life for a while, he recovered and, apparently liking what he had seen of Colorado, decided to stay. Foster sent for his wife and set up a rural practice in the tiny San Luis Valley town of Hooper. Like many others, he moved from rural practice to Denver where, apparently hoping to supplement his practice, he opened a pharmacy. Denver's medical climate was highly competitive and, apparently unwilling to move away from the metropolis, the Fosters moved to the "suburb" of Arvada. The doctor purchased the home and practice of a physician who, like himself, had come to Colorado because of tuberculosis and who had also combined practice and pharmacy. Foster did quite well in the "suburbs" and, in addition to his successful private practice, contracted with the Denver Tramway company, one of the railroads, and a nearby coal mine. Dr. Foster died in 1960, his professional life having spanned six decades.

In his "bio-ethnologicial" survey, Dr. Charles Spivak provided some interesting background on Colorado's early twentieth century physicians.[28] The average age of the respondents was forty-seven. More than 90% were born outside of Colorado, the majority in six states in the

9.13 The automobile was soon adopted by city and country doctor alike.

Northeast (New York and Pennsylvania) and the Midwest (Ohio, Illinois, Iowa, and Missouri). Nearly 10% were foreign-born, all Canadian or European, with the exception of one Japanese. Nearly one out of every three Colorado physicians had been raised on a farm. Other paternal occupations included medicine (14%), business (11%), religion (4%), and law (4%). About one in fifteen came from working class families, including those of a butcher, a baker, and a cheesemaker. They tended to come from large families, the average physician having four or five siblings. Nearly 75% had graduated from non-Colorado medical schools, including, in order of frequency, Rush and Northwestern (both in Chicago), Jefferson, the Universities of Michigan and Pennsylvania, Harvard, and Bellevue (now New York University). Two-thirds had attended college prior to medical school, and the same proportion had completed an internship before entering practice.

Like everyone else, doctors were quite varied in their temperaments and personalities. In Dr. Cathell's allegorical prose,

> the door to the Aesculapian temple is open, wide open, to every variety of individual . . . not only to Dr. Merryman, Dr. Fair, Dr. Ettykett and Dr. Warmgrasp, but also to Dr. Growler, Dr. Sneerer, Dr. Crusty, Dr. Showoff, Dr. Frigid, Dr. Gall . . .[29]

Despite the shortcomings they might observe in their fellows, physicians were advised to "avoid all quarrels, bickerings and disputes with your medical brethren."[29] Nevertheless, ugly encounters arose. The *Denver Medical Times* noted that "Jealousy . . . is said to exist to a greater extent among physicians than any other body of men".[30] *Colorado Medicine* asked whether "it is any wonder that rival physicians," competing in a crowded profession, "distrust, dislike and even hate each other?"[31] Such conflicts, it added, were most likely to arise within the confines of a small town. Often, disputes were kept quiet and resolved by the state or county medical society. When a colleague challenged the credentials of Trinidad's Dr. Michael Beshoar, the Colorado Medical Society found the charges to be baseless and censured the complainant.[32]

Much to the chagrin of a profession which preferred to settle its disputes privately, occasional disputes became public. In 1875 Georgetown's Dr. J. Van De Voort posted the following broadside:

> To the Public: On Friday, the 12th, I returned from Denver City and learned . . . that while absent . . . reports had been industriously circulated derogatory to my character, not only as a gentle-

man, but as a member of the medical profession. I hereby . . . denounce the Authors and Propagators of these—As—Liars, Cowards, and Scoundrels, and challenge them as to the proof. I am personally responsible for what I say, and all know where to find me.[33]

Family and Home

According to Dr. Spivak's study, nearly all of Colorado's physicians were married, and divorce was rare.[34] The average physician had a small family, averaging less than two children each. In her popular 1890s book, *The Physician's Wife*, Mrs. E. M. Firebaugh pointed out that a doctor's wife had to be a special type of person.[35] Physician's wives, she claimed, "Watch and wait." With her husband away for long and unpredictable hours, "no one outside the profession can ever know how many breakfasts and dinners and suppers have been spoiled in the waiting . . ."[35]

Nighttime at the physician's home was equally unpredictable and "different from what it is at other people's houses. Other people can retire and sleep in undisturbed repose . . . while at the doctor's they never know what an hour may bring forth." The doctor was likely to be called at any time and, if he wanted to make a living, he had better respond. Although all men are "absent-minded and forgetful," said Mrs. Firebaugh, "physicians are particularly so . . .," and the loyal wife had to be tolerant of this foible.[36] The physician's wife was likely to learn many confidential things about friends and neighbors, but she had to be tactful and discrete. Furthermore, knowing that "when the doctor comes home, he will enjoy talking about something else than what has occupied his mind at the office," the doctor's wife should turn the conversation to other topics.[37]

The doctor's wife was expected, by her friends, never to get sick. When she did become ill, unlike other women, she had no choice of physician—it was expected that her husband would treat her.[37] Perhaps her greatest challenge, however, came when the doctor himself was ill. Accustomed to having his own way in the sickroom, the doctor, merely an "autocrat" when well, became a "tyrant" when sick. Mrs. Firebaugh summarized her image of the role of the doctor's wife:

> We, the wives, cannot do the good in the world that our husbands have it in their power to do . . . and so, our real usefulness to those around us . . . may be likened as shadow unto form. But it is good to know that shadows, too, have had their mission in the world . . . It is thus that we may

work. Quietly, unostentatiously . . . with cheerful heart . . . doing the little that we may in this world.[38]

As the social and economic status of the American physician improved, he began to be considered a good "catch" for the daughters of successful farmers, businessmen, ministers, and lawyers. By the turn of the century, many of Colorado's physicians' wives came from middle class, or sometimes even upper class backgrounds.

Working day and night, the physician sometimes had to be reminded that:

> [you are] mortal and should get as much out of life as you can, by seeking proper relaxations and amusements . . . An occasional day's sport with rod or gun, or a summer trip, or an evening at a convivial gathering or at the theater, etc . . . .will lessen the worries, frets, tumults, jarring and cares of practice, break the monotony of life . . . and remove brain-weariness and the result of overwork . . . [39]

Some doctors did a great deal of travelling and did not mind having their travels chronicled in the "news notes" of the medical journals. Perhaps this was a sign of status, an indication that their professional position was secure. Occasionally, public notice was taken of a physician's non-medical pursuits or interests, a hobby or an intellectual or cultural activity. When Denver's Dr. J. M. Perkins visited the poet, James Whitcomb Riley, it was duly noted in *Colorado Medicine*, along with the fact that the doctor could recite most of Riley's poems from memory.[40] Another "item" reported that Dr. C. K. Fleming had written the music for "The Bryan Marseillaise," a popular political tune which espoused the presidential candidacy of William Jennings Bryan.[41]

In the cities, physicians and their wives had an opportunity to

> visit the theater, where they saw the dark Othello rant or the fair Ophelia rave. They were enlightened in conversations with the learned and invited to the entertainments of discriminating wealth.[42]

In rural areas, opera, theater and literary groups were unavailable, and physicians had to be satisfied with less lofty, if perhaps, equally satisfying, extra-curricular activities:

> Dr. Burgin of Delta is an accomplished ventriloquist and, while on the Gunnison River this week, kept the fishermen startled by strange voices apparently coming from bushes or rock crevices . . . Dr. Burgin gets much amusement from his talent in this way.[43]

Women Physicians

There are many new factors in the practice of medicine which he who would benefit his fellow man must take into account. One of these is woman as a trained physician. I believe she had demonstrated her fitness and capacity for good work in our profession.
        Minnie C. T. Love, M.D., 1902[44]

Thus far, little mention has been made of women physicians in Colorado. To a large extent, this is a reflection of the fact that women formed a tiny minority of Colorado's, and the nation's, physicians during the nineteenth century. It was not until less than a decade before Colorado's Gold Rush that a woman graduated from an American medical school. Having been awarded the M.D. in 1849, Elizabeth Blackwell and her early successors were shunned by many men physicians and excluded from hospitals and medical societies. Even as small, but increasing numbers of women were being accepted by medical schools, women physicians were still being referred to as "doctoresses" or as "Mrs. Dr. So-and-so," and their practices often limited to women and children.

This was the situation when the first women physicians came to Colorado. The earliest reference available to a woman physician in Colorado was to a "Mrs. Smith—Doctress and Female Nurse" in Georgetown in 1869.[45] Her card, published in *The Miner*, noted that "Ladies and children's diseases [were] particularly attended to" and that her office was located at the residence of Reverend Peter J. Smith, presumably her husband. There is no indication that Mrs. Smith had a medical degree. She was followed in Georgetown in the 1870s by Mrs. Helene Anderson and a Mrs. Pratt.[46] The latter advertised herself as an "Accoucheuse and Physician" and later as a "Ladies Physician."

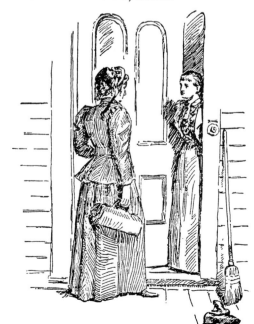

9.14 In the early days, most women physicians limited their practices to women and children.

A few years later, in his presidential address to the Colorado Medical Society, Dr. W. H. Williams advocated equal rights for women physicians. Acknowledging that his opinion was unpopular and likely to result in "acrimonious criticism" from his male colleagues, he stated his belief that men and women should have the same opportunity to either succeed or fail in their professional ambitions:

> I do not propose that ignorance nor incompetency shall escape behind petticoats [or] through the observance of . . . foolish gallantry . . . If they fail, the failure is theirs, not ours; and if they prove competent, permit them to enjoy the immunities of the profession co-equal with us . . . That a woman should not practice medicine because she is a woman, is absurd and intolerant.[47]

With the enactment of Colorado's new licensing law in 1881, we find the registration of several women who can be clearly identified as graduates of legitimate medical schools. The first woman to receive a license to practice medicine in Colorado was Dr. Edith A. Root of Denver.[48] Dr. Mary H. B. Bates was also licensed that year. A graduate of Woman's Medical College of Philadelphia, Dr. Bates came to Leadville in 1878 and practiced in that hectic mining camp for two years before moving to Denver. She became one of Denver's leading women physicians and practiced there for thirty years.

In 1881 Colorado's first medical school, the Denver Medical College, opened its doors—to male students. By 1887 it had awarded an M.D. to the state's first woman medical graduate, Dr. Eleanor Lawney.[49] In 1883 in its first catalogue,

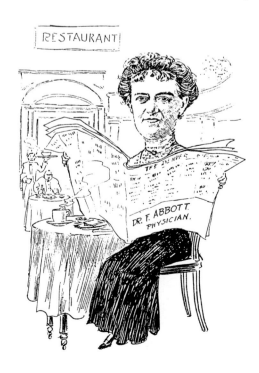

9.15 Dr. Frona Abbott was one of the first women to be a faculty member at a medical school in Colorado. She was acknowledged to be "all right . . . and can't be scared" by her students.

the University of Colorado's medical school announced that it was open "to all persons of either sex who are qualified for admission."[50] This policy was not popular at a time when Harvard and other prestigious eastern schools were refusing to admit women. The *Journal of the American Medical Association* predicted that the new school's attempt at medical coeducation would be unsuccessful.[51] In fact, it was not until 1891 that the University of Colorado awarded its first M.D. to a woman, Dr. Nelly Frances Mayo. In the next two decades, however, a relatively large percentage of the School's graduates, more than 10%, were women.[52]

It was not easy to be a woman medical student. In addition to the usual academic challenges of medical school, the "hen medic" had to face the resentments and hostilities of some of the male students and faculty. Dr. Agnes Ditson felt that she had more problems as a woman medical student than later as a woman in medical practice.[53] The female medical student was not without her supporters, however, as reflected in this male student's comments in 1895:

> We have the new woman here studying medicine. She will succeed because she is so preparing herself that it is almost impossible to fail . . . There is no reason why the new woman should not study medicine and be just as handsome and just as good as she could be in any other respect.[54]

A little patronizing, perhaps, but undoubtedly well intended. Women faculty members were much scarcer than women medical students. For those few, again, it must not have been easy. One early woman professor probably had to pass a few tests of her own before her students were willing to acknowledge that "she is all right, up-to-date in every way and can't be scared."[55]

In 1875 the issue of admitting "regularly educated females" to the Colorado Medical Society was raised. The society's president, Dr. Henry K. Steele, asked his fellow members:

> How can we reject them? . . . They have studied the same textbooks that we have; have been educated at the feet of the same great teachers with us; their aims and aspirations are as ours. There are female physicians in our own land whose education, acquirements and judgement are acknowledged with the greatest respect by some of the best of our fraternity.[56]

This was followed by a motion to invite women physicians to attend the society's meetings. After intensive discussion, "pro and con," the motion was tabled. A committee was then appointed to report on the "propriety of admitting female practitioners, graduates of orthodox medical colleges, to fellowship in consultation and membership in the society." The committee decided that it was too big an issue for it to decide and that the matter should be put to the membership for a vote. There is no indication of such a vote having been taken, and the issue remained unresolved for a decade. In the meantime, in 1881, Denver's medical society admitted Drs. Bates, Root, and other women to membership.[57] Finally, and without fanfare, in 1888, the State Medical Society accepted Dr. Rilla G. Hay as a member. Dr. Hay had impeccable credentials, having graduated from the University of Iowa (1873), been licensed to practice in Colorado (1885), and having established herself as a reputable practitioner in Pueblo.[58] She was soon followed by other women members, and as one prominent woman physician put it, the members of the State Medical Society "more than atoned for their early coolness toward women by electing them to office."[59]

Having been accepted into the men's medical "club," some of Denver's women physicians apparently now felt the need for a women's medical society. In 1895 they founded the Denver Clinical Society, the nation's sixth women's medical society.[60] In 1896 the society's outgoing president, Dr. Lawney, noted that " . . . years ago, a woman practicing medicine in Denver was in a very lonesome business."[61] Often, she recalled, she dared not accept a difficult case, because, unlike a man, when she failed to cure a patient, it was likely to be blamed on the fact that she was a woman. In such cases, it had been advisable to transfer the case to a male physician. Dr. Lawney added:

> You do not need to be told why a woman is less able than a man to bear this opprobrium. We have not the prestige of custom, and we have not here a school or hospital where the work of men and women under obviously like conditions is open to the public for comparison . . . A good deal of 'hedging' is still the 'better part of valor,' but a woman may now take more chances with fewer risks than she could when I began.[61]

In 1901 Dr. Minnie C. T. Love cited the advances that had been made by Colorado's women physicians. She mentioned staff appointments at the Arapahoe County (Denver General) Hospital, the State Hospital for the Insane at Pueblo, and various dispensaries, missions, and "homes" for unwed mothers.[62] With the exception of National Jewish Hospital and a brief appointment for Dr. Lawney in obstetrics at St. Luke's Hospital, however, she made no mention of hospital appointments at any other

private hospitals. Dr. Love did note that a woman had been appointed as county physician in Pueblo and that Denver's commissioner of health had appointed women as medical inspectors for the city. Dr. Love herself had become the first woman in Colorado to be appointed "a state officer" when she was named to the State Board of Charities and Corrections, and others had since been named to various institutional and school boards.

By 1901, 106 women had been licensed to practice medicine in Colorado. Women were being admitted to the medical schools and the medical societies and were gradually making some inroads into hospitals and governmental institutions and agencies. Occasionally, some men physicians expressed resentment against their women colleagues. In 1900 the editor of the *Colorado Medical Journal* voiced his concern that Colorado's women physicians were insufficiently active in the medical societies and uninterested in academic activities.[63] He commented that few medical papers were written by women. A response, signed "M," was not long in coming.[64] Since it would be unfair to assume that the rest of the profession shared the editor's ignorance, wrote "M," "the women physicians of the Rocky Mountain region will not trouble themselves to state in print what 'they are doing in and for their profession'." As for writing papers,

> The editor must have a strangely perverted view of the value of contributions to the advancement of the general medical profession if he measures them only by papers written . . . Is it not really a matter of congratulation that the women physicians, at least, have not yet wholly succumbed to the *cacoethes scribendi*, now almost epidemic?[64]

In the first two decades since licensure (1881 - 1901), the 106 women who had been licensed in Colorado had published a total of seventeen papers.[65] In the subsequent two decades, Colorado's women physicians published about fifty papers.

Other complaints occasionally surfaced. A special concern of some men physicians was a perceived incompatibility between medical practice and wifely and motherly duties. The *Denver Medical Times* reprinted an article which stated that "medical women" should not marry.[66] The article proposed that, if a woman physician did marry, she should do so only if she would "consent to a childless union, or perhaps if she would devote herself to some narrow specialty that makes only short and specific demands on her time." Some men physicians continued to believe that women physicians should limit their practices to women and children. In a "turn-about is fair play" comment, Dr. Love predicted that "the two departments of the medical profession which the future will see closed to the male practitioner are those of obstetrics and gynecology."[67]

In the early 1870s Boulder's Dr. Mary Solander was convicted of manslaughter in an illegal abortion-related maternal death. As a result, she became the first woman to be sentenced to the state penitentiary at Canon City.[68] A number of Boulder's citizens felt that she was innocent and the victim of prejudice. Although she was ultimately pardoned by the governor, her career was ruined and she left the state. Over the years, there appears to have been an impression that many, if not most, abortionists were women. Abortion was considered to be an unethical practice by the medical profession and women physicians were sensitive to this charge. When one of her male colleagues commented, in public discussion at a state society meeting, on the inordinate interest of his female medical students in the methods of abortion, Dr. Love sarcastically responded:

> I am sorry the doctor's experience has all been with women students. I think some of us [women physicians] do try to prevent abortions.[69]

Such male-female confrontations occasionally appear in the otherwise bland discussions of papers presented at medical society meetings. When Dr. Mary E. Bates presented a paper on the medical aspects of women's clothing and blamed the use of corsets and other "irrational" dress on the predominantly male medical profession, she engendered heated protests from some of the men in the audience. One doctor felt that her "commentary on the male part of the profession is uncalled for," adding he had always hated the term "emancipated women" because

> women have always been emancipated. Man has been her friend, and no country can boast of having a greater friend to woman, than can America.[70]

Another physician, a visitor from Kansas, probably thought he was calming the waters when he remarked:

> I admire the women of Denver . . . When visiting the city some years ago, I called the attention of my son to their well developed waists and clear complexion. They have much better waists than the women of the great Mississippi Valley and farther East . . . Does your altitude compel a larger use of lung tissue?[70]

Dr. Bates had fought for women's, children's and animal's rights and against saloons and gambling. She had endured the challenges of being the first woman intern at Chicago's Cook County Hospital and had taken on Denver's redoubtable Judge Benjamin Lindsey over the issue of "companionate marriage." Ignoring the Kansan's naivete, and with the dignity to be expected of a no-nonsense woman bachelor who would later sit on the boards of large corporations, she responded quietly:

> I must confess that I was not surprised by the discussion . . . I rather expected something of the kind. I rather expected that there would be somebody, even a professional somebody, who was not capable of understanding my remarks. I am very glad to know that there are but a few.[70]

And so it went. The attitude of men physicians towards their women colleagues varied over a wide spectrum—ranging from indifferent to benevolent to patronizing to hostile.

In addition to the women physicians already discussed, a number of others should be mentioned. In Colorado's mountains, there was Dr. Susan Anderson.[71] In her twenties, "Doc Susie" had set up practice in Cripple Creek in 1897.

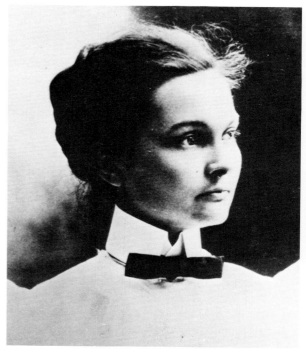

After ten years in that mining camp, she moved to a log cabin in the tiny community of Fraser. Here, along the "Moffat" railroad, she practiced for the next fifty years, caring for railroadmen, ranchers, and lumberjacks, and making calls on horseback, snowshoes, or in the cab of a locomotive. On the plains, in Weld County, there was Dr. Ella Mead, who, for many decades, initiated programs in public health, care of the handicap-

9.16 After ten years of practice in Cripple Creek, Dr. Susan Anderson moved to a log cabin near tiny Fraser on the Moffat railroad. Here for more than half a century, she cared for the area's trainmen, ranchers, and lumberjacks.

ped, mental health, birth control, the public schools, and so on.[72] In Denver, there was Dr. Sarah J. Fearing. From a wealthy New England family and a graduate of private schools, Dr. Fearing developed tuberculosis and came to Denver. Here she devoted "her every energy to medical work among the poor." After suffering a massive pulmonary hemorrhage at the age of thirty-six, Dr. Fearing died.[73] Drs. Lucy Passover in blood transfusion, Elizabeth Newcomer in radiotherapy, and Margaret Long in clinical pathology were local pioneers in their fields.[74] Dr. Emma Drake wrote lay medical guides (*What a Young Wife Should Know, Maternity without Suffering*), Dr. Lida B. Russell promoted a "milk diet" for tuberculosis, and Drs. Madeline Marquette and Josepha Williams ran a private sanitarium in Denver.[75] When the Spanish-American War broke out, Dr. Rose Kidd Beere, ineligible, as a woman, for an appointment as military surgeon, volunteered as a Red Cross nurse.[76] Accompanied by seven nurses, she sailed for the Philippines and was placed in charge of a military hospital in Manila. Dr. Mary H.B. Bates was responsible for Colorado's public school health law, a model of its kind in the early twentieth century.[77]

Dr. Minnie C. T. Love was, perhaps, the most remarkable of early Colorado's women physicians.[78] Dr. Love was born in Wisconsin in 1855 and received her M.D. in 1887 from Howard University, the only white student in her class. She and her husband came to Denver in 1893. After a long bout with tuberculosis, he died, leaving her with three young children. At about the same time, Dr. Love became involved in a variety of activities. She helped organize the State Industrial School for Girls, ran the Florence Crittenden Home (for unwed mothers), and was a major medical force behind the founding of Denver Children's Hospital. She was an

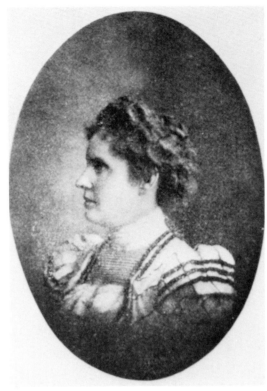

9.17 Dr. Minnie C.T. Love was perhaps the most remarkable of early Colorado's women physicians.

activist in women's, children's, and public health movements and served on Denver's Board of Education, the State Board of Health, and various other boards and agencies. In the 1920s she was elected to the state legislature. She was described as "a handsome woman, with a ringing voice and a gift of sound logic, who could speak any cause she espoused to success and at the same time never failed to recognize the value of being completely feminine."[79] Unfortunately, one of the causes she apparently "espoused" was the Ku Klux Klan, which supported her legislative campaigns in the 1920s, an ironic twist for a person of such major accomplishments, not to mention a graduate of Howard University. Dr. Love died in 1942, at the age of 86.

10 ORGANIZED MEDICINE

For the advancement of our profession, and our common advantage, and the cultivation of harmony and good feeling, a complete understanding is necessary between the members of the profession relating to fees, ethics, etc . . .

By-laws, Jefferson Medical Society, 1860
(Colorado's first medical society)[1]

IN JUNE 1860, COLORADO'S handful of physicians organized the Jefferson Medical Society. The purpose of the society was to advance the profession and to establish some uniformity with regard to medical ethics, fees, and other aspects of medical practice. With the coming of the Civil War, according to Dr. Bancroft, many of the members enlisted, and "the embryo society, left to itself, perished from inanition."[2] In 1864 the Denver Medical Association was formed, but its existence was even briefer.[3] Bancroft recalled that another society was established in 1868. Like the others, it was subject to "internal dissensions" and lacked "cohesiveness and durability," and virtually nothing is known about it.[4]

Denver Medical Society

Finally, in April 1871, eleven physicians, most of Denver's medical profession, met in Dr. W. F. McClelland's office to organize what would become Denver's, and ultimately, Colorado's, permanent medical societies.[5] These physicians included some remarkable men: Frederick Bancroft, Arnold Stedman, Richard Buckingham, Henry K. Steele, John Elsner, and Eugene Gehrung. During the next two weeks, the newly formed Denver Medical Association met several more times and adopted a constitution, by-laws, and a list of medical fees. It also passed resolu-

tions to improve Denver's sanitary condition and to promote harmony with the town's pharmacists. Dr. Buckingham was elected the society's first president. The new president described the association as

an organization of intelligent and educated physicians who meet together semi-monthly for friendly and social intercourse, to interchange views, and to discuss the various subjects connected with the profession, thereby cultivating pleasant and friendly relations and enlightening each other with their mutual observations and experience, upholding the honor of the profession, and showing to the community that . . . we are determined to be indefatigable in the pursuit of that knowledge which will enable us to render the assistance they so much need in their hours of sickness and distress.[6]

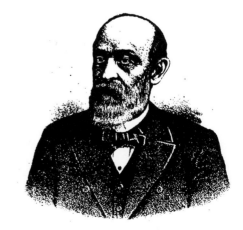

10.1 In 1871 Dr. Richard Buckingham became the first president of Denver's newly organized medical society.

Gradually, however, the character of the association changed, and the emphasis shifted almost entirely to politics. A later president described it as an organization which could

> wield a power over the morals and general welfare of the city, county or state and who can, when necessary, for self or public protection, enter the arena of politics to assist the right and defeat the wrong . . .[7]

Indeed, the activities of the Denver Medical Association had became so political as to alienate some of its members. New applicants had to wait a year for membership, "with the object of ascertaining and influencing [their] professional politics . . . The methods of wire-pulling politicians were resorted to in choosing officers."[7] Meetings had become "unattractive and tedious . . ." and devoted to "medical politics and ethical wrangling" rather than topics of scientific and clinical interest.

In 1883 a splinter group formed the Araphahoe County Medical Society, named for the county in which Denver was located. Its goal was to restore to society meetings science and medicine: the "encouragement . . . of that department of physical sciences which has for its objects the preservation of human health, the restoration from disease or injury, and the prolongation of life."[7] The new society's meetings emphasized the presentation of papers, clinical cases, and pathologic specimens. The formation of a medical library was encouraged by the purchase of " a suitable book-case."

Not surprisingly, the old and the new societies and their members were soon at odds, but within two years, the president of the new society was pleased to report that "the feeling of antagonism is rapidly dying out."[8] In 1889 the societies merged to form the Denver Medical Association and Arapahoe County Medical Society, and in 1892, the name was shortened to the Denver and Arapahoe Medical Society.[9]

As with any long-standing organization, Denver's medical society alternated between periods of activity and interest and periods of inactivity and apathy. The latter appears to have been the situation in 1896:

> This society seems to have a natural tendency to attacks of debility. In spite of the most heroic tonic treatment by its officers, its revival of spirits and strength has been only for a short period of time, after which its defects again manifest themselves and there seems a likelihood of complete prostration . . . Our membership numbers nearly 150, it should be 250, and our average attendance is less than 30.[10]

· · THE · ·

Denver & Arapahoe Medical Society.

A REGULAR MEETING WILL BE HELD AT THE

Brown Palace Hotel,

Tuesday Evening, January, 26, 1897.

PROGRAMME:

1. Surgical Shock at High Altitude. By Dr. H. G. Wetherill.
   Discussion by Drs. Rogers, Powers, Freeman, Parkhill, Eskridge, Sewall and Hall.
2. Report of Cases. By Dr. W. C. Bane.
3. The advisability of inviting the American Medical Association to Denver in 1898 will be considered by the Society. In view of the importance of this question, it is desirable that there shall be a full attendance.

The Board of Directors have provided for the delivery of messages telephoned to No. 1280 for physicians in attendance upon these meetings.

10.2 Denver's medical society has undergone a series of name changes over the years.

One difficulty was finding a meeting place. The society was grateful to the Brown Palace Hotel for "extending to us gratuitously the use of the club room . . .," but

> still we are pushed about from pillar to post on the top of the hotel, in rooms that are very poorly ventilated and where we are constantly disturbed by the great noise always existing in places of this character . . . [It] is the reason for the absence of a great many of our members from the meetings.[11]

By 1912, the renamed Medical Society of the City and County of Denver was thriving, having increased its membership in one year by twenty-seven percent.[12] It maintained a large medical library, played an active role in public health and other medical legislation, and provided a forum for the presentation of "the gratifying . . . amount of research and practical [medical] work being done in Denver." The society invited its members to the Friday night meetings of the Post-Graduate Club, where they might "refresh their previous studies," and to use the newly acquired "balopticon" to display their interesting medical specimens. Its president envisioned even greater things for the society—that it "should be a big and all-powerful body of medical men, liberal in its views and having on its roll every legitimate practitioner in this city."[12]

Colorado Medical Society

In 1871, soon after its formation, the members of the Denver Medical Association called for a convention to form a territorial medical society. In September physicians from various parts of Colorado gathered in the district courtroom

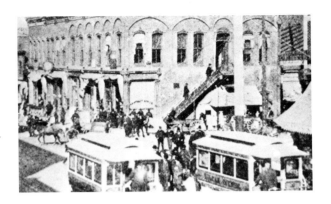

10.3 In the fall of 1871, a handful of Colorado's physicians met in Denver's district courtroom, above a store on the corner of 15th and Lawrence Streets, to organize the territorial medical society. Afterwards, they walked over to Barney Ford's restaurant for "a bountiful repast."

above a store on the corner of 15th and Lawrence streets in Denver. Dr. G. S. M. McMurtrie of Central City was chosen President pro tem. Dr. Buckingham, as president of the association, delivered the major address. He began:

> Gentlemen of the Medical Profession: You have been called together today from all parts of our Territory . . . to deliberate upon the propriety of establishing a Territorial Medical Society . . .[13]

Buckingham reviewed the accomplishments of the Denver Medical Association, the role of the physician in society, and the growth of Colorado and its medical community. Finally, he offered the hope that

> the time [would] soon come when the Territorial Medical Association of Colorado will rest upon as firm a basis as the grand old mountains before us, that lift their snow capped summits to the clouds.[13]

After lunch, the group considered the proposed constitution and by-laws. The goals of the society were to be

> the improvement of its members in scientific and professional knowledge; the association of the profession for purposes of mutual recognition and fellowship; the promotion of the character, interests, and honor of the fraternity by maintaining union and harmony and by aiming to elevate the standard of medical education.[13]

It was decided that "any regular graduate of Medicine and Surgery may become a member of this Society" as long as they adhered to the Code of Ethics of the American Medical Association and that the initiation fee would be five dollars.[14] In the evening, the group reconvened and voted to adopt the fee schedule of the Denver Medical Association, "subject to such changes in different localities as the local societies may deem proper." They then concluded their business and congratulated themselves on having created the Colorado Medical Society. Apparently, during the day, additional physicians had joined the group and, finally, twenty-six charter members signed the completed document. In

addition to fourteen physicians from Denver, there were representatives from Central City, Black Hawk, Georgetown, Idaho Springs, Laporte, Golden, and Pueblo.

The long day's business concluded, the doctors walked over to Barney Ford's restaurant on Larimer Street, where they partook of "a bountiful repast [which] did credit to the well-known skill of the caterer." Supper was followed by a series of toasts . . . to the A.M.A., the Colorado Medical Society, "legitimate" medicine, the press . . . and to "The Ladies." The press, who had apparently been invited to share in the festivities, reported that "other remarks were made, some good stories told, and, at a late hour, the guests separated."[15] It is tempting to imagine the doctors finally leaving Ford's establishment in the wee hours, staggering down Larimer Street, perhaps singing a bawdy song or two . . .

A year later, the Society held its second annual meeting in Denver's First Presbyterian church.[16] Several more names had been added to the rolls, but only fourteen members showed up, and they must have looked lost in the commodious church. Despite the year's expenses, $51.25, the treasury held a healthy surplus of more than $40. The members approved the finance committee's recommendation of one dollar in annual dues. One of the charter members was expelled from the society, "he being considered unworthy of membership." Dr. W. F. McClelland was elected president, and about one-third of the membership was appointed to one office or another. Finally, the evening was concluded by the reading of a paper by Dr. M. J. Davis of Golden. The paper, on "persistent catarrh and its treatment," called forth a "spirited and highly instructive discussion." The next day, the meeting was devoted to "scientific" sessions, including a paper by Denver's Dr. Elsner on the materia medica of Colorado, another by Georgetown's Dr. Pollok on "Diseases Peculiar to High Altitudes," and the demonstration of several pathological specimens by Central City's Dr. S. B. Davis. Dr. Steele's young son, Master Robert, was thanked "for his services and attention to the comfort of the members," for which he was rewarded by "a substantial testimonial."

By 1874 the third year of its existence, the society was having financial problems.[17] The chairman of the finance committee reported that "the only report I have to make is on the emptiness of the treasury—with the exception of 75 cents." The problem was corrected at the next year's meeting, by raising the annual dues by three hundred percent, to four dollars.[18] In his presidential address, Dr. McMurtrie cited the two objectives of a medical society—first, a united body which would provide

> strength and self protection for the members of a profession peculiarly open to the malicious attacks of the charlatan and . . . to the misapprehension and sneers of a considerable class of our fellow men.[18]

and second,

> the encouragement and advancement of science; not only for its own sake, but for a purely humanitarian purpose . . . We must encourage scientific research.[18]

Dr. McMurtrie's call for unity was not met with unanimous support. Resisting the dominance of his colleagues in Denver and the northern part of the territory, Trinidad's Dr. Beshoar and a handful of other physicians from southern Colorado joined with some of their fellows in northern New Mexico to form the Rocky Mountain Medical Association.[19] The association held its first meeting in 1874, drew up by-laws and a fee schedule, and sent its president, Beshoar, to Chicago carrying a caged eagle as a gift to the A.M.A.'s president.[20] The association itself, however, was not united, allegedly excluding foreign-born physicians from membership.[21] Whether or not this was true, the Menger brothers, who were Jewish, and Dr. Jules Le Carpentier, who was French, formed the rival Trinidad Medical Society. Within a few years, the Rocky Mountain Medical Association had dissolved, its membership absorbed into the state society.[22]

By the fifth meeting, the society had demonstrated its viability; the membership was up to fifty-six and the treasury was able to report a surplus of $64.75.[23] A number of learned papers were presented, including one on blood letting. Dr. William Williams presented "a specimen of fracture extending into the knee joint necessitating amputation," a new obstetric forceps was demonstrated, and a patient with congenital cataract was presented, the last "showing, unmistakably, the benefit of scientific treatment . . . " A motion to use the society's surplus funds to purchase a bookcase was rejected. A motion to accept the Denver Ale Brewing Company's invitation to visit their establishment was approved.

Colorado achieved statehood in 1876, and the sixth meeting saw the Territorial Society renamed the State Medical Society.[24] Membership for women physicians was considered and tabled at the seventh meeting. The eighth meeting was the first to be held outside of Denver; it, and the subsequent three meetings were held in Georgetown, Colorado Springs, Leadville, and Pueblo. By the 1880s, the annual proceedings had become sufficiently complex to warrant the adoption of Robert's Rules of Order, and a half-day was designated for the meeting of separate "sections [to] permit a greater dispatch of business."[25] By now, some of the society's early pioneers had become senior citizens, and at the sixteenth annual session, in 1886, the members congratulated Dr. Buckingham, the society's first president, on his fiftieth year of practice. In addition, "as a mark of respect, a carriage was ordered to be placed at his disposal."[26] The society had not become too big for such personal touches, or for that matter, to refuse the kind offer, by Denver's Mr. Scholtz (of Scholtz's Drug Store), of a box of cigars for the "immediate use" of the members.

By 1885 there were murmurings about the quality of the society's scientific sessions. At the last meeting, the *Denver Medical Times* complained, "there were numerous papers read, the major portion of which were mere re-hashes of the work of men that are foreign to Colorado." The essence of a society meeting, the *Times* declared,

ADDRESS

DELIVERED BY

Dr. F. J. Bancroft,

PRESIDENT OF THE COLORADO STATE
MEDICAL SOCIETY,

AT ITS

ELEVENTH ANNUAL CONVENTION,

Leadville, September 13, 1881.

DENVER, COLORADO:
C. J. KELLY, BOOK AND JOB PRINTER, 433 LARIMER ST.,
1881.

10.4 The president's address has been the highlight of the Colorado Medical Society's annual meetings.

should be original investigation, work, discussion . . . and not banquets and the election of officers . . . Why is it that Colorado physicians cannot of themselves contribute to the world's literature the results of personal experience and investigation? We are certain that every member of our Society could, if they would.[27]

The problem appears to have been a chronic one, and ten years later, a society spokesman was telling the members:

We not only want you to be present at the meeting, but we want the products of your labor at the bedsides . . . whether in the mountains or on the plains, in the country or in the city, in hospitals or private homes. Give us the benefit of your researches with the microscope and culture tubes.[28]

By the turn of the century, the quantity, if not necessarily the quality, of papers presented at the annual meeting was such that the published transactions were several hundred pages in length. Guest speakers were also invited to present papers. Dr. W. T. Councilman, the distinguished professor of pathology at Harvard, was the honored guest at one meeting.[29] At the same time, what was felt to be a growing emphasis on esoteric topics was decried by a "country doctor" from Montrose who complained about the "absence of papers treating of the common diseases."[30] Another disgruntled member complained about society politics and alleged "cliques, gang rule, and star chamber proceedings."[31]

The annual gathering of Colorado's physicians was not all science, business, politics, and "star chamber proceedings," however, and many an otherwise staid and serious physician used the yearly meeting as an opportunity to unwind from the daily tensions of medical practice. Dr. J. N. Hall recalled:

After a good dinner . . . and after a cocktail and two or three varieties of wine, we were ready to listen to toasts proposed by Dr. E. C. Rivers, the perpetual toastmaster of that day. By eleven o'clock, he would be standing on the table with a wreath of flowers on his head and a champagne glass in his hand . . . No one wanted to go home.[32]

Hall recalled that another toastmaster, "one of the most scientific men of our profession . . . drank a full glass of champagne at every proposed toast. About midnight, he fell asleep and gradually . . . slid under the table." None of the others at the table noticed and the festivities continued. The annual banquet of 1886 was reported in rapturous terms:

From the setting of the table at the Windsor Hotel, to the last speech and the last glass of wine, every

part of the entertainment . . . was like a poem. Ministers, judges, railroad men, pharmacists, and doctors, all in harmony. There was evidence on every hand of Falstaff's philosophy.[32]

The society's meetings were well received by the host communities. On welcoming the doctors to Pueblo in 1902, the mayor awarded them the key to the city and an "Open Sesame to everything in Pueblo, for there is nothing too good for our doctors."[33] To add to the welcome, a poem was read. Entitled, "To the Medicine Men," it began:

All hail to the doctors that 'bide in the West.
In fair Colorado, of all states the best,
They come from the canons, the mountains and plains,
To discuss the new methods of subduing pains.[33]

Sometimes the festivities dominated the proceedings. At the 1910 meeting in Colorado Springs,[34] in addition to the banquet, dinners, and luncheons, and the president's reception in the grand ballroom of the elegant Antlers Hotel (where "the dancers thronged the floor and prolonged the festivities until the wee sma' hours"), the doctors "betook themselves to a grand old Barbecue Jungle Party". Not only was there a barbecue, but the party also included a "fake bulldog and badger fight," a boxing match, a "clever exhibition of buck-and-wing dancing," a tightrope walker, bagpipes, and "a pillow fight." The last event was not described in detail, but it was noted that Dr. Gerald Webb won the prize. The doctors' wives were also kept busy with railroad excursions, motorcar tours, a "bridge tea" at the Golf Club, a banquet at the El Paso Club, and while their husbands were at the Jungle Barbecue, a vaudeville show. Colorado Springs has always been a gracious host to its guests!

The State Medical Society's activities were not limited to its annual meetings. Benefiting from a long list of distinguished presidents and other officers, the society played a major role in the political, economic, and ethical aspects of medical practice in Colorado. In time, however, its involvement in the "scientific" aspects of medicine contracted, and the the medical school's faculty, no longer identified with the society's leadership, took over this role.

The Denver Meeting of the A.M.A.

For a few days in 1898, Colorado was the focal point of American medicine. During that brief time the American Medical Association held its annual meeting in Denver, and 1,500 physicians converged on the Queen City. The Colorado Medical Society had campaigned actively for the honor of hosting the association and sent Dr. L. E. Lemen, in 1897, to lobby the delegates at the A.M.A. meeting in Philadelphia.[35] Lemen thought he had garnered sufficient votes only to find, when the issue came to the floor, that many of his supporters had been pursuaded to switch to Columbus, Ohio. Rather than plead his case, Lemen, a former mining camp doctor of imposing proportions, rose and recited an anecdote for the assembly. The story was about a merchant in Georgetown who had been doublecrossed by the town's bankers. He ended with the merchant's words to the bankers: "Individually, you are some of the finest men I ever knew [but] collectively, you are a set of ——s." At that point, Lemen sat down. After some nervous silence, a motion was made to hold the next meeting in Denver. It was unanimously approved.

THE AMERICAN MEDICAL ASSOCIATION

DENVER MEETING, JUNE 7-10, 1898

GENERAL SESSIONS: 10 A. M.
                    Tuesday, Wednesday, Thursday.

BROADWAY THEATRE

PLEASE SHOW THIS TICKET AT THE DOOR

After "a year of tedious detail work and much anxiety," the the delegates arrived in Denver.[36] The Brown Palace Hotel served as the meeting's headquarters. Some 500 papers were presented at the Broadway Theater and other halls, including Dr. J. B. Murphy's classic on the induction of collapsed lung to treat pulmonary tuberculosis. Other papers were presented by such national medical luminaries as Mayo, Kelly, Billings, and Solis-Cohen.[37] The exhibition hall was filled with displays of the latest in medical technology, books and journals, instruments, and pharmaceuticals. The most popular exhibit was a medical-electrical device which provided a fifteen inch spark and "marvelous . . . X-ray effects."[38]

The homes of Denver's social elite were opened to the visitors, and the Hills, Campions, and Kountzes hosted receptions. A railroad excursion was made over the spectacular Georgetown loop (where the "Kodak fiend was kept busy") to Idaho Springs. The town provided a brass band and "pretty maidens" to wait

on luncheon tables in a huge tent erected near the train station. Other trains were provided by the Colorado Midland and the Denver and Rio Grande railroads to transport 1,500 doctors and their guests to Colorado Springs, Pike's Peak, and a grand ball at Manitou.

When the last of the visitors had finally departed, Colorado's doctors breathed a sigh of relief. The meeting had been a great success, and the nation's doctors returned to their homes proclaiming the medical, economic, climatic, and scenic advantages of the state. Indeed, the visitors had been impressed, and the *Colorado Medical Journal* took pleasure in publishing their rave reviews. To the *Philadelphia Medical Journal*, for example, the Denver meeting had demonstrated that " 'the Wild West' had lost whatever rawness and crudity it may have illustrated [but] a few years ago."[39] Such praise, although somewhat condescending in its tone, was music to the ears of Colorado's doctors. To them, it was a stamp of approval, a sign of acceptance by the eastern establishment, and worth all of the enormous work it must have taken to host the A.M.A. meeting of 1898.

County Medical Societies

In the same way that the state societies formed the units of the American Medical Association, the county societies were the backbone of the state medical societies. In Colorado, it was a county society, the Denver Medical Association, that had preceded and stimulated the formation of the state society. By 1881 medical societies had been organized in Boulder, El Paso, Fremont, Lake, Pueblo, and Las Animas counties.[40] Each of these counties had at least one large town that served as a focus for medical meetings. In the rest of the state, however, small populations and large distances worked against any formal organization of physicians. Even in 1907, the state society's journal reported that

the Clear Creek Medical Association, like so many other county societies, is greatly hampered by having their members living far apart. The district includes . . . Georgetown, Idaho Springs, Central City, Black Hawk, besides outlying villages and [mining] camps, and as a consequence it is impossible to get all the members to attend a meeting.[41]

At other times, disagreements among physicians prevented the formation of a county society. When Chaffee County attempted to organize a society, the outcome was compared to what

is observed when some chemicals are united—the mixture attempted, gave rise to much warmth . . .

10.5 In 1898 the A.M.A.'s meeting put Denver on the national medical map.

and at length an explosion which smashed the embryo society into smithereens.[42]

In La Plata County, the state society's councilor, Dr. Tracy Melvin

> found the disorganization at Durango to be complete and that there was no hope of getting them together . . . It is unfortunate that among the eleven physicians in Durango one cannot be found who is willing to devote some time to the promotion of harmony in the medical ranks.[43]

One society physician listed the reasons why some of his colleagues remained "unaffiliated" with their county society: "conceit, carelessness, indifference and ignorance."[44] The state society's secretary, Dr. Melville Black, urged such "medical gentlemen to remember that the community at large has no more respect for them than they have for themselves . . . They must bury their jealousies and meet one another."[45] County societies played an essential role, he felt, and he suggested that, even "if it is not possible to arrange a medical program, then let some member give a dinner. Two or three such dinners a year, for small societies, at which an informal presentation of cases and exchange of ideas is the order of the evening, will serve to cause [medical] rivals to have more respect for each other".

Despite the bickering, most county society meetings were relaxed and convivial. For example:

> The Lake County Medical Association held its annual meeting on the 4th of January. After the discussion of numerous clinical cases the society adjourned at 2 A.M., and it was the general opinion . . . that the meeting was almost, if not quite, as pleasant as playing checkers and gossiping at Si Perkins' corner grocery, from which we assume that our meetings will be more numerous the coming year.[46]

Sometimes professors from Denver were invited to address a county society. In 1905 Drs. J. N. Hall and Leonard Freeman were invited to Cripple Creek.[47] The mining camp's physicians were delighted that "both addresses were very practical and especially adapted for such a company of general practitioners as was present." The subsequent banquet was accompanied by much banter between the two visiting professors. Dr. Freeman's "Christian disposition," it was noted, "was severely taxed in trying to restrain Dr. Hall," who, in turn, "told of some wonderful experiences" he had had in Cripple Creek, experiences which, if repeated to his Denver friends, "will dumbfound the wise."

The state and county medical societies did not provide sufficient professsional fellowship for some physicians, especially in Denver. In 1892 Drs. Robert Levy and Carey Fleming founded the Denver Clinical and Pathological Society.[48] This was a small group of bright young doctors who gathered every month for an evening of social conviviality and the presentation of "obscure, interesting and instructive cases . . . patients, and new instruments." Initially limited to forty members and meeting in such pleasant surroundings as the Brown Palace and the Denver County Club, over the years the society's membership came to include many of Denver's most prestigious medical names—a professional and often socially elite roster. The Denver Clinical and Pathological Society served as a model for several other medical clubs , including the Clinical Club of Colorado Springs and The Colorado Clinical Club. In 1903 the need for still another type of medical society was met in the form of the Denver Academy of Medicine.[49] Its prototype was the New York Academy of Medicine, an organization devoted to the growing view that medicine should be founded on scientific investigations and principles. With Denver's prominent clinician-scientist, Henry Sewall, as its president, in two years the academy had nearly one hundred "Resident Fellows."[50]

Licensure and the Board of Medical Examiners

One of organized medicine's major goals was to restrict the practice of medicine to those it felt were qualified to practice, i.e. bona fide M.D.s. There had been no regulation of medical practice in colonial America, and virtually anyone had the right to "doctor" his fellows. After the Revolution, medical societies came into being, and the states provided them with the authority to examine and certify medical practitioners. In essence, membership in the state medical society was the equivalent of a medical license. The societies, however, were ineffective in enforcing their own rules and standards, and in the early part of the nineteenth century, the states took over. The states, however, proved equally ineffective, and in mid-nineteenth century America, hordes of poorly educated "physicians," with or without the official imprimatur of a license, were practicing medicine. After the Civil War, with the enormous increase in medical schools, many of them "diploma mills," even an M.D. was not proof of an adequate medical education. By the 1870s, many physicians were agitating for the meaningful regulation of their profession. In 1875 the president of the Colorado Medical Society, Dr. H. K. Steele, pointed out that

> The regular profession have been striving for years to have the people allow their legislators to enact laws requiring those who offer to practice medicine to be educated in their profession.[51]

In 1871 neighboring Wyoming enacted legislation regulating medical practice. Wyoming was soon followed, in the West, by Montana, Arizona, and Nevada.[52] Finally, in 1881, Colorado joined the now rapidly growing list of states with regulatory statutes. That year, the legislature established the State Board of Medical Examiners and charged it with the responsibility of evaluating candidates for medical licensure in Colorado. The board, appointed by the governor, was composed of ten members representing the three "schools" of medicine—six "regulars", three members of the homeopathic sect of physicians, and one member of the eclectic sect (Chapter 21).[53] Candidates with a diploma from a "well accredited medical college" were automatically granted a license.

Without an approved degree, the candidate was required to pass an examination. In 1883 Dr. Jesse Hawes reviewed the board's examination questions and cited examples of answers provided by some of the examinees.[54] He did this, he said, in order to demonstrate the "class who, previous to the [new licensure] law, were in practice in Colorado . . . but who are now prohibited from practicing . . . The amount of injury that might be wrought by these men . . . is left to your computation . . . In some answers the original spelling is preserved in its native rugged strength." He also provided a few editorial comments. Some examples:

> Question: "Name the organs found in the thoracic cavity." Answer: "Liver, hart, loungs, stomack, splen and pancreas." Comment: "Note the spelling. Liver, stomach and pancreas are not found in the thoracic cavity."

> Question: "What is the surgical treatment of nose bleed?" Answer: "Ligate an artery in the neck; the name I have forgotten." Comment: "Ligating any artery in the neck would do no good, but harm."

> Question: "Treatment of post-partum hemorrhage." Answer: "Use the tampon." Comment: "Almost certain death."[54]

The great majority of licenses were issued without any examination. Licensee No. 1 was Dr. C. M. Parker of Denver, and during the next seven years, more than one thousand additional licenses were issued.[55] During the next two decades, many states tightened their requirements for medical practice, but in Colorado, the medical law of 1881 (with minor modifications in 1885, including the recognition of another sect, the "electro-paths"), remained unchanged.

In 1891 the board's president, Dr. Hall, reviewed its past decade's activities.[56] In one year, nearly 95% of the 226 candidates for licensure had been approved by the board, the great majority on the basis of diplomas received from recognized medical schools. In addition, 4% had been licensed after passing the written examination. The board felt that the state's stringent requirements discouraged "the most notorious candidates" from even applying—hence the low rejection rate.

The board often found itself in the middle of conflicting interests and opinions. There was continuous pressure from all sorts of quacks, healers, and sects, backed by lawyers and a few legislators supposedly concerned with personal freedom and alleged medical monopolies, to liberalize the licensure law. On the other hand, many "regular" physicians wanted to tighten the law to exclude such unorthodox M.D.s as homeopaths, eclectics and electropaths. Some felt that the board's main goal should be to control the number of physicians in the state. Many physicians, already licensed, simply didn't care and were apathetic to the board's work. Dr. Hall complained that the board "has never received the support which should have been accorded it from the state society."[56] The board had to walk a fine line between opposing groups. In general, it favored reformist attempts by the American Medical Association and the American Association of Medical Colleges to improve licensure criteria and standards.

Some of the board's harshest criticism came, not from the quacks it tried to exclude from practice, but from "regular" physicians. In 1895 in line with the recommendations of the American Association of Medical Colleges, it declared that it would accept diplomas only from four-year medical schools. This was too much for the *Denver Medical Times*, which accused the board of "usurping authority which they neither legally nor equitably possess."[57] The *Times'* editor used the opportunity to state his overall opinion of state medical boards and their members:

> In the medical profession . . . we have cranky, fanatical, misanthropic, disgruntled and "disjointed" individuals; their chief pleasure in life

seems to consist in doing the disagreeable. When placed in a position of power . . . they invariably go to the extreme . . . It is unfortunate that we have such men connected with medical examining boards.[57]

During the 1890s there was increasing pressure by Colorado's physicians to tighten licensure requirements. In 1899 after enormous effort, a new medical bill was passed by the legislature and promptly vetoed by Governor Charles Thomas. Four years later, a second bill was passed by the legislature, only to be vetoed by another governor, James H. Peabody. The doctors were furious and the governors were denounced in no uncertain terms: "gubernatorial gabbler . . . peurile . . . disqualified for any position of honor and trust . . . ," and so on (Chapter 11). The pressures for medical reform were unrelenting, however, and finally in 1905, a new medical law was enacted. The bill was a compromise ("spineless, tendonless, and nerveless," said the press), which left it up to the board to decide whether or not an examination was to be required of each applicant.[58] The new law defined the practice of medicine and the use of the terms "M.D, surgeon, and doctor," and specifically prohibited certain practices which the profession had regarded as quackery. It did not, however, prohibit medical activities based on religious tenets or church activities, so long as those practices did not involve the use of drugs.[59]

The Colorado Medical Society was generally pleased, its journal noting that, "while the law is not exactly as an expert would write it, nevertheless, when one thinks of the numerous influences which we were compelled to consider, the people and the profession of Colorado should rejoice in such a superior law."[60] Some of the society's rank-and-file, however, were less pleased with the law—and with the board. Greeley's Dr. W. F. Church complained that more physicians had been granted licenses in Colorado during the first six months of its enactment than had been granted in an entire year in Minnesota.[61] This, despite the fact that Minnesota had three times as many people as Colorado and a much lower physician-to-population ratio. Dr. Church proposed that "nine out of ten medical men [in Colorado] . . . do not care to have their state called 'the dumping ground for the refuse of other states.' " There were already too many physicians in Colorado, said Dr. Church, and, unless the board insisted upon a written examination for licensure, the state would be swamped by medical immigrants. He pointed out that

the physician in New Jersey afflicted with weak lungs can come to Colorado and have his license endorsed . . . [without having to pass a written examination], while the doctor in Colorado can go to New Jersey . . . and spend the rest of his days waiting for [their] board to endorse a license.[61]

The Weld County Medical Society felt so strongly about the issue that they passed a resolution urging Colorado's board to require a written examination of all candidates for licensure.[62] The board's Dr. S.D. Van Meter responded that

however acute and chronic may be the congestion of the physician body [in Colorado], our duty is to license all persons qualified—not to restrict the number of persons entering the profession . . . Because other states are prostituting their medical law, and making a closed corporation of the practice of medicine within their borders, is not reason to follow in their footsteps.[63]

Finally, although the board certainly did not want to deny their Weld county colleagues the right to criticize their actions or to "in any way cast reflection upon the quality of the gray matter of the Greeley profession," the board stated that it was not about to see Colorado's medical law tainted by anything that smacked of "trade unionism." To Colorado's basically conservative medical community, the union label was anathema and the board's critics were quieted. Within a few years, however, even Dr. Van Meter, who had defended the 1905 law, acknowledged that "the present medical law has not put a stop to all the evils which it was intended to eliminate."[64] Ultimately, the board did require a written examination for applicants from other states, and organized medicine turned its attention towards osteopaths (who had been specifically excluded from the Medical Act of 1905), chiropracters, and other practitioners of "alternative" medicine (Chapter 21).

Journals

Fortunately for the student of Colorado's medical history, quite a few medical journals were published during Colorado's early years. They provide a wonderful source of information on the evolution of medical concepts, ideas, technologies, and therapies, and glimpses into the medical challenges and problems which faced early Colorado's physicians. Some of these journal were short-lived, while others have survived, despite successive name changes.

There were four major journals. The first, the *Transactions of the Colorado Territorial Medical Society*, began publication in 1872. "Territorial" was replaced by "State" in 1876, and in 1903 the journal's name was changed to *Colorado Medicine*.[65] In 1880 the *Rocky Mountain Medical Review* was founded. Two years later, it became the *Denver Medical Times* and for many years was published and edited by the colorful and literary Dr. Thomas Hawkins.[66] In 1896 a third statewide publication was launched, *The Colorado Medical Journal*.[67] In 1911 the Denver Medical Society's *Denver Medical Bulletin* appeared.

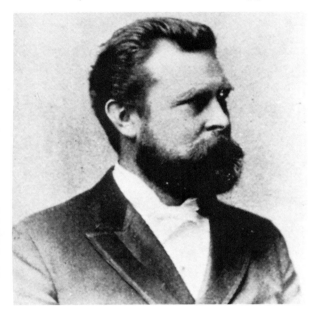

In addition to these four, there were two homeopathic journals, *Critique* (1897) and *Progress* (1903), and journals published by some of the tuberculosis sanitaria and the medical schools. Finally, there were two short-lived journals written by physicians for the lay public, Dr. Beshoar's *The Medical Educator* and Dr. P.D. Rothwell and colleagues' *The Health Monitor*.[68]

The editors of some of these journals included some of the best known and most outspoken of Colorado's physicians. At times, their editorial pages fairly burned with anger, invective, and sarcasm directed against certain politicians, journalists, and clergymen, and, less discriminately, against virtually all "irregulars," faith healers, charlatans, and quacks. Emotional and intense, such editorials were generally couched in colorful Victorian prose. For example, from *Colorado Medicine*:

> Our urbane and pornographic friend Robinson is not pleased with our opinion of his nasty little book . . . Dr. Robinson goes so far as to say that the editor of Colorado Medicine is a liar. Tut, tut, Willie! We would not throw discredit on you for the world—just a little chloride of lime occasionally, to take away the worst of it.[69]

Chloride of lime, the early Colorado reader did not have to be reminded, was routinely used to neutralize the contents of cesspools and pit toilets!

Occasionally, one medical journal would direct its barbs against another. *Colorado Medicine*, for example, pointed out:

> As the woman of questionable virtue becomes most noisy and vituperative in defense of her reputation, so the [*Denver Medical Times*] becomes aggressive and abusive in proclaiming its independence.[70]

Physician's feelings may remain as intense today, but the prose is just not the same.

HEAVEN PITY THE DOCTOR
who has time to read every thing that comes to his table.

To be UP-TO-DATE, however, he must read some things.

..TRY..

The Denver Medical Times
THOS. HAYDEN HAWKINS, M. D., LL. D., Editor.

10.6 Dr. Thomas Hawkins, founder and editor of the *Denver Medical Times*. His editorial style was colorful and outspoken.

10.7 The abundance of medical journals in Colorado led to some aggressive competition for subscribers.

11 MEDICAL PRACTICE: ECONOMIC, ETHICAL, SOCIAL

The careful, conscientious physician will always charge for services—and not for results.

C. F. Shollenberger, M.D. (Denver) 1895[1]

Ethics treats of right conduct and character. Medical ethics treats of the physician's duty to his patients, the public, and himself.

W. J. Rothwell, M.D.(Denver) 1902[2]

[The doctor] is looked upon more or less as a member of an unfair and prejudiced class.

Colorado Medicine, 1923[3]

THE ECONOMIC, ETHICAL AND social aspects of medical practice are closely related. Many economic issues, for example, have major ethical and social implications. As such, we will begin with some of the economic aspects of practice in early Colorado, and gradually develop some of the ethical and social considerations.

Making a Living

With the exception of a few doctors employed by the mines, railroads, and a few other industries, the great majority of Colorado's early physicians practiced independently and charged the patient a fee for their services. One of the major functions of organized medicine was to establish a list of approved fees for specific medical services. Such a listing served two purposes: it provided information to the public, and it prevented competing physicians from undercutting each other and undermining the economic foundations of the profession. Thus, in 1860, one of the

first actions of the Jefferson Medical Society, was the formulation of a fee "bill" or "schedule." The approved fees for many services and procedures varied over a wide range, and physicians could charge different fees for the same procedure, depending upon their locale, clientele, type of practice, and other factors. Nevertheless, the suggested fees served as guidelines. Members of a medical society were expected to adhere to the fee bill, and deviations were considered unethical practice.

Looking at successive fee bills over a half century of early Colorado medicine, it is remarkable to find how little change there was in physician's charges (Appendix). A "complicated delivery," for example, cost anywhere from $50 to $200 in 1860 and the same in 1909. The good news for the consumer was that physicians' fees were stable. Furthermore, the doctor's charges comprised, by far, the major portion of the cost of medical care. Most medical care was provided in the patient's home, and even when hospitals became generally available, their charges were relatively small. A week's stay in the hospital might cost anywhere from $10 to $25, including all of the ancillary costs.[4] The bad news was that doctors' fees represented a considerable outlay for the average American wage earner. By the early 1900s, a coal miner earned $2.50 to $4.00 a day; a plumber, $4.00; and a nurse, $2.00 to $5.00.[5] Also by way of comparison , a hundred-pound bag of flour cost $2.10. Given the low level of wages and the correspondingly low cost of living, physicians' fees were relatively high. The cost of a minor surgical procedure, such as suturing a laceration or lancing a boil, might take three days of a worker's wages. Thus, physicians' fees, combined with the spectacular financial success of a few physicians, led to the public's perception of the "rich doctor." Most agreed with the early Colorado pioneer-poet who had complained:

OFFICE PRACTICE.

Prescription in office..	$2 00 to $5 00
Physical examination..	5 00 " 10 00
" " for Life Insurance Co..............	4 00
Vaccination at office..	2 00 " 5 00
Written opinion or written advice to patient............	10 00
Prescription for Gonorrhea (in advance)....................	5 00 " 10 00
Treatment of Gonorrhea (in advance)........................	25 00 " 30 00
Treatment of Syphilis (in advance)..........................	40 00 " 100 00

GENERAL PRACTICE.

For single visit in city, in ordinary cases.................	$4 00
For two or more visits, same day (unless more than ordinary attention is required)............................	5 00
Single visit from day to day....................................	3 00
" " at night, from ten p. m. to six a. m........	5 00

A myriad shams on every hand we see; Doctors grow rich, though they disagree.[6]

Half a century later, a rural Colorado newspaper editor compared his financial status with that of the physician:

One good, strong, healthy doctor's bill will run this [newspaper's] office six months. An editor works half a day for $4 . . . A doctor looks wise and works ten minutes for $200 . . .[7]

The doctors, on the other hand, did not feel that their fees were exhorbitant—especially when they compared themselves to another group of professionals:

The lawyer thinks nothing of charging $100,000 in a suit involving a million dollars, and yet the physician who charges $1,000 in saving the life of a millionaire would be considered a first-class wholesale robber.[8]

A professor at a Denver medical school, Dr. Charles Shollenberger, advised his students:

Tell patients that it is not that you charge the rich more but the poor far less than what your services are really worth.[8]

He added some practical advice:

Some [bills] should be sent by mail, others . . . by a collector, while with others, you will have better success if you see to them personally.

It is not good business policy to furnish itemized accounts—unless requested.

The careful, conscientious physician will always charge for services, and not for results.

Finally, Dr. Shollenberger illustrated how he dealt with the eternal complaint of "so high a fee for so little time spent":

In a case of confinement, the father complained of the size of my bill, because I was only in the house for one hour. I answered him [that] I presumed he would pay the bill much more cheerfully if I had allowed his wife to suffer 24 - 48 hours.[8]

A few physicians had grand homes, fine carriages, elegant clothes and hobnobbed with bankers, brokers, and mining magnates. Most did not. Nationally, in the 1890s, the average annual income of a big city doctor was about $2,000 —about twice that of the aforementioned plumber. In the smaller towns and rural areas it was $1,200.[9] In 1902 it was estimated that beginning physicians earned less than $500 in their first year of practice. At the other end of the scale, it was reported that less than half of one percent of doctors earned more than $15,000 a year.[10]

Often, the modest financial status of many doctors was not apparent until their death. Dr. Shollenberger, in advising his students, found that:

Many a physician, after working hard for 25 or 30 years, goes to his grave, to get his first actual rest, leaving his family unprovided for and compelled to struggle along as best they may.[11]

This was probably true of Dr. Thomas Rosebrough of Hooper, Colorado. Rosebrough, the only physician in his part of the huge San Luis Valley, also maintained a pharmacy. When he died, this poignant notice was published in one of Colorado's medical journals:

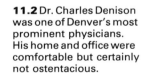

11.1 Some of the suggested medical fees from the Denver Medical Association's fee bill of 1871.

11.2 Dr. Charles Denison was one of Denver's most prominent physicians. His home and office were comfortable but certainly not ostentacious.

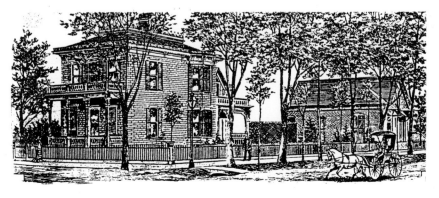

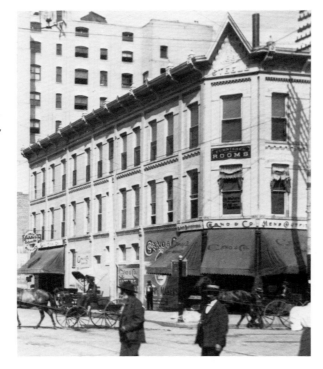

11.3 Some doctors did well financially. Dr. Henry Steele built this building, the Steele Block, in downtown Denver.

[Dr. Rosebrough's] widow is desirous of disposing of the drug store, together with the home, office and drug room. The valuation she places upon the whole is $2,500.[12]

Many city physicians were not any better off financially. One Denver doctor, having endured the perennial big city blight—a mugging—complained to his colleague that his assailant had taken all of his money—fifty cents.[13]

Although their fees were high, most physicians' incomes, as we have seen, were low. Several reasons accounted for this discrepancy. One was the failure to abide by the medical society's recommended charges. Half of the state's physicians did not belong to the Colorado Medical Society and the other half, having to compete with their fellows, often reduced their fees accordingly. Many physicians worked out arrangements with patients, often adjusting their fees to the family's financial situation, accepting fifty cents or so each week until a bill was paid. Often, physicians were paid "in kind", i.e. in produce, goods, or labor. This practice was not limited to rural areas, apparently. One of Denver's most prominent surgeons recalled receiving, in lieu of a fee, a book, *The Evolution of Christian Hymnology*.[14]

In general, the collection rates of Colorado's early physicians appears to have been quite low. This, despite the fact that some of the earliest doctors were quite strict about their fees. One early pioneer even suggested that "M.D." really stood for "money down."[15] In establishing its fee bill in 1860, the Jefferson Medical Society stated:

11.4 A physician's view of a medical "deadbeat."

Every member is expected to close the account due him immediately on the recovery of the patient, either by having the money paid or taking a note drawing interest at the rate of at least ten percent per month.[16]

Physicians, and even the medical societies, could sympathize with the financial difficulties of honest, hard working people. They were much less tolerant of the "deadbeat," the individual the *Denver Medical Times* defined as: "A person [male or female] who does not pay his debts, though he could do so."[17]

The *Times* went on to describe the species. He or she had a characteristic physiognomy, or

facies deadbeatica . . . A sort of air of indifferent effrontery, of obnoxious comraderie, a look of I'm-just-as-good-as-you-are-even-if-I-don't-pay-my-debts. Almost pathognomonic is the deadbeat's recital of his previous [doctor's] mistakes and failings.[17]

Some doctors took action. The Clear Creek County Medical Society prepared a list of "deadbeats" for the use of its members, and the doctors of Yuma, Colorado, resolved that "all past due accounts must be settled in full before any of the undersigned physicians will render further services."[18] The practitioners of the Cripple Creek district formed the Teller County Physicians' Business League, joined forces with the Retail Credit Men's Association, and announced, "by systematic publication in the daily papers, and in language easily understood," that services would be refused to any "deadbeats" unless delinquent accounts were settled.[19]

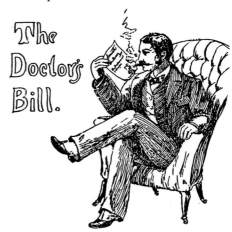

The Doctor's Bill.

Deadbeats sometimes resorted to innovative means in order to deprive the doctor of his fee. This example made the national medical press:

A druggist of Denver is said to have refused to pay a local surgeon who removed his appendix until the surgeon produced the appendix. The surgeon is said to have thrown away the appendix and to have brought suit against the druggist.[20]

Some physicians took more drastic action in order to collect their fees. One doctor had a writ filed against an old woman who owed him forty-eight dollars.[21] Unable to secure bond, she was placed in jail. The judge, finding both the claim and the action to be unjust, dismissed the case, apologized to the defendant, and expressed regret that he could not take action against the doctor. Even more extreme was a doctor in Sterling who, unable to collect a fee from a young man,

> hammered him with a broomstick. This failing, he used a heavy club. The doctor, having concluded the job to his satisfaction, left the young man semiconscious and, it is said, with a fractured skull. The doctor is under $500 bond.[22]

Although physicians were justified in complaining about non-paying patients, their patients would have been equally justified (had they been aware of the practice) in complaining about fee-splitting. The classic example of fee-splitting was the surgeon who returned part of his surgical fee to the general practitioner who had referred the patient to him. Though organized medicine considered such "payoffs" unethical, it was widely practiced and quietly tolerated by many in the profession. As expressed by a Denver surgeon:

> It is nobody's business what I do with a fee, so long as I do not overcharge. If I want to give half of it away, that is my affair, and does not concern the patient or anyone else.[23]

On the other hand, a particularly blatant example of fee-splitting was deplored by another physician:

> A country doctor arrived [in Denver] with a half-dozen celiotomy cases, which he endeavored to farm out to the highest bidder. We were glad that he [eventually] took his cases to another city.[24]

In 1917, Colorado made fee-splitting illegal—a misdemeanor punishable by fine and/or imprisonment.[25]

Medical Manpower

In 1896 one of Colorado's medical journals noted: "At the last meeting of the Board of Medical Examiners, seventy-eight physicians were licensed to wait and starve in Colorado while a practice was forthcoming."[26] Colorado has always been blessed with an ample supply of physicians. As early as 1859, one pioneer observed:

> Signs of "Dr." stick out from cabins, shanties, tents, and wagons, and the title is heard in almost

every company in the diggings. A wag at Cherry Creek called out "doc" in the street, and eighteen men turned around in response.[27]

After the Civil War, physicians continued to pour into the state, and by 1885 it was noted that only one out of three Colorado physicians had been in the state for more than four years.[28] A few years later, the *Denver Medical Times* reported:

> Physicians have been coming to the city at a rate of two and three a week, looking over the ground . . . A six months sojourn [convinces] many that Colorado air is a great purifier of the blood, but that it is not a blood maker—they must have food and shelter too . . . Many cases of genteel poverty in the profession abound . . .[29]

The State Board of Medical Examiners received daily inquiries "as to the prospects of speedy prosperity in the line of medical practice."[30] The mining camps were as crowded as Denver. Cripple Creek, for example, had more than fifty physicians, and when two physicians died in Leadville, there was a sudden influx of medical men into that camp.[31] As has always been the case, however, some communitites had difficulties in attracting doctors. The same year that the *Times* was bemoaning Denver's physician glut, Meeker, in northwestern Colorado, and Lamar, on the eastern plains, were advertising for a doctor.[32]

Nevertheless, even Colorado's non-medical promotional brochures, which normally encouraged immigrants, warned: " If you are a doctor . . . do not think to find an office open and waiting for your arrival. There are people ahead of you. The good, easy places are all taken."[33]

And still, the doctors came:

> There seem to be more doctors here [in Denver] than anything else. Every other house is a doctor's house . . . Everyone is extremely discouraging about the prospect of making a living . . . I was never so horribly impressed with the struggle for existence.[34]

The doctor who made these remarks recalled that he had earned a total of thirty-two dollars in his first three weeks of practice in Denver in 1902. Actually, that was better than another newcomer who had earned twenty-eight dollars in three months. That year there were 457 physicians in Denver, about one for every 300 citizens—a very high ratio! In Colorado Springs the ratio was about 1:190, and in Boulder it was 1:230.[35] At the same time, there were whole counties without a single physician, and twenty counties in Colorado had only one, or at the most, several, physicians.[36]

Part of the problem, according to the *Denver Medical Times*, was: "Though the demand for physicians is more than supplied, our colleges continue to graduate vast numbers every year."[37]

Advertising

Physicians have always been concerned about the propriety of advertising themselves and their services and skills. Garish advertisements were regarded as the hallmarks of the charlatan and quack. M.D.s, on the other hand, were expected to behave in a restrained and dignified manner. Any deviation from the advertising standards established by organized medicine was considered unethical practice.

Colorado's earliest physicians advertised by placing their "professional card" in the local newspaper. For several decades, the placement of such advertisements, discretely stating the physician's name, degree, office address, and type of practice, was considered acceptable by the medical societies. Office window signs were also expected to be tasteful and modest. Those who expanded upon such principles were subject to the ridicule and wrath of their colleagues. The editor of the *Denver Medical Times*, for example, compared "a certain member of the State Board of Medical Examiners" to the great showman P. T. Barnum:

> In his office are four windows, and on each is a sign, the letters of which are only limited in size by the size of the window pane . . .
> No. 1 - Dr. Blank—Diseases of Women
> No. 2 - Dr. Blank—Nose, Throat, and Chest
> No. 3 - Dr. Blank—X-ray and Electricity
> No. 4 - Dr. Blank—General Practice
> In the interest of professional modesty, we are glad he didn't have any more windows, but he would have saved a lot of paint had he used but one sign: Diseases of the Skin—and Everything Inside.[38]

W. H. WILLIAMS, M. D.,

Room No. 5, Evans' Block,

Southwest corner 15th and Lawrence sts.

DENVER, COLORADO.

R. G. BUCKINGHAM, M. D.,

378 Larimer Street,

Between 15th and 16th,   Office, Cole's Block,

Denver, - Colorado.

11.5 In the 1870s, the placing of a doctor's "card" in a business directory or newspaper was considered acceptable. In later years, the medical societies declared this practice to be unethical.

Physicians who specialized in diseases of the "private" (i.e. sex) organs and venereal diseases had special difficulties when it came to informing the public of their expertise. One such physician wrote to a medical journal for advice:

> Will the editor . . . please tell a Denver specialist, his specialty being venereal disease, how he may advertise it on his sign, and what kind of sign to use, size, etc.?[39]

The editor was not about to miss such a heaven-sent opportunity for a bit of medical humor. He suggested that the specialist:

> Procure from Paris a large wax model, flesh-colored, representing the organ of choice, about five or six feet long, and protrude this from his [office] window. Have painted on either side of this—"Diseases of . . . " and, on a flag floated from the end of this modest little sign, have printed—"A Specialty."[39]

Having had his bit of fun, the editor became serious, noting that, indeed, "this is a specialty difficult of modest advertising on sign or card." No such considerations, however, inhibited the explicit advertisements of quack remedies and cures for "lost manhood" or "depraved womanhood" by non-physicians, the "sizzling slough of nauseating obscenity [which] appeared daily in the press of Denver."[40] Years later, Colorado banned "advertisements of private diseases."[41] The following year, the State Board of Medical Examiners revoked the licenses of three physicians who had "caused the publication and circulation of advertisements relative to a disease of the sexual organs."[42]

Eventually, the medical society banned virtually any kind of advertising by physicians, even the insertion of a "card" in the local newspaper. Anything which smacked of publicity for a doctor was discouraged, no matter how distinguished the physician or newsworthy the event. Thus, when Pueblo's Dr. Richard Corwin, one of the state's most prominent surgeons, performed a new operation for a congenitally dislocated hip, and the event was featured in a newspaper—together with a photograph of the doctor—some members of Pueblo's medical society voiced their disapproval. No action was taken, but the issue was important enough to be commented on by J.A.M.A.[43] Doctors whose accomplishments were frequently reported by the press were often referred to by their more fastidious colleagues as "newspaper doctors."[44]

The Poor and the Free Dispensaries

It must be recalled that throughout the period covered by this book, there was no welfare system in the United States. There was no Medicare, Medicaid, or Social Security. Colorado had a few city and county hospitals—derived from poorhouses, identified with pesthouses, and, even later, clearly labeled as "charity" institutions. In some areas, the local government paid a physician, usually part-time, to care for the indigent. Some private physicians donated their time and efforts to "charity" cases and some of the private hospitals designated a few of their beds for non-paying patients. Physicians and hospitals took care not to establish a reputation for unrestrained generosity, lest they tarnish their professional reputations and sink into financial oblivion. The sisters who ran many of the private hospitals must have been tormented by the perpetual conflict between moral and fiscal responsibility.

In the late eighteenth century, many eastern cities had established free dispensaries. These were, essentially, outpatient clinics where the poor could obain medical care for no charge. They were variously supported by municipalities, churches, medical schools, or philanthropic organizations. By the 1870s, New York City had twenty-nine free dispensaries and Philadelphia had thirty-three.[45] Thus, it was to

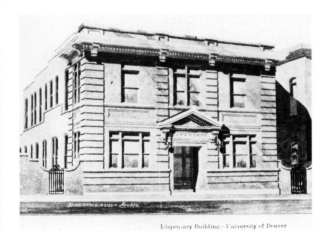

Dispensary Building – University of Denver

NO.............

Denver University Free Clinic.

............*Oct 1*............189*8*...

M...*Report of Dispensary*............

for Dr. *Univ of Denver*............Clinic

on............*for Sept 1898*............at............P. M.

Always bring this Card and show it to the Dootor.

the dispensary that many immigrants, blacks, other minorities, and street people would come to have a fever treated, a boil lanced, a broken bone set, or a tooth pulled. The physicians in attendance were usually volunteers and, in those dispensaries associated with medical schools, faculty or students. The latter situation provided a traditional medical *quid pro quo*—free medical care for the poor in exchange for clinical experience for students and young physicians.

The private practitioner had no quarrel with providing medical care for "the truly needy." Denver's Dr. H. G. Wetherill, for example, pointed out that: "The dispensaries connected with our medical schools are doing good work . . . and we believe they are doing it within their legitimate field."[46] What concerned the doctors was the impression that many dispensary patients could, in reality, afford to pay for their medical care, and that their practices were being depleted of a significant number of paying patients. The *Denver Medical Times* had warned the medical community against the dispensaries or "medical shops." By 1884, it concluded:

> It is too late. These fungi are firmly established, and their roots sucking the earth's more modest plants, the "private doctors." These latter are now opening their eyes, rudely awakened from their dream of fancied financial security . . . Unless something radical is done, [the private doctors] will have to fry in their own fat.[47]

By the turn of the century, the *Colorado Medical Journal* was complaining:

> In Denver, the abuse of the free dispensaries . . . is fast assuming vast proportions . . . Unite all the dispensaries in one building [and] excercise a rigid supervision over the applicants . . . so that none but deserving poor persons shall be treated. Let [the dispensaries] be . . . FOR THE POOR, AND FOR THEM ONLY![48]

Any attempt to establish a non-medical school affiliated dispensary was met with stiff opposition from the doctors. When Reverend Uzzell attempted to open his "politico-religious-medical dispensary,"[49] the *Denver Medical Times* suggested:

> Let religious philanthropic fanatics launch their dispensaries as they like, but let the medical profession refuse positively to give them any aid or support.[50]

The *Times* urged that "any medical gentleman connecting himself with a free dispensary not attached to a medical college should be considered 'irregular,'" i.e. one notch above a quack.[50] Finally, with the eventual elimination of three

11.6 Free dispensaries were accepted as long as they were affiliated with a medical school such as the University of Denver.

of Denver's four medical schools, a single Municipal Free Dispensary was opened in 1914. Its volunteer staff included a number of specialists and it had its own laboratory:

> One of the first cases . . . was a child suffering from an appendiceal abscess which had been overlooked . . . Another was a little girl with a sore throat [in whom] a culture was taken and found to be positive for diphtheria . . . These cases prove the necessity of a free dispensary for the city's indigent.[51]

Health Insurance and Lodge Doctors

Even in the early days, a significant portion of Colorado's labor force was covered by some form of health insurance. In general, the CF&I's steelworkers, hardrock and coal miners, and railroad employees had a dollar deducted from their monthly wage to insure them against future doctor's fees and hospital charges. No such coverage was available for other workers, farmers, and small businessmen. They were expected to pay for medical care for themselves and their families as the need arose. A bout with pneumonia, a complicated delivery, an appendectomy—these were not only life-threatening events, they could also devastate a family's finances. Medical bills of one hundred dollars might represent a breadwinner's earnings for a month. Combined with lost wages and the lack of any welfare benefits, an illness could leave a family penniless.

In many areas of the eastern United States, a form of health insurance developed which became known as "lodge" or "club" medicine. Originating in fraternal organizations and then spreading to factories, mills, and labor unions, a group would contract with one or more doctors to provide medical services to the members and their families. The concept was expanded to private "lodges" and "clubs" whose sole purpose was to provide health insurance for a small monthly or annual payment. Entrepreneurs contracted with doctors to provide their services, generally for a fee which was far below the minimum stipulated by medical society fee bills. For the lodge doctor, the contract provided a guaranteed income and many newly graduated M.D.s, fighting for survival in an overcrowded profession, were happy to sign up.

Organized medicine saw lodge doctors as a serious threat to private practice. In 1897 Dr. Carrol Edson reported to Denver's medical society:

> There is at present an evil even greater than the dispensary abuse, one which is the outgrowth of commercialism in medicine. I refer to the medical clubs and unions which . . . have already become dangerously common . . . They should be prevented at all hazards, and those already started, eradicated.[52]

Edson warned the young, innocent physician, tempted "by dire necessity" into signing a contract, that he was entering "medical slavery." Furthermore, predicted Dr. Edson, as middle-class and even wealthy people joined the "clubs," and the number of clubs and lodges proliferated,

> the contagion of underbidding [would] begin. The dollar a month club is followed by the 75-cent union, and that by the 50-cent association. The competition [for physicians] has not been avoided, but the field narrowed into securing the chance of slaving for a club.[52]

Lodge doctors and contract medicine were major topics for discussion at medical society meetings. Dr. Will Davis told the Pueblo Medical Society that "we have been so unrelentlessly and continuously shorn by the contract doctor, it is beyond human patience and forbearance to further sit in lamb-like meekness," and called for "sweeping reforms."[53] The Clear Creek County Medical Society, meeting in Central City, condemned contract medicine as "unfair and unprofessional" and voted to ostracize any members who engaged in such activities. They carefully excluded from their denunciation the "time-honored contract work" which involved mines and railroads. On the other hand, they felt that private individuals and families were not entitled to prepaid health plans. Clear Creek County's physicians were either unaware of the inconsistency of their actions or considered it irrelevant. Their attitude may have been influenced by the fact that many of them depended on their contracts with mines and railroads.[54] At any rate, several months later, the Society preferred charges against an Idaho Springs physician "for doing contract work."[55] Ultimately, of course, prepaid health plans were accepted by organized medicine, and physicians' fees are now dictated by government accountants and insurance company managers. The threat of "contract medicine" has been resurrected, and the private practitioner has become an endangered species.

Images

In his 1871 address to the organizational meeting of the Territorial Medical Society, Dr.

Richard Buckingham delineated his image of the physician—a role which he envisioned as combining service, devotion, and sacrifice:

> By a timely and judicious application of remedies we [physicians] are instrumental in snatching some sufferer from the jaws of death; our nights of bliss are the nights of toil and sympathy for the distressed and dying. There is no social pleasure physicians do not willingly forego when summoned to the couch of pain; no scene of mirth or amusement is too attractive to detain us when our services are demanded . . . Not even the sacred worship of the Sabbath.
>
> What is our recompense for all these sacrifices? Is wealth an object? . . . Do you seek for fame? . . . Is it honor that you strive for?[56]

No, concluded Dr. Buckingham. These are not the goals of the physician. "Why then," he asked, "all this sacrifice of your time, rest, pleasure, social enjoyment, home comforts?" Because, he answered,

> There is an inward voice whispering to your heart—I delight to do good; I love to visit the sick; to relieve the distressed. And when the means I employ in the relief of my fellows accomplish the desired end, there is an inward joy that swells the fountain of love within the heart; and that great fountain would burst its walls but for the tears that flow and fill the breast with peace and happiness.[56]

A bit corny, perhaps, but *some* of Dr. Buckingham's sentiments were undoubtedly applicable to *some* physicians . . . at least *some* of the time.

Colorado's physicians were as heterogeneous a group of doctors as anywhere in the country. We have seen that they came to Colorado for a variety of reasons—some to practice, some to mine, some to explore the frontier, and some for their health. Some had never gone to medical school or had graduated from diploma mills, while others had attended the finest medical schools in the East or in Europe. By 1883 the image of Colorado's physicians was of sufficient stature for the esteemed *Boston Medical and Surgical Journal* to proclaim: "Colorado, though a new state, [has] . . . in medicine, as in other departments, many workers of first-rate ability."[57]

Indeed, Colorado's physicians were presenting papers at national meetings, publishing in important national (as well as local) journals, and playing an active role in national societies. In 1885 Dr. Charles Denison became the first Colorado physician to appear in print in the J.A.M.A.[58] His comments on the stethoscope were followed in the A.M.A.'s journal by articles by Drs. J. W. Brown of Silverton (on

pneumonia) and S. E. Solly of Colorado Springs (on "temperament").[59] The first edition of *Who's Who in America*, published in 1899, included seven Colorado physicians among its luminaries.[60] By 1914 the Colorado Medical Society, in commenting on the fact that several Coloradans had become officers of national medical societies that year, used the occasion to congratulate the state on the quality of its physicians:

> We are not overshooting the mark in asserting that some of the best medical men of the country are located in our midst and that our medical men in general compare favorably with those located in the center of medical education.[61]

The contributions of Coloradans to the medical literature accelerated rapidly. By 1916 there were more than 500 such citations in J.A.M.A. and by 1921, nearly 5,000 in other medical journals.[62]

The self-image of Colorado's doctors had evolved from Dr. Buckingham's heroic portrait to a more realistic view of imperfect human beings using an imperfect science to help an imperfect mankind. The doctors were proud of their profession, its remarkable progress, and its contributions to humanity. They resented what they regarded as, at best, the indifference and ingratitude, and at worst, the hostility, of their public.

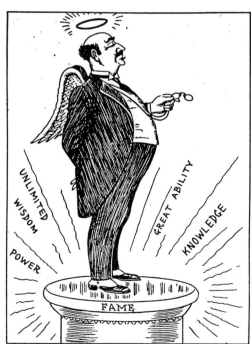

11.7 The doctor's self-image was not always the same as the public's image of him.

The public's image of doctors had always been mixed. By the very nature of his profession, the doctor was identified with some of life's worst moments—pain and injury, illness, and death. Doctors performed painful procedures, prescribed unpleasant medicines, made mistakes, and disagreed with each other. As for the patient who recovered, a popular homily stated—"God cures, and the doctor collects." The social reformers and the socialists denounced doctors as part of the moneyed establishment and as uninterested in poor people. The "know-nothings" and populists accused them of maintaining a medical monopoly and stifling free enterprise. The doctors were not spiritual enough for the religious, and they were not scientific enough for physical scientists. The anti-vaccinationists accused them of being against free choice and the anti-vivisectionists of being cruel to animals. The doctors were too conservative . . . they were too liberal. As for the "average" American, he or she probably agreed with the rural Colorado journalist who wrote:

> The doctor goes to college for two or three years, gets a diploma and a string of words that the devil himself could not pronounce, cultivates a look of gravity that he pawns for wisdom, gets a box of pills, a cayuse and a meat saw, and sticks out a shingle.[63]

The doctor's image of his patients was sometimes less than exhalted as well. The editor of the *Denver Medical Times* described the "average patient":

> *The average patient* likes to be humbugged. Any old fad will do so long as it has a new name.

> *The average patient* believes that the os humerus is the funny bone and that the seat of all the finer emotions is in the heart, but he thinks he knows more than the doctor.

> *The average patient* sends for the doctor in haste and repays him at leisure.

> *The average patient* . . . will take a bottle of Rotgut's Relief, or a box of Poopendike's pills, and to these he will give all the glory, and 'the doctor be damned.'[64]

Religion and the Clergy

Much of the lack of confidence which physicians have in preachers comes from the fact that preachers are . . . not educated in the simplest matters concerning the physical being of man and of the whole natural world. Hence they are continually making the most absurd and irrational arguments.

Denver Medical Times, 1893[65]

Most of the time, Colorado's doctors and clergymen worked together, ministering to the respective physical and spiritual needs of humanity. Physicians and clergymen who cared for the rich had much in common with each other and their clients, as did those who worked among the less fortunate. Their work often cut across religious boundaries—the Episcopalian priest working with the Methodist physician, the Jewish doctor admitting patients to the Catholic hospital.

There was also the potential for friction between the professions—not surprising considering that one group emphasized faith and ancient ideas while the other had come to stress reason and modern concepts. Most were pragmatic in their attitudes toward each other's profession, but some physicians were outspoken in their view that religion had no role in medical care, while some religionists used their pulpits to proclaim that disease was a purely spiritual phenomenon and that doctors were superfluous. Problems arose when some members of the clergy allied themselves with anti-medical fringe groups such as those who opposed vaccination or with faith healers who opposed rational medicine in general.

Alcohol provided a focus for several disputes between the doctors and the clergy. In 1878 some of the more ardent prohibitionists among Denver's Protestant ministers attacked the medicinal use of alcohol, especially its widespread use in tonics of various types. This led to a major confrontation which required the intervention of some of the more senior, and cooler, heads of both professions (Chapter 18). Fifteen years later, some of Denver's ministers supported attempts to provide state funding for several "cures" for alcoholism—programs which the physicians had denounced as quackery. The *Denver Medical Times* was outraged and accused the clergymen of "having trailed their ministerial robes in the gutter of ignorance."[66] The editor spoke of preachers

> continually becoming the victims of the most shameful and ignorant charlatans, who have found . . . that nothing is too irrational to obtain the sanction of the pulpit . . . Quacks of all descriptions . . . thrive and grow fat because of fulsome pulpit eulogies and more fulsome testimonials from preachers.[67]

Even "establishment" clergy were not immune to an occasional lambasting by the doctors. In 1903 the target was the Reverend John H. Houghton, rector of St. Mark's Episcopal Church in Denver. The minister's transgression was his plan to establish, within St. Mark's, what the doctors referred to as a "Christian Science-Clairvoyant-Magnetic-Faith Cure Clinic."[68] That plan was soon sidetracked by the Bishop, but soon after, Reverend Houghton was described as having "broken loose" again. In a talk to a group of nurses, the minister commented:

> I am heartily in favor of the nurses. They do more good than the physicians. But, one thing in that connection which has always aroused me, is the fact that ministers are not allowed in the sick room . . . A minister can do a sick person more good than all the pills and medicines any physician ever poured down one's neck . . . I want you nurses to remember this and get us in to see the sick . . . [69]

The doctors were furious and spoke of "professional dishonesty [and] pernicious teaching by the clergy." One medical editor wrote: "If all ministers were built along these lines it would be little wonder if physicians should bar the door against their admission."[69]

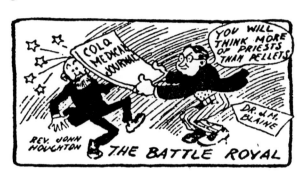

Newspapers and the Press

Our profession is at the mercy of the press . . . How long will the members of our noble profession submit to the tyranny of this monster . . . Let us gird ourselves with the armor of truth and go forth as David of old.

P. D. Rothwell, M.D. (Denver), 1899[70]

Most of the time, Colorado's newspapers supported the doctors in their efforts to improve and modernize medical care. In public health matters, for example, most of the newspapers backed movements for improved sanitation, pure drinking water, quarantine, vaccination, and so on. On the other hand, the press periodically reminded the doctors that they, like everyone else, were subject to their editorial scrutiny. Dr. Bancroft, for example, must have winced when his friend William Byers's *Rocky Mountain News* complained that Colorado's physicians' fees were "far above the average."[71]

Sometimes, individual doctors were subjected to scrutiny—and criticism. When that happened, the profession would generally close ranks and defend their colleagues. When the *Denver Evening Times* published an editorial entitled, "Those Careless Surgeons," the Colorado Medical Society's journal responded:

> The editor . . . must have been very hard up for a subject . . . The tone of the editorial is undignified and tends to discredit the surgical profession in general. [He] would have us believe that such mishaps [leaving a pair of scissors in the patient's abdomen] are of common occurrence.[72]

The doctor went on to remind the *Times's* publisher, who also happened to be Denver's mayor, of the many civic contributions made by the city's doctors. For good measure, he added a subtle warning to the politician-publisher:

> We are reminded that the former management of the *Times* made a special effort to secure the support of the medical profession . . . Is it possible that this support is no longer desired? Surely the tone of this editorial would indicate that such is the case.[72]

The most heated confrontation between the doctors and the press involved John C. Shaffer, publisher of the *Rocky Mountain News*. Shaffer's son, Kent, had come to Colorado for his health, and the father, a millionaire Chicago financier, had followed his son and moved to Denver.[73] Shaffer already owned several newspapers and he added the *Rocky Mountain News* to his holdings. Unfortunately, the younger Shaffer held a number of bizarre views on health and disease, and these soon began to appear on the newspaper's editorial pages. Denver's Dr. H. G. Wetherill took the publisher to task for

> permitting your son to use the editorial columns of the *News* to preach, in his feeble and puerile way, his religious opinions and medical beliefs . . . That he makes himself ridiculous is immaterial . . . To employ the power of the press to promulgate propaganda against the employment of modern scientific methods of disease prevention is an atrocious and an abominable thing to do . . . Can you conscientiously ignore your accountability to humanity? Can you sleep o'nights with this thing on your conscience?[74]

In more recent times, there have been other occasions when Colorado's press and physicians have disagreed—but the literary qualities of those differences are just not the same.

Politics and Governors

The very life of a doctor does not fit him to be a good lobbyist. He is too busy with his practice and too much occupied . . . to defend his position clearly and convincingly.

S. D. Van Meter, M.D. (Denver), 1909[75]

As with the press, Colorado's doctors were generally succesful in working with municipal, county, and state officials on public health and

11.8 Reverend Houghton's comment that nurses do more good than doctors was not appreciated by Colorado's physicians.

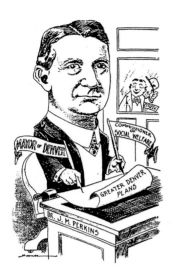

11.9 Former Denver mayor, Dr. J.M. Perkins, complained that his term of office had ruined both his stomach and his finances.

other purely medical issues. Some physicians played an active role in politics and were elected and served as state legislators, as mayors of many cities and towns, and in other governmental offices. Some were active behind the scenes in the Democratic and, especially, the Republican parties. A few espoused the political views of some of the more transient, and sometimes radical, political parties and organizations. Most doctors preferred to leave politics to the politicians. Those who didn't sometimes found themselves politically dyspeptic. The former mayor of Denver, Dr. J. M. Perkins, commented that under no circumstances would he be a candidate for re-election, declaring that "his term of office had ruined [both] his stomach and his finances."[76]

The major conflict between the doctors and the politicians was over attempts to reform Colorado's medical licensing law. At the turn of the century, organized medicine had succeeded in having the state legislature pass reform bills, only to have them vetoed by governors. The first was a Democrat, Governor Charles Thomas, who infuriated the doctors not only by his veto, but by his "vaporous discourse [and] malicious misrepresentation of the medical profession."[77] Medical editors spoke of "a shameful act by a petty politician . . . , cheap palaver characteristic of the demagogue . . . , [and] the gubernatorial gabbler who prates of trusts and insists on the immemorial right of the American people to be humbugged." Letters to the editor denounced a governor who would "prostitute his high office to the level of a low ward politician [and] make an honest prevaricator blush for shame."[78] A medical banquet toast began with the refrain, "There once lived a cat named Thomas . . ." and ended with:

> Every dog his his day, as so has the cat,
> And Thomas will find where he's at;
>   We'll give him a whack,
>   So he'll never come back,
> Sic semper tyrannis Tom Cat.[79]

The doctors planned their revenge. Two years later, when the governor failed in his attempt to obtain his ulitmate political goal, a seat in the U.S. Senate, the *Denver Medical Times* gloated:

> The medical profession remembered . . . He failed because of the opposition of the doctors of Colorado. He signed his political death warrant [when he signed the veto] on April 24, 1899.[80]

Then, in more colorful terms:

11.10 The battles over medical licensure laws showed Colorado's doctors the need for some political clout. A few, like Creede's Dr. John Biles, became politically active and even served in the legislature.

> How the flighty have fallen! Wipe your eyes and noses ye hoboes and pluguglies, for the glory of the inimitable Charles is departed forever. Weep, ye harlots, and lament, ye tin horns; tear your hair and grind your teeth, ye 'healers,' for your patron saint is not more. He is politically defunct, not to say decayed and deodorized. May we never see his like again![80]

Unfortunately for the doctors, his like was seen again, in the form of Governor James H. Peabody. This time it was a Republican governor who vetoed the hard-fought medical bill. Again, the veto message was offensive to the physicians, and again the doctors voiced their anger and frustration. Finally, however, the doctors had become aware of their political ineffectiveness. One physician confessed his own naivete to his colleagues:

> I was in politics two weeks ago. I went with the best intentions in the world . . . to the Democratic party, ready to spew out all the dead-beats and grafters . . . I went in, and I came out. I found out that I had not as much influence as a four-year old boy. The matter had been all fixed beforehand.[81]

Within a few years, however, the doctors were beginning to exert some political clout. By 1910 there were five physicians in the state legislature and all sorts of medically significant laws had been enacted.

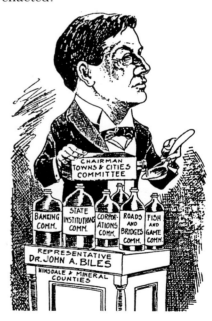

Lawyers and Malpractice

In Colorado, any worthless vagrant may bring an unjust and vexatious suit against a physician who has attended him . . . provided he can find a lawyer who will take his case on a contingent fee.

    H. G. Wetherill, M.D. (Denver), 1897[82]

Relations between Colorado's doctors and lawyers appear to have been generally peaceful until the 1890s, when malpractice suits began to become fashionable. In the past, such suits had been uncommon, but by 1892, Greeley's Dr. G. Law was warning his colleagues of things to come.[83] The targets of malpractice suits, he had found, were not incompetent or negligent physicians, but "worthy and competent men who, by long years of careful and faithful work, have accumulated some property."

The plaintiff attorney will . . . adroitly lead [physicians] to commit themselves against their brother practitioners . . . Twelve men selected by lot will be called upon to decide medical and surgical points. It is obvious that the odds are against the defendant doctor.[83]

A few years later, several noteworthy malpractice suits were brought in Colorado and the *Colorado Medical Journal* exclaimed, "The malpractice fad is upon us."[84] The first was against a prominent Denver surgeon, W. W. Grant, and involved an orthopedic problem.[85] The plaintiff claimed that Dr. Grant had failed to diagnose a fracture which another doctor had found by using a new diagnostic tool—X-rays. This was the first time that X-rays had been introduced as evidence in court.

Soon after: "The prediction made by some of the knowing ones that the suit against Dr. Grant was but a forerunner of other damage suits . . . was verified."[86] . . . and continues to be verified.

Opinions

Like everyone else Colorado's early physicians had a variety of "social" opinions on topics which ranged from such serious issues as crime, abortion, and bigotry, to matters of lesser moment. Many of these opinions are expressed elsewhere in this book. Here are a few additional comments:

Smoking:

Smoking: [At medical meetings] half of the doctors are smoking . . . They go out into the night air reeking of tobacco smoke. Might we not practice what we preach? . . . Are not those of us who smoke at such meetings intensely selfish and inconsiderate of the rights and comfort of others and of the true welfare of all?
H.G. Wetherill, M.D. (Denver), 1909[87]

Women:

The knowledge that will enable a young woman to make good bread, cook foods, keep her house in a neat and orderly condition, feed a baby without poisoning it . . . is of far greater value . . . than a knowledge of Greek, Wagnerian music, or any number of [similar] accomplishments could be.
E. Stuver, M.D. (Fort Collins), 1902[88]

Social Welfare:

[I deplore] any measures of taxation which impose an undue and excessive burden upon the mentally superior, the efficient, the successful, and the self-sufficient, in order to ameliorate the living conditions of the dull-witted, incompetent, inefficient, timid, and self-indulgent.
A.C. McC . . . ., M.D. (Victor), 1922[89]

Heredity:

I am satisfied that the newly awakened interest in eugenics will . . . accomplish nearly as much for the betterment of the human race as it has done in the betterment of our horses, cattle, hogs, and dogs.
A. L. Stubbs, M.D. (La Junta), 1913[90]

Fashion:

A South African Hottentot is more modest in his or her wearing apparel than the girls who dress according to modern fashion.
Colorado Medicine, 1916[91]

Bigotry:

Let the white man . . . remember that the negro is a human being [and] of the same origin as the white man, and that he is under the same moral and physical laws . . . Let us give the black man a square deal and a fair chance . . .
J. M. De Weese, M.D. (Denver), 1910[92]

Exercise:

One of the commonest errors that health seekers make is in the matter of exercise. They usually carry it to excess.
S.E. Solly, M.D. (Colorado Spings), 1883[93]

Religion:

Practitioners of medicine are usually cautious in their treatment of religion . . . There is no surer method of giving offence, and of rendering yourself obnoxious, than by announcing peculiar views on the subject of religion.
J. W. Exline, M.D. (Denver), 1892[94]

Higher education:

Dwelling on the lasciviousness, indecency, and immorality of Greek and Latin literature, with an occasional plunge into the foul stream of modern aristocratic amours, is it any wonder that the modern college student . . . has sunk to the depths of degradation? . . .
E. Stuver, M.D. (Fort Collins), 1902[95]

12 MEDICAL SCHOOLS AND MEDICAL RESEARCH[1]

[In Colorado's early days] a medical school . . . required much less than a block of ground. A room for lectures, another for dissections, and strong influence with the County undertaker who was to furnish bodies for dissection, were the primary requirements.

Dr. C.S. Elder (Denver), 1895[2]

Upon what stem of character and intellect the [University of Colorado School of Medicine] was founded and through what vicissitudes of poverty, stimulation and opposition it has emerged . . .

Dr. Henry Sewall (Denver), 1925[3]

I N THE EARLY 1800s, a medical education was obtained either by going to medical school in Europe, attending one of the few American schools, or, as most did, apprenticing with a practicing physician for a year or two. By 1840 there were some thirty medical schools in the United States, and after the Civil War, the number continued to increase steadily. Some were associated with universities (e.g. Harvard, Columbia) and others were proprietary, that is independent and sometimes profit-making institutions founded by a group of practicing physicians. Regardless of their status, most medical schools were supported by the tuition and fees of their students. Requirements for admission were minimal; a high school diploma usually sufficed. In exchange for tuition, students were given tickets admitting them to lecture series in the medical disciplines—Anatomy, Physiology, Chemistry, Botany, Materia Medica, Medicine, Surgery, Obstetrics, and Diseases of Women and Children. There was no orderly progression of courses or curriculum. The lectures were repeated yearly, and the stu-

dent could attend them at his pleasure. The faculty consisted of doctors whose first responsibility was to their patients. Part of the year was spent in the classroom and the balance as the equivalent of an apprentice with a preceptor, or practicing physician. Laboratories and teaching hospitals were virtually non-existent. At the end of two years, the M.D. was awarded and this served as the sole basis for certification and licensure. In 1871 Harvard Medical School introduced a three-year graded curriculum, i.e. a course of study which proceeded from the basic to the clinical sciences in a systematic and progressive fashion. The same year, the Colorado

12.1 The medical student's tuition paid for his ticket admitting him to classes.

Denver and Gross College of Medicine

PHYSIOLOGICAL LABORATORY TICKET

Session of 19 06 19 07

Admit M⟨r⟩. L. L. Patterson

Robert Levy

Secretary.

This is to certify that the holder of this ticket has satisfactorily completed the work in this Laboratory.

Territorial Medical Society was formed. In his address at its organizational meeting, president-elect Buckingham predicted that Colorado would soon have its own medical school.[4]

Colorado's Four Schools

It was not until 1881, however, that Colorado's first medical school opened its doors—at the University of Denver. Why did a remote, frontier state need a medical school? Probably to satisfy a need by Colorado's physicians for the kind of academic environment that a medical school would generate and, perhaps even more important, the professional prestige and status that a faculty appointment would imply. The proponents of the new school were part of Denver's establishment: men such as Bancroft, Denison, Steele, and Stedman, and it was probably they who pursuaded their fellow non-medical establishment members on the University of Denver's Board of Trustees to accept their proposal. Indeed, the University's founder and most influential board member was a physician, John Evans. Although he hadn't practiced medicine since coming to Colorado as its second territorial governor, Evans had previously been one of Chicago's leading physicians and a professor at Rush Medical College. At any rate, the trustees accepted the plan, and the Medical Department was installed in the main university building in downtown Denver.

Two years later, in 1883, a second medical school was opened—at the University of Colorado in Boulder. The reasons for its establishment are less clear. Perhaps it was to make use

of the fact that the university's president, Dr. Joseph Sewall, was a physician. Certainly, the new school's goals were noble and impressive:

> [Since] the Regents believe that the lives and health of the people of Colorado are not second in importance to any other interest . . . the object of the [medical school] is to secure a higher standard of medical education for those who may, in the future, be entrusted with the lives and with the health of our citizens.[5]

The goals may have been grand, but the institution was not. The school consisted of two rooms in Old Main, two professors, and two students. Dr. Sewall served as dean and Professor of Chemistry.

Tuition at C.U. was free, and women were to be admitted on an equal basis with men. The entrance requirement was a high school diploma. In lieu of a diploma, successful completion of a written examination was acceptable. Although "students from the moral, educated and intelligent youth of Colorado . . ." were sought, non-residents were also encouraged to apply. Stressing Colorado's salubrious climate, the school's prospectus noted that Boulder was a "most desirable location for young men of the more eastern states who seek to improve their health."[5]

Lest anyone become too concerned about the costs of educating physicians "entrusted with the lives and the health of our citizens," the Board of Regents reassured the taxpayers that "the most considerate and scrupulous regard influences [our] actions in the expenditure of public funds . . ."[5] The *Journal of the American Medical Association* wished Colorado's new school

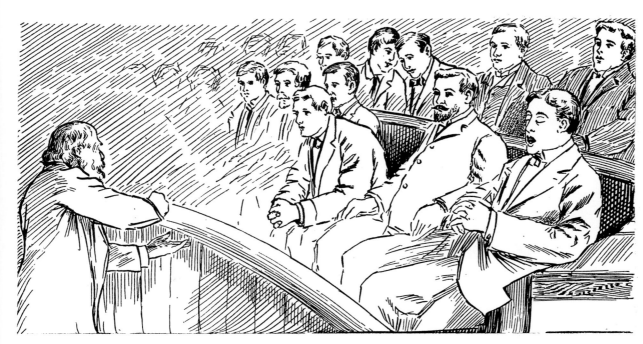

12.2 Most classes were in the form of lectures. Since the faculty were part-time practitioners whose livelihood depended on their private patients, classes were often canceled—when the lecturer was called to see a patient.

well, despite reservations over its policies of free tuition and coeducation.[6] The University of Denver was not pleased with the upstart in Boulder, the state medical society's journal took no notice of it, and the *Denver Medical Times* referred to its establishment as symptomatic of the "medical college craze in Colorado."[7] It predicted that additional schools would soon be forthcoming.

The prediction was accurate. A number of Denver physicians had not been invited to join the University of Denver's faculty. Having been ignored by the establishment, in 1887 they organized Colorado's third medical school, the Gross Medical College. Named for a famous Philadelphia surgeon, Samuel Gross, the new school was located in downtown Denver and admitted twenty-one students to its first class. If less "establishment" than its downtown neighbor, the Gross's faculty was no less distinguished professionally. Furthermore, while the trustees of the University of Denver included a governor, a senator, and a former chief justice of the state supreme court, the Gross had H.A.W. Tabor as one of its trustees. Tabor, a former storekeeper, was now the biggest of Colorado's silver millionaires. Finally, in 1894, Colorado's homeopathic physicians opened their Denver Homeopathic College to 26 students. Thus, by 1894

there were no less than four medical schools in Colorado, three in Denver, and one in Boulder.

Things had been looking fairly good for the state school in 1885. The faculty had been expanded and a university hospital had been opened. Suddenly, that year the legislature tightened the University's purse strings, and the regents responded by cutting the medical school's budget to $2,600. Even in 1885, that sum did not go very far. It looked as though the school was about to disintegrate when one of its new professors, Dr. J.H. Kimball, proposed that the institution rely entirely upon the voluntary services of practicing physicians. The regents found this "free-ride" hard to resist, and the

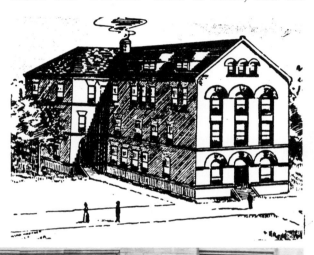

12.3 In the 1890s, Denver's private medical colleges outclassed the University of Colorado's school in the quality and size of faculty, facilities, and clinical resources. Below: The impressive chemistry laboratory at the University of Denver. Right: Students in front of the University of Denver's medical college. Right above: Gross Medical College.

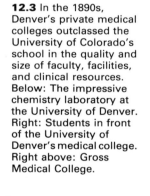

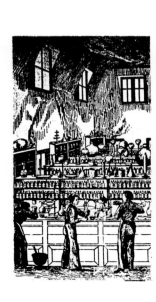

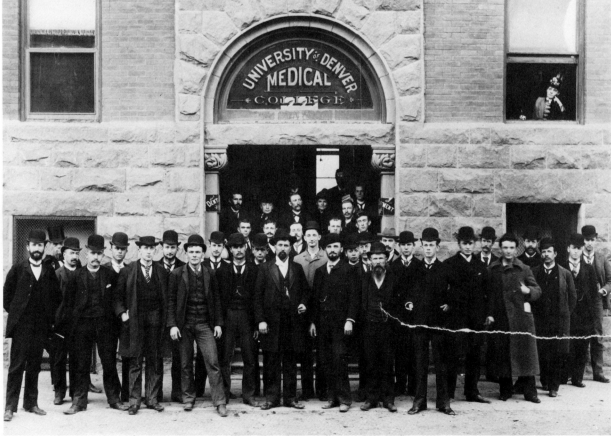

school survived. Two years later, Dr. Sewall was fired from his jobs as president, dean, and professor—charged with ineptitude and fiscal mismanagement. In subsequent years, there were more ups and downs. The school was able to recruit some excellent faculty and acquired its own building. On the other hand, a legislative commission recommended that " . . . the medical school be discontinued and the hospital be turned into some practical use."[8] The recommendation was not implemented, but the lack of financial support continued, there was no medical libary, and clinical teaching facilities were inadequate. While Denver's schools had access to the large County (later Denver General) Hospital and several private hospitals for their students, C.U. had to rely on its thirty-bed University Hospital in Boulder.

In the meantime, the University of Denver's school, now the Denver Medical College, had acquired a large building, extended its curriculum to three years, and was apparently doing well. Similarly, the Gross Medical College had constructed a four-story building near the County Hospital, complete with an ampitheater seating 125, well-equipped laboratories, and a museum. By the 1890s, both schools felt so secure that they were able to charge $100 tuition. C.U., however, was having trouble attracting students, mainly because of its inadequate hospital facilities. In 1893 it made a bold move by arranging to have its students receive their training in Denver at the County Hospital. This was a brilliant idea which, unfortunately, had overlooked one small technicality—it was illegal. The Denver Medical College helpfully pointed out, in court, that the state school was required by Colorado's constitution to do all of its teaching in Boulder. C.U. cried "foul" and arguments were aired in the newspapers and the medical journals. The issue finally went to the state supreme court which ruled that the move to Denver was, indeed, unconstitutional.[9] The Denver physicians who had joined the faculty promptly resigned and the demoralized medical students returned to Boulder and its tiny hospital. Boulder's citizens contributed to the building of a new and slightly larger University Hospital, but the problem persisted.

The Denver-Boulder issue was symptomatic of the intense competition for students among Colorado's three regular medical schools, a local manifestation of the national over-abundance of medical schools. Hostilities were often expressed publicly. The *Denver Medical Times*, whose editor was an active supporter of the Gross Medical College, deplored, for example, the fact that the

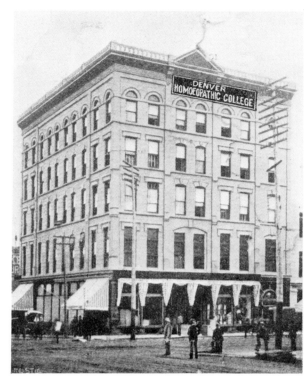

12.4 In 1894 the Denver Homeopathic College became the state's fourth medical school.

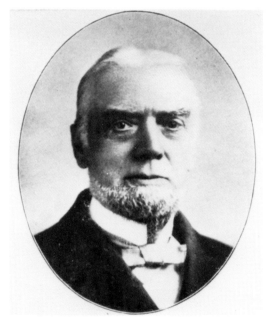

12.5 When the University of Colorado's medical school was established in 1883, Dr. Joseph Sewall became its first dean. He was subsequently fired.

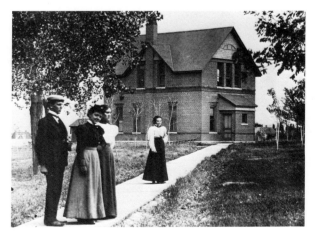

12.6 This unpretentious building on the Boulder campus served as the medical school's home during its early years.

Denver Medical College "is up to its old tricks again, viz: advertising itself . . . in the daily press. This is wrong, unethical, and in very bad taste."[10] Referring to C.U.'s attempts to justify its move to Denver, he asked "Can any man, coming out of such a school ever come to any good end? . . . Any institution backing itself up by lying, deception, and 'shenanigan' will, or at least should, come to grief."[11] Proponents of the other schools were equally vocal, and the homeopathic school liked to tweak all three of its regular rivals. In his president's address to the Colorado Medical Society in 1894, Dr. Edmund Rogers summarized the situation:

> The jealousies and antagonism between these schools in their scramble for the few students that could be found in a State so sparsely settled as this could only lead to harm. Instead of the profession being elevated and honored, it was lowered and split up into petty factions.[12]

Furthermore, the four schools were dividing the state's resources, preventing any of them from becoming truly outstanding. The president of the Denver Medical Society observed that, "the united laboratories of the whole four schools have not sufficient equipment for one good laboratory." The schools, he complained, with their

> incomplete facilities for instruction [and] inadequate endowment and income . . . are pretending to teach medicine when their instruction is little more than a travesty upon real medical education judged by modern standards.[13]

By 1902 the situation had become so difficult that two of the former rivals, the Denver Medical College and the Gross Medical College were forced to merge and form the Denver and Gross College of Medicine. The pressures toward consolidation continued. In 1909 the Denver Homeopathic College closed. The same year, under the auspices of the Carnegie Foundation, educator Abraham Flexner went on a whirlwind tour, inspecting every medical school in the country. His visit to the Denver and Gross was not auspicious. Flexner's report, the enormously influential *Medical Education in the United States and Canada*, described the Denver and Gross as " . . . a proprietary school, managed by its own faculty . . . with a total absence of scientific activity, . . . a few cases of books in the college office behind the counters, and no full time professors."[14] The dean, referring to Flexner's observations as "unadulterated cussedness, . . . raw malice, . . . and percolated venom," attempted to answer each of the charges. Finally, he asked, "Why is Mr. Carnegie butting in anyway? Why has he assumed that it is his royal perogative to decide what are the best methods of medical teaching?"[15]

And Then There Was One: C.U. Medical School

The University of Colorado, on the other hand, was given a passing grade. More importantly, Flexner suggested that it alone, "can

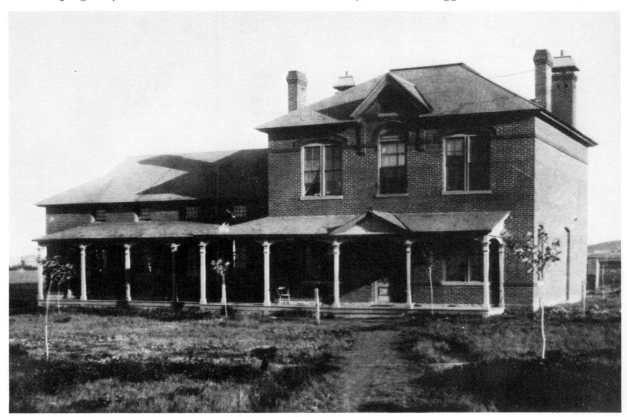

12.7 The first of the University of Colorado's University Hospitals was opened in Boulder in 1885. The present-day University Hospital is on the Health Sciences Center campus in Denver.

hope to obtain the financial backing necessary to teach medicine in the proper way, regardless of income from fees, and to it a monopoly should quickly fall."[16] The die had been cast, and by the end of 1910, Denver and Gross was absorbed by what had become, and would remain, the only medical school in the state, the University of Colorado School of Medicine. As one physician noted:

> Thus ended the early period in medical education [in Colorado] . . . Its history shows how strangely strength and frailty, wisdom and folly, are compounded in human character. There were great and good men in each of the schools.[17]

Another major problem for C. U. was solved that year—the inadequate clinical facilities. In 1910 a constitutional amendment was passed which allowed the School to move the clinical portion of what had become a four-year curriculum to Denver. The first two, or "basic science," years would continue to be taught in Boulder, and the last two, the "clinical years," would be taught in Denver. The old Archer mansion downtown was purchased as the school's Denver facility, and hasty arrangements were made with the County Hospital for clinical teaching.[18] The euphoria over the medical school's triumphs was, unfortunately, only temporary. The Archer mansion soon proved to be inadequate as the site for lecture and demonstration rooms, offices, outpatient clinics, and, on the third floor, a clinical laboratory. Furthermore, from the very beginning, conflicts began to emerge between the politically oriented administrators and staff of the County Hospital and the academically oriented administrators and faculty of the medical school. The school complained that medical and academic decisions at the hospital were being made without its input and for purely financial and political reasons, while the city charged that the school was meddling into its affairs and that its attitudes and demands were impractical and unrealistic. The situation became so heated that the dean was dropped from the hospital's staff. At the same time, there was little improvement in the status of the basic science facilities and faculty on the Boulder campus. Soon after his appointment in 1916, the new dean, Dr. Charles Meader, realized that the only solution to the medical school's problems was to consolidate the basic and clinical sciences on a single campus, include its own university hospital, and locate the whole complex where the population was, i.e. in Denver. For nearly a decade, Meader

devoted much of his time and effort towards that goal, one that would finally be fulfilled in 1925 (Chapter 22).

Deans, Faculty, and Students

In the meantime, there were additional problems for the deans of the medical school. The legislature and the community tended to be indifferent towards the school, the regents were sympathetic but impecunious, and the medical societies were concerned about the continuing pressure of newly graduated physicians on what they considered to be an oversupply of doctors in Colorado. There were disputes with the affiliated hospitals, and indigent patients were frequently "dumped" at the school's free dispensary. On the other hand, the availability of free care at the dispensary was deplored by some private physicians who complained that it also siphoned off some of their paying patients. There were disputes among the faculty, threatened resignations, and difficulties in recruiting new professors to a school which offered a maximum salary of $2,500 a year.[19] In his first year, Dean Meader complained to the president of the university about his office furniture ("for $55 they could be replaced by handsome pieces . . . of permanent value") and had to obtain the president's permission to spend six dollars for a new textbook for the library.[20] Students complained about faculty and faculty complained about students.

Nevertheless, despite its problems, the school continued to attract some outstanding faculty, especially to its departmental chairs. These were talented people who were willing to exchange some of their private practice income for the excitement and challenges of academics. Still, they were part-time faculty, and "if it happened to be inconvenient to give a lecture at the appointed time, the professor was absent."[21] The student newspaper reported such absences—such as the time when classes were cancelled so that two of the professors could take the train to one of the mining camps to perform an appendectomy.[22] Faculty attitudes towards the goals of medical education ranged over a wide spectrum, from those who were interested in graduating scientifically oriented physicians who, "breathing the spirit of pure science . . . point the way to our most brilliant successes in clinical medicine," to those who wanted to see more practically oriented family physicians, rather than "laboratory cynics and deadroom nihilopaths."[23] Discussions on curricular matters also reflected different approaches—some favoring lectures and others opposing lectures, some favoring emphasis on research, and others urging early exposure to clinical problems.[24]

As in most medical schools:

> The students came from every walk in life, some illiterate, many with a fair education. Some were rich, some poor . . . All came, on fire to be doctors.[25]

Of the twenty-nine medical students matriculated at the University of Colorado in 1889-1890, eighteen were Colorado residents, nine were from other states, and two were foreign.[26] At first, the great majority were men, generally of Anglo origin. Gradually, eastern and southern European and Jewish names began to appear on the roster. The first Hispanic surname is that of Tobias Espinosa (Class of 1902) and the first Oriental one is that of Sosuke Ochiai (Class of 1911).[27] The first woman to receive an M.D. from the University of Colorado was Dr. Nelly Mayo, in 1891, and in the years prior to 1910, twelve percent of the school's degrees were awarded to women.[28] Some of the male students were hostile to their female classmates, but the majority attitude seems to have been expressed by this student's somewhat patronizing but obviously well-intentioned comments in 1895:

> We have the new woman here studying medicine. She will succeed because she is so preparing herself that it is almost impossible to fail. God helps those who help themselves, and the new woman is helping herself just as rapidly as she can to everything she can lay her hands on. There is no reason why the new woman should not study medicine and be just as handsome and just as good as she could be in any other respect.[29]

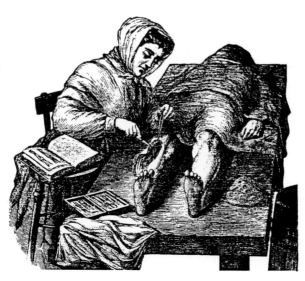

12.8 "We have the new woman here studying medicine."

Some of the out-of-state students had come to the state school in order to combine a medical education with the hopefully therapeutic effects of Colorado's climate on their tuberculosis.

Tuition was free in the early years and the cost of room and board was estimated at four to six dollars a week. By the 1920s, there was a quarterly tuition charge of forty dollars, and room and board had risen to eight to fourteen dollars a week. Many of the male students made ends meet by working part-time for the Denver Tramway Company, usually as conductors. Some had accumulated savings prior to entering medical school. Ridgway's Dr. B. B. Slick had worked as a railroad machinist and watchman in the roundhouse in Como, Cripple Creek's Dr. John Smith as a pharmacist's assistant in Black Hawk, and Breckenridge's Dr. A. Arbogast as a ditch tender at the Gold Run ditch in that mining camp.[30] Then, as now, medical school was demanding and the students worked hard. One student groaned: "The other day I was asked: 'Do you folks study hard?' Oh! Ye Gods!"[31]

There was time, however, for an occasional diversion—football, a picnic, or a dance, and, as a student noted one spring, "The practical study of the game of quoits is proving more interesting than books just now to our tired students."[32] Another student, apparently burnt out, sought refuge "in the shadow of Pike's Peak. The turmoil of Denver became too much for me and now I am trying to forget that I ever saw such a thing as a medical book or another medical student."[33]

Medical Research

[At the medical school] there are now 6 guinea pigs and 20 rabbits which are being carefully nurtured. These are to be used in experimental work . . .

Silver and Gold (University of Colorado), 1908[34]

In the early days, medical research in Colorado was pretty much limited to physicians reporting their interesting cases or, perhaps, a series of cases. The introduction of a new technique, instrument, or therapy provided the basis for many papers. The data was empirically derived, controlled studies were unheard of, and the opinions of one's peers formed the major basis for evaluation. Hundreds of such papers were published, mainly in Colorado's, but also in national, medical journals; and some physicians accumulated large bibliographies. In addition to the usual areas of clinical interest, Colo-

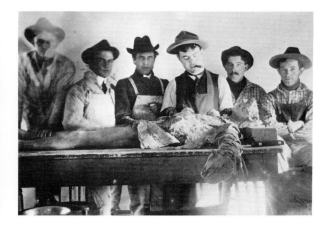

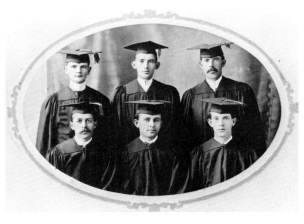

12.9 A medical student was asked: "Do you folks study hard?" He responded: "Oh! Ye Gods!" The University of Colorado's Class of '05 in the anatomy laboratory and, four years later, at graduation.

rado's early medical authors published numerous articles on tuberculosis and climatology.

There was almost no experimental work in the early years. One notable exception was the work of Gerald Webb, an outstanding clinician who, for many years, studied the role of lymphocytes and immunologic phenomena in tuberculosis at his Tuberculosis Institute in Colorado Springs.[35] Webb examined the effects of lymphocytes on tubercle bacilli and the effects of altitude on these white blood cells. Observing that altitude increased the number of circulating lymphocytes and that lymphocytes destroyed tubercle bacilli, Webb concluded that he had found evidence for a mechanism by which Colorado's high altitude exerted its beneficial effects on patients with tuberculosis. Although some of his findings were later determined to be incorrect, and his search for an immunologic means to

combat tuberculosis was unsuccessful, Webb's research has been said to have contributed "the basis for many subsequent discoveries" by other scientists.[36] Dr. Webb may have been the first investigator in Colorado to have been awarded a research grant, a thousand dollars from the A.M.A.[37]

Webb had been influenced by the work of a young physiologist at the University of Michigan, Henry Sewall. Sewall had found that repeated inoculations of small doses of snake venom resulted in the eventual immunity of the host to a large dose. In 1887 Sewall proposed that the same principle might be used to protect the host against bacterial toxins.[39] This hypothesis, although unacknowledged, was the basis for the diphtheria, tetanus, and other antitoxins which were introduced to a grateful world a few years later. Within two years, however,

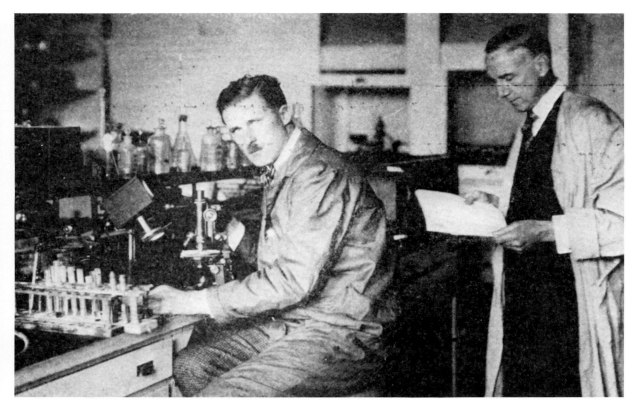

12.10 The pioneer research of Dr. Gerald Webb and his colleagues in pulmonary diseases is continued today at the Webb-Waring Institute at the University of Colorado's Health Sciences Center. Dr. Webb is on the right.

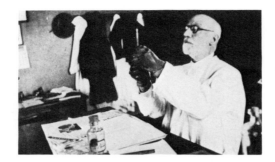

12.11 Medical school faculty had to support themselves through practice, leaving little opportunity for research. Dr. Henry Sewall, who began his career in research at the University of Michigan, returned to the laboratory in his later years at the University of Colorado.

Sewall was recovering from tuberculosis in Colorado. In exchange for teaching physiology, he was allowed to enroll, tuition-free, at the Denver Medical College and subsequently received his M.D. For the next two decades, Sewall devoted most of his attention to his extensive practice in Denver, specializing in cardiology, and serving as Professor of Medicine at the University of Colorado. In 1915 he resumed his research. It was said that he maintained a colony of several hundred guinea pigs in the attic of his home during this time, and he continued his research activities virtually until his death in 1936 at the age of eighty-one.

There were other scattered attempts at research in Colorado, and not always by well-known scientists and professors. A railroad surgeon, for example, Dr. F. Gregory Connell, investigated the effects of different kinds of intestinal sutures in experimental animals while employed by the Denver and Rio Grande Hospital in Salida. His work was published in the *Journal of the American Medical Association* in 1906.[40]

Although more than 100 papers were published by the University of Colorado's medical school faculty in 1911-1912, none of them involved experimental work. One basic scientist recalled that the large teaching load "left little time for research" and the *Regent's Report* for 1919-1920 noted that "the conduct of research is seriously hampered by insufficient personnel and equipment."[41] It was not until the 1920s, particularly after the move of the basic science departments to the new Denver campus, and the appointment of several distinguished scientists to the faculty, that experimental work was undertaken to any significant degree at the medical school.

13 SPECIALISTS AND SPECIALTIES

There is as much difference between work on the eye and gynecology as between the nose and throat and dentistry. The problems of diagnosis, with the uncertainty of drug action, makes one man like internal medicine, while the quick and certain results of operative works makes a surgeon of the other.

W.A. Kickland, M.D. (Fort Collins), 1909[1]

Don't think that we [family practitioners] are lowering our standard when we admit that certain doctors, who have fitted themselves for special work, do that work better than we.

W.W. Harmer, M.D. (Greeley), 1912[2]

NEARLY ALL OF Colorado's earliest physicians were generalists. They were expected to be able to diagnose and treat dropsy, whooping cough, and mountain fever, perform a difficult delivery, pull a tooth, set a fracture, and amputate a limb. In the tiny ranching community or the isolated mining camp, the solo practitioner had no choice. In the larger town, with several physicians, competing generalists had little choice. If his own limited skill or lack of expertise was perceived by his patient, the case might wind up in the willing hands of his ambitious colleague down the street. A physician could not long survive the loss of patients or of reputation.

Gradually, especially in the cities, a few physicians became known for their expertise in specific areas. A few took post-graduate training in eastern or European medical centers. The development of new instruments, methods and procedures in the second half of the nineteenth century contributed to the development of medical specialties and the specialties were soon formalized by the organization of societies. The American Ophthalmological and Otological Societies were formed in the 1860s; they were followed by neurology, dermatology, gynecol-

ogy, surgery, urology, orthopedics, and pediatrics. Most of Colorado's specialists were concentrated in Denver. By the early 1900s, the growth of specialization had made some general practitioners wonder about the future of their professional status. Dr. H. B. Whitney was only half jesting when he told the Colorado Medical Society:

We find the good old family doctor prophetically deposited upon the junk heap of the not too distant

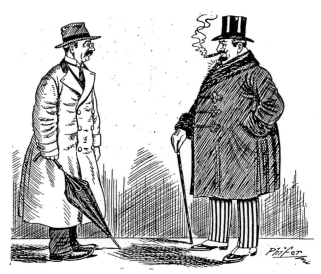

13.1 The general practitioner and the city specialist. The caption reads: "Which do you think is which?"

future . . . Many of us can manage to subsist only by the aid of speculation, participation in the drug business, or growing beans in the back yard.[3]

However, he quickly reassured his audience,

> Let no one fear that the day of the family physician is really past. More than ever before, there is need of the man of broad attainments and far vision; if for nothing else, to protect the public against the specialist.[3]

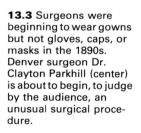

DAVID McCAW,
——Physician and Surgeon——

Treatment of Diseases of the Eye, Ear and Throat
a Specialty.

Office, Dutton's Block,   *OURAY, COLO.*

13.2 Specialization was not limited to the big cities. This advertisement appeared in a Colorado business directory in 1889.

Surgery and the Appendectomy

In the twenty years following the Civil War, surgery was little changed from pre-bellum times or, for that matter, from previous centuries. Despite occasional heroic attempts, and the introduction of general anaesthesia in the 1840s, abdominal surgery was essentially limited to an occasional gynecologic operation or a drainage procedure. The thoracic and cranial cavities remained virtually untouched.

The major impasse to internal surgery was the danger of post-operative infection and the resultant high mortality. In the 1860s antiseptic measures, such as the use of carbolic acid sprays and other disinfectants were introduced. This was followed, later in the century, by such fundamental aseptic techniques as the washing of hands, the sterilization of instruments, and the wearing of gowns and gloves. Even with these improvements, in the 1880s centuries of accumulated experience continued to make surgeons hesitate to enter the body cavities. In 1889, of 402 operations performed in one of New York's major hospitals, only thirty-two were abdominal, and a significant number of these were gynecologic. Most had been done to drain abscesses. There were no instances of surgery for gall bladder disease or intestinal cancer that year and only one appendectomy.[4]

Actually, the emergence of the appendectomy in the last two decades of the nineteenth century marks the beginning of modern surgery. Surgeons had long been aware of the clinical pattern of right lower quadrant abdominal pain, fever, and prostration which occurred predominantly in young people and often progressed to shock and death. In the occasional case subjected to surgical exploration, the right lower quadrant and its contents were encased in pus, and, if the condition had been present for some time, within a mass of adhesions and abscesses. The primary site of the disease, then termed "typhilitis" or "perityphilitis," was uncertain. Most cases were treated medically, and the only accepted surgical procedure was to incise the abdominal cavity and allow the infected area to drain. Occasion-

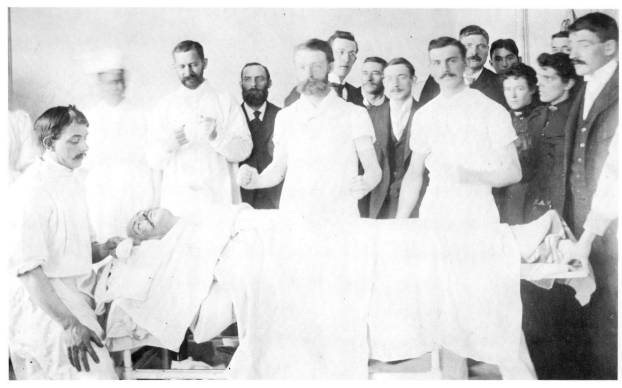

13.3 Surgeons were beginning to wear gowns but not gloves, caps, or masks in the 1890s. Denver surgeon Dr. Clayton Parkhill (center) is about to begin, to judge by the audience, an unusual surgical procedure.

ally, the infection dissected its way throught the adjacent soft tissues and skin, forming a chronically infected fistulous tract.

Such was the case in December 1882, when Dr. W. W. Grant was called to the home of a twenty-two-year-old woman school teacher in Davenport, Iowa. Grant, who later became a prominent surgeon in Denver, recalled the case years later.[5] By January there had been no improvement, and Grant decided to enlarge the fistula. In probing deeply into the tract, he encountered a prune pit and concluded that the source of infection was enteric, probably a perforated appendix. Although he knew that an appendectomy was indicated, he felt obliged to follow standard medical procedures and continued to irrigate and drain the wound. This approach was approved by a leading surgical consultant from Chicago who "declined to sanction the operation [appendectomy] on account of the 'great danger.'" The patient's condition did not improve, however, and "worn out with failure and deferred hope, [she] now gave me [Grant] unlimited discretion to perform the operation I had urged for a year." On January 4, 1885, Dr. Grant, assisted by two of his colleagues, operated on a kitchen table in the woman's home. He "deliberately opened the abdomen over the cecum, . . . inserted two fingers in search of the appendix . . . " and went on to perform what appears to have been the nation's first appendectomy. Subsequent attempts to close the fistula were unsuccessful, but the patient did well and moved to a new job in South Dakota. Six years later, Dr. Grant, now located in Denver, received a letter from his long-lost patient. She wrote, "If you think you can now close up the opening, I will come to Denver at once." The procedure was done in Denver's St. Luke's Hospital in January 1892. Twelve years later, Dr. Grant heard that she was alive and well.

Dr. Grant did not report his appendectomy until 1892, in the *Colorado Medical Journal*.[6] In the meantime, the eminent Harvard pathologist, Reginald Fitz, had introduced the concept and the term "appendicitis," and the New York surgeon, Charles McBurney, had made appendectomy an acceptable procedure. Grant's accomplishment, published in remote Colorado several years after Fitz, McBurney, and others had brought the lowly appendix into the surgical spotlight, remained unrecognized.[7]

As with so many "new" diseases, appendicitis evolved, virtually overnight, from a nonentity to a common disease. The excitement was summarized in a poem published in the *New York*

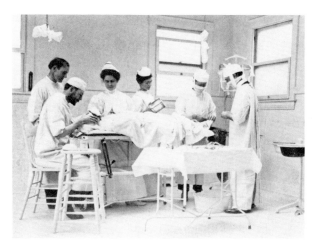

13.4 By the early 1900s, caps, masks, and gowns were being used, by at least some members of the surgical team.

World, "Appendicitis—The Latest Fad." It began:

> Have you got the new disorder?
> If you haven't, 'tis in order
> To succumb to it at once without delay.
> It is called appendicitis—
> Very different from gastritis
> Or the common trash diseases of the day.[8]

Appendectomy had broken the barriers to abdominal surgery, and, by the turn of the nineteenth century, many surgeons were doing large numbers of abdominal operations. Denver's Dr. I.B. Perkins reported 173 abdominal operations which he did over a two-and one-half-year period.[9] In addition to a large number of gynecologic procedures, he had done forty-five appendectomies, sixteen herniorrhaphies, eight gall bladder operations, and eleven exploratory laparotomies. Surgery was quickly moving beyond hernias, appendices and gall bladders, and surgeons were rapidly expanding their horizons to the cranial and thoracic cavities as well.

Psychiatry, Insanity, and the State Insane Asylum

In the nineteenth century, the major domain of what we now call "psychiatry" was the care of the insane. According to Colorado's General Laws of 1879, any "reputable" individual could file a complaint, in court, alleging that a "person is a lunatic or insane person."[10] The court then ordered the sheriff to apprehend and confine the alleged lunatic pending an inquest. The inquest consisted of a jury of six citizens appointed to "ascertain whether such person is so insane or distracted in mind as to be incapable and unfit to care for and manage his or her estate." Insanity was not defined for the jurors. Provision for medical input was not specified, although physicians were often called to provide expert testimony. If the jury found that the person was insane, the court committed "such insane person . . . to the county jail or other convenient place," or to the custody of a "suitable and proper relative or friend." Included among the insane were people with psychosis, chronic alchoholism or drug addiction, dementia, mental retardation, and various forms of organic brain disease—all treated alike.

Although primitive by later standards, late nineteenth century management of the insane can be considered to have been enlightened when compared to earlier times. Previously, the insane were considered bewitched or possessed by demons, and such spirits were exorcised by a variety of violent means. Not much better was the view of moralists who considered insanity to be the natural consequence of a stern Providence meting out punishment for immorality, weakness, or original sin. In the early nineteenth century, society often sequestered its poor, criminals, and insane together in public institutions—combination jails, hospitals, and poorhouses. In 1848 an emerging social conciousness in the United States was highlighted by the Congressional testimony of reformer Dorothea Dix. The unremitting scrutiny of Miss Dix and other humanitarians revealed a scandalous litany of inhuman treatment of the insane—of chains and beatings, filth and cages. States began to build asylums for their insane, and some semblance of medical care and research was begun. In Indiana, for example, Dr. John Evans, then a a small-town practitioner, campaigned for a State Asylum for the Insane.[11] Evans was successful, became the asylum's first superintendent, and was commended by Miss Dix. Years later he became Colorado's second territorial governor.

Prior to 1879 Colorado's insane were housed in county hospitals, jails, or the homes of relatives or friends. In the fall of 1879, the State Asylum for the Insane was opened near Pueblo, Colorado. The superintendent during the asylum's first two decades was Dr. Pembroke R. Thombs, a Civil War veteran who had come to Pueblo in 1866 to practice medicine and surgery.[12] Dr. Thombs read about mental and nervous diseases to prepare himself for his new job. The asylum was a former estate which was remodeled to include, in the main building, ten 6x8-foot "cells" and two bathrooms. There was room for thirty-eight men and women.[13] The State Board of Health reported:

> A cheerful, healthful condition pervades the whole institution. Dr. Thombs has evidently made a success of the Asylum . . . The only real objection . . . is want of room.[13]

Gradually, additions were built, and by 1896 the asylum's census was up to more than 400 patients. Nevertheless, there was always a shortage of space, and that year it was said that there were many persons, especially women, who were "confined in the county hospitals and jails . . . waiting vacancies."[14] By paring expenses, Superintendent Thombs was able to keep costs down to forty cents per patient day. For years, Thombs continued to be the only physician on the premises. The president of the State Board of Lunacy Commissioners complained:

> How one medical man, no matter how skillful, conscientious and faithful he may be, can attend to 400 or 500 patients each day is beyond my comprehension. Such a state of things makes an insane asylum a place of detention, rather than a hospital for the treatment of the mentally ill . . .[14]

In addition, there were only eleven attendants during the day and just a night watchman in the evenings.[15] Complicating matters was the fact that the institution provided virtually unrestricted access to visitors, mainly "sightseers and curiosity hunters."[16] By 1898 things were so bad that the board reminded the state:

> Beyond a certain point, economy is criminal in the management of this institution. This class of people is the last class for pinching and a stringent economy to be practiced upon. A careful investigation . . . discloses no extravagance.[17]

Unfortunately, the same year saw "sensational charges . . . against the management of the asylum, . . . charges of neglect of the institution and patients as well, besides immorality among the attendants . . ."[18] Although the charges were never made public, and the superintendent was cleared of all responsibility, Dr. Thombs was burnt out and he resigned in 1900.[19] Problems of overcrowding and inadequate care continued to plague the asylum. By 1916 there were more than 1,200 patients, and the legislature had changed the institution's

13.5 When it opened in 1879, the State Insane Asylum in Pueblo had 38 patients. By the 1920s, its census was up to nearly 3,000.

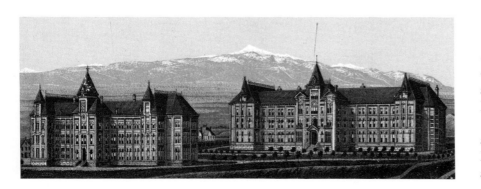

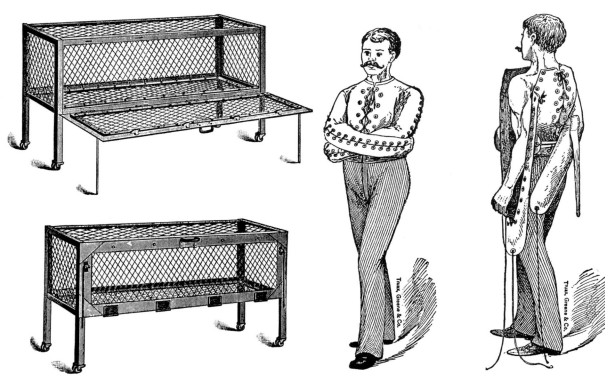

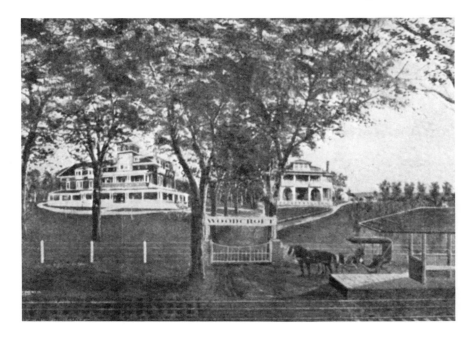

13.6 There was little opportunity for treatment at the state asylum. With one physician and a handful of attendants, restraints were used frequently. Left: "Protection bed for the insane." Right: Typical straightjacket.

name to the Colorado State Hospital. By the late 1920s, there were nearly 3,000 patients.

In the latter half of the nineteenth century, concepts of mental illness were undergoing a transition from medieval precepts to the fundamental tenets of twentieth century psychiatry. In its report on "Insanity" in 1877, the State Board of Health adopted the new and somewhat radical view that:

> A diseased mind is proof of a diseased body, and conclusive evidence that the principal disturbance is located in the nervous system, usually the brain . . . Every action of our body is brought about upon mechanical properties and is amenable to its laws.[20]

So much for demons and original sin. Instead, said the Board of Health, mental illness was due to a loss of "nerve power," and just as overstrain of a muscle results in "fatigue, pain, and refusal of the muscle to do its work, the same holds good as to our brain and nerves—fatigue, inability to fix the attention, defective memory, irresolution, irritablility, despondency, incoherence, [etc] . . ." Dr. Thombs, in his presidential address to the Colorado Medical Society in 1883, called for research into the causes of "insanity" (i.e. mental illness), as well as such other societal afflictions as mental retardation, criminality, and "pauperism."[21] Like many of his contemporaries, Thombs supported an organic and genetic basis for insanity and invoked the then popular theory of biological determinism.

Not far from the state asylum, Dr. Hubert Work ran a private sanitarium, the Woodcroft

Hospital for Nervous and Mental Disease. Unlike Thombs's huge understaffed and underfunded asylum, Work's sanitarium housed a small number private patients. Here then, a therapeutic approach was possible.[22] Many of Dr. Work's patients were depressed and refused to eat. Such patients would probably have starved at the asylum, but at Woodcroft adequate staffing allowed forced feeding by nasogastric tube—a routine meal consisting of four raw eggs, a quart of milk, a little salt, and a bit of whiskey. Dr. Work encouraged his patients to sleep and, when awake, to engage in exercise, e.g. "a brisk walk in the grounds between strong attendants." Chloral was used as

13.7 Dr. Hubert Work's Woodcroft Hospital was a private institution. Its therapeutic approaches to managing the insane patient reflected late nineteenth century psychiatric concepts and teachings.

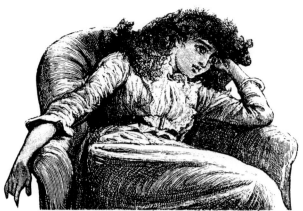

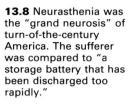

13.8 Neurasthenia was the "grand neurosis" of turn-of-the-century America. The sufferer was compared to "a storage battery that has been discharged too rapidly."

a "hypnotic," bromides to induce sleep, ergot for "cerebral congestion," and cannabis Indica for "melancholia." Work pointed out that "the insane should never be punished, but restraints are often necessary . . . The room of an insane patient should have no furnishing except a bed on the floor, and one chair so heavy that it cannot be used as a weapon . . ." Firmness mixed with kindness was an essential part of treatment, but friends and relatives were not permitted to visit the patients. Dr. Work's hospital and management program was the prototype for care of those of the mentally ill who could afford it at the turn of the century in Colorado.

As psychiatry began to emerge as a discipline, in addition to articles on "the insane," Colorado's psychiatrists began to contribute papers dealing with such topics as neurosis and psychotherapy. Some authors dealt with the postulated effects of Colorado's climate and altitude on mental illness. As one early psychiatrist, Dr. H. T. Pershing, pointed out, "There has been a widespread popular belief in Colorado that the altitude in some way causes functional nervous disorders to be far more prevalent than at sea-level."[23] Many early physicians had suggested that, while serious mental illness was no more common or severe in Colorado, neurotic illnesses were—especially in women. As Dr. Pershing put it, this concept had "originated with the pioneers in pre-neurological times [and] was sometimes qualified by the remark that the climate was not so bad for men, but hard on women and horses." His own opinion on the matter was quite clear: "I have come to regard it as a baseless error, which the medical profession should actively oppose." Another distinguished neuropsychiatrist, Dr. J. T. Eskridge, stated the prevailing opinion—"There is little doubt that those with inherent nervous temperaments are made more nervous by a prolonged residence in Colorado."[24]

What many of these physicians were referring to was the grand neurosis of industrial age

America, neurasthenia. Dr. Pershing described neurasthenia, or "nerve weakness," as the result of an excessively active nervous system that had become exhausted, "like a storage battery that has been discharged too rapidly or for too long a time."[25] The disorder was felt to be a by-product of modern culture and due to the excessive brain work demanded by an industrialized society. Symptoms included irritability, insomnia, dyspepsia, palpitations and flushing, paresthesias, absent-mindedness, and impotency. Neurasthenia was a fashionable disorder, one which identified its victim as an active participant in business, professional, and cultural endeavors, i.e. the nineteenth century equivalent of a Yuppie. It was especially prevalent among educated and emancipated women.

Hundreds of different therapeutic approaches were offered, including all sorts of quack remedies and devices— hydrotherapy, magnetic belts, massage, vibrators, electrical machines, and so on. Dr. Pershing suggested a regimen of oxygen, a diet rich in meat and eggs, stimulants (e.g. strychnia), codeine or small doses of opium, and lots of sleep. Denver's Dr. Bernard Oettinger felt that enemas were the key to eliminating neurasthenic toxins while Grand Junction's Dr. H. S. Day preferred bromides, ergot, tonics, and laxatives.[26]

In the meantime, the concepts of Sigmund Freud and his colleagues were being widely disseminated, and even in Colorado, general practitioners and country doctors were beginning to encounter the vagaries of psychoneurosis. Neuropsychiatrists such as Denver's Dr. Edmund Rogers were forever reminding the practitioner that "the mind is constantly playing an active part in influencing the results in all medical treatment."[27] Somewhat bewildered, somewhat skeptical, many Colorado doctors must have chuckled when they read Mr. Dooley and his friend Hennessy's discussion of "psychotherapeutics" in the pages of *Colorado Medicine:*

'But what does sycotherapewticks ra-ally mane?' asked Hennessy, with a dazed expression.

'That's what no wan seems ter clearly undherstan,' replied Mr. Dooley. 'As near as I can make out, it's a spacies iv spiritool flim-flam . . .'[28]

Internal Medicine: Diagnosis and Treatment

In the early nineteenth century, what we now regard as internal medicine was pretty much the province of general practitioners. As the century progressed, some physicians began to eliminate surgery and obstetrics from their practice and concentrated on those areas which we now regard as the medical subspecialties, e.g. cardiology, pulmonary diseases, gastroenterology, renal diseases, neurology, and infectious diseases. The premier internist in early Colorado was probably Dr. J. N. Hall. Hall, whom we encountered earlier in this book as a pioneer country doctor in Sterling, Colorado, moved to Denver in 1892 and served as Professor of Medicine at the University of Colorado for many years. During this time, he wrote papers in virtually every medical subspecialty and a two-volume opus in internal medicine which emphasized diagnostic skills and techniques.[29]

Hall was an inveterate record keeper. In his huge practice, for example, he analyzed some 600 cases of heart disease, providing us with a cross-section of turn-of-the-century Colorado cardiology.[30] The art of auscultation and the clinicopathologic correlation of cardiac murmurs was in ascendance, and nearly three-fourths of Hall's patients were diagnosed as having lesions of the cardiac valves. On the other hand, there was little understanding of the relationship between coronary artery obstruction and myocardial ischemia. Myocardial infarction was generally regarded as a form of inflammation. Hall did ascribe several cases of cardiac death to "arteriosclerosis." In a contemporary paper, a lesser known Denver physician made two prescient remarks with regard to the soon-to-be evident onslaught of coronary artery disease. In commenting on the post-mortem lesions of what we would now recognize as myocardial ischemia, Dr. E. C. Hill observed that "the heart is often starved because of thickening . . . of the coronary arteries."[31] He also remarked that "arteriosclerosis [now] occurs earlier than in former times, owing to the hypertension of modern life."

Pulmonary diseases such as asthma, bronchitis, pleurisy and pneumonia, and influenza and tuberculosis were common and readily diagnosed, but in the pre-cigarette era, emphysema was hardly mentioned, and lung cancer was a rare disease. The various forms of arthritis were generally lumped together as "rheumatism," and most renal diseases were termed "Bright's disease." Peptic ulcer was recognized, but a variety of gastroenterologic disorders were classified as "dyspepsia." Jaundice was usually ascribed to "bilious fever" and cirrhosis was infrequently alluded to, despite the frequency of alcoholism. Generalized edema, whether of cardiac, renal, or hepatic origin, was termed "dropsy." Specific

hematologic diseases such as pernicious anemia were being recognized, but leukemia was just beginning to be diagnosed with any frequency. Diabetes mellitus was said to be a rare disease in Colorado, one Denver internist noting only a single case in his large practice.[32]

The latter half of the nineteenth century was marked by improvement in pathogenetic concepts and diagnosis, but medical treatment was still primitive. The ancient techniques of cupping, purging, and bloodletting were being discarded, but slowly and not without resistance. From a Central City, Colorado, newspaper of 1871, for example:

> J. H. McMurday has been in a succession of convulsions since yesterday. Wednesday afternoon he manifested some signs of recovery and today he is much better. One half gallon of blood was taken from him.[33]

The pharmacopoeia was filled with the same drugs that physicians had been using for the past century or in some instances, since ancient time. A page in a standard medical supply catalogue included such standbys as:

> Bronchitis compound—belladonna, Dover's powder, ipecac, and quinine
>
> Brown Mixture—licorice, camphor, benzoic acid, anise, opium, and tartar emetic.
>
> Carminative—strychnine, black pepper, ipecac, gentian, oleoresin capsicum.
>
> Cold medicine—camphor, quinine, morphine, atropine, and glycyrrhiza.

A pharmacological revolution was in the making, however. The organic chemists were becoming more adept in their molecular manipulations and syntheses, and biochemistry was emerging as a science. The foundations of immunoprophylaxis were being laid and applied, as in the production of an antitoxin to diphtheria. A physician in Pueblo was using "an extract of suprarenal capsule" (corticosteroids) as an anti-inflammatory agent.[34] In the 1880s, oxygen was being manufactured in Denver and touted as "one of Nature's remedies."[35]

Radiology and the Radium Boom

Unlike other medical specialties which evolved gradually, radiology appeared virtually overnight with Dr. Wilhelm Roentgen's demonstration of the X-ray in Germany in December 1895. Less than two months later, two professors from Colorado Springs' Colorado College traveled to Denver to demonstrate the

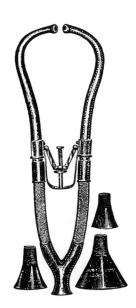

13.9 This "new, improved" stethoscope was designed by Denver's Dr. Denison. Then as now the stethoscope was a symbol of the physician, especially the internist. Nowadays, it is often artfully draped around the medical student's or resident's neck.

new marvel. More than 300 physicians packed the grand ballroom at the Brown Palace Hotel to view the array of glass tubes and huge batteries, to hear the crackling sounds and see the eerie lights, and finally, to witness for themselves the "power of the mystifying and mysterious X-rays."[36] Two months later another meeting was held, this time including not only physicians but "their ladies, scientists, and the curious."[37] The evening's high point was a "live" demonstration by the president of the Mountain Electric Company. The subject was Dr. W. F. Hassenplug, specifically the doctor's right hand. After three minutes of X-ray exposure, the plate was developed, and the resultant "skiagraph" clearly demonstrated a piece of buckshot between the third and fourth metacarpals. The doctor explained that he suffered a gunshot wound several years before and had always wanted to know exactly where the shot had lodged. Since it didn't cause him any pain, he was "perfectly" satisfied to continue to wear it as a memento."

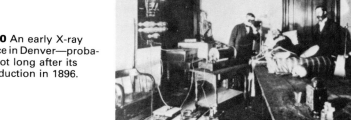

13.10 An early X-ray device in Denver—probably not long after its introduction in 1896.

Although there was some resentment over all the hoop-la (public demonstrations were held in churches and department stores and patients were clamoring for the new procedure), its clinical value was soon demonstrated when X-rays were used to locate a swallowed toy wheel in a child (after ten minutes exposure) and a bullet near the spine of a gunshot victim (after thirty minutes exposure).[38] Another celebrated case occurred in March 1896. The patient was Central City's marshal, Mike Keleher. The marshal, who had been shot in the line of duty, had been sent to Denver, and Dr. Chauncey Tennant's X-ray machine showed the bullet to be lodged in the mediastinum. Ironically, the marshal had been shot by a man who had objected to a court order to pay a physician's bill.

In 1898, less than three years after Roentgen's work, Madame Curie, analyzing the uranium ore pitchblende, discovered its even more radioactive derivative, radium. The powerful

13.11 An early chest X-ray taken by Denver radiologist Dr. S.B. Childs.

new element was soon put to medical use.[39] Even the richest ore contained minute amounts of radium, and tons of rock were required to obtain a single gram—making radium one of the rarest and most expensive materials on earth. The world's entire annual production was measured in ounces, at more than a million dollars an ounce. Its rarity, expense, and therapeutic potential excited the public and the press, and radium was a "hot" topic in the early 1900s. Colorado was the world's major source of radium during this time. Pitchblende, the ore in which radium had originally been discovered, had been found in the area around Central City back in that mining district's early days. Later prospectors discovered vast quantities of another radium ore, carnotite, in the Paradox Valley and nearby sites on Colorado's western slope. A Colorado radium "boom" developed, not unlike the later post-World War II uranium "boom." Several large radium mining and refining enterprises emerged. The Flannery brothers, one-time Pittsburgh undertakers, made their first strike in 1911 near present-day Uravan on the Dolores River and formed the Standard Chemical Company. Another outfit, the Radium Company of Colorado, set up a laboratory and an extraction plant in central Denver.[40] In addition, the National Radium Institute, organized in 1913, set up an extraction plant in South Denver. The institute was formed by Dr. Howard A. Kelly, the famed Johns Hopkins gynecologist. By 1917, the institute had extracted enough radium from Paradox Valley ore

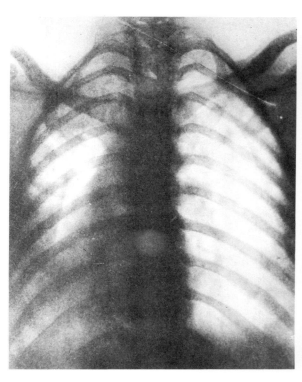

to provide Baltimore's Kelly Hospital with what may have been the largest amount of radium (five and one half grams) at any single location in the world.[41]

Radium wasn't just mined in Colorado. As in the rest of the country, it was widely used medically. In 1914 a Colorado physician reviewed the medical status of radium for the Colorado Medical Society:

> That radium has, within the past few years, come to be a therapeutic agent of great importance, to be reckoned with by the medical man, no one will deny ... No one can follow the work of [those studying the medical uses of radium] without catching the enthusiasm and anticipation of what is in the near future for us along this line.[42]

Denver's Dr. George Stover was one of the first physicians in the country to actually limit his practice to radiology.[43] Stover was a pioneer in the therapeutic use of X-rays and radium. Like many early radiologists, he tended to minimize the harmful effects of radiation. In 1902 he wrote:

> I have a dermatitis of the left hand of some five years standing, and I believe it is better than it used to be, though I am using the rays more and more every day and I take no precautions to prevent dermatitis.[44]

Several years later Stover was in Boston, having multiple small cancers excised from his hands. Despite skin grafts, the lesions healed poorly, and "it was a common sight to see the doctor with his left arm in a sling."[45] In the meantime he served as dean of the Denver and Gross Medical College, Professor of Roentgenology at the University of Colorado and editor of the *Denver Medical Times*. At the age of forty-four, after more than 150 skin grafts, he went to Johns Hopkins to have a finger amputated. He was found dead in his Baltimore hotel room. Stover's attitude towards the high price he paid for his research is reflected in his comment, made a few years before his death, that "A few dead or crippled scientists do not weigh much against a useful fact ..."[46]

Perhaps Stover and his colleagues should have known better. A doctor in Central City, where pitchblende had originally been mined, had told the story of

> a miner [who] came to him one day with an intractable ulcer of some weeks' duration ... situated just under the watch pocket of [his] ... trousers ... In a few days, another miner came in, with a duplicate ulcer! Then the doctor's native shrewdness came to his help. He knew ... that [miners]

always carry the choicest bit of ore that they have found in that identical pocket ... He said to the miner, "Jim, what kind of ore are you at work in lately?" Then he learned that it was pitchblende, and the miner told him that he had carried the best piece of ore he had ever found in that pocket for weeks.[47]

Gynecology and "Women's Diseases"

The first report of a gynecologic operation in Colorado was presented at the second meeting of the Territorial Medical Society in 1872 by Dr. S.B. Davis of Central City.[48] Davis's patient was a forty-two year-old woman who had a large, rapidly growing uterine tumor. "Believing that she could live but a few months unless relieved by an operation," Davis and six other physicians gathered on September 2, 1872, to perform the surgery. A supracervical hysterectomy was done and the resected uterine corpus contained a "fibroid tumor ... the size of an adult head." Unfortunately, two days later, the woman died.

By 1875 Dr. Eugene Gehrung, Colorado's pioneer gynecologist, had reported several successful uterine and vaginal procedures.[49] In 1884 Dr. H. A. Lemen reviewed the twenty-three cases of abdominal surgery for "the relief of ovarian cystoma, morbid growths connected with the uterus, and other diseased conditions of the pelvic viscera" which had been done in Colorado up to that time.[50] The results were not good— only nine of the twenty-three patients had survived, and Lemen suggested that it might be wise for women who needed gynecologic surgery to go East. Denver's Dr. Thomas Hawkins, whose Hospital for Women had several patients awaiting gynecologic surgery, felt otherwise:

> I shall not hesitate to operate on any or all of them, just so soon as I can get their consent. Why send patients East? I believe that we have as good talent in the medical profession of Denver, as can be found anywhere in the world.[51]

Much of gynecologic treatment was non-surgical. Many so-called "women's problems were ascribed to uterine displacements. The treatment was replacement, accomplished by the insertion of pessaries, rubber rings, and other devices. Dr. Josiah Slick, a physician in the railroad town of Como, reported a case in which a pessary, placed five years earlier and subsequently forgotten, was discovered and removed, thereby relieving the patient's severe discomfort.[52] Other therapies, less common though more exotic, were also used—including the application of leeches to relieve "congestion" of

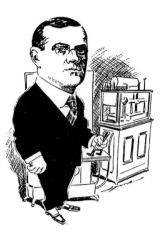

13.12 Like many other pioneer radiologists, Denver's Dr. George Stover paid a high price for his unprotected exposure to radiation. He felt that the benefits justified the cost.

the cervix. Denver's Dr. S. Cole described an unusual example from his own practice:

> I threw in two leeches and, after having unsuccessfully spent about a half hour in trying to induce them to bite, I crammed a wad of cotton into the speculum to maintain them in position against the cervix. Hardly had I completed this manoeuvre when my patient complained of an intense colicky pain. I withdrew the cotton at once, and found but one leech in the speculum. My missing leech had evidently made its way up into the cavity of the womb.[53]

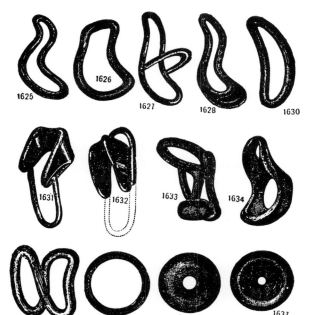

13.13 Pessaries, in innumerable sizes and shapes, were available to the nineteenth century gynecologist.

Dr. Cole next passed a probe into the uterine cavity, "stirring up his lordship to such an extent, that his quarters became uncomfortable," and the errant beast "made his appearance, slowly crawling from the os."

Dysmenorrhea and menstrual disorders were highly controversial topics, and innumerable means were used in their treatment. All sorts of tonics and other medicines, manipulations and exercises, and techniques and procedures were advocated by physicians and quacks alike. Electricity was one of the more popular means of therapy, and one of its best known proponents was Denver's Dr. Minnie C. T. Love. She described her patients as "women and girls who [have] suffered for years [and] who have been

dosed and 'built up' without relief from suffering until they are completely discouraged."[54] Typical was Miss K., age 21, to whom Dr. Love gave twenty applications of 'faradism and galvanism to the abdomen and endometrium." Dr. Love described her satisfaction as she watched the "decidedly blue uterus grow pink under the application of electricity to the [uterine] neck."

Obstetrics, Childbirth, Puerperal Fever, and Abortion

In a four year period, 1868-1871, Denver's Dr. Richard Buckingham delivered 286 babies.[55] In his series, he had only ten abnormal deliveries—including two breech presentations and five instances of prematurity or stillbirth. Buckingham must have been an excellent doctor—and a lucky one!

Typically, delivery was done in the patient's home. There was little in the way of pre- or postnatal care, and although the physician could assist in labor, apply forceps, and even attempt to correct an abnormal fetal presentation, there was little he could do about eclampsia, hemorrhage, or shock, and few physicians would attempt a Caesarian section. Most medical schools taught obstetrics by lecture, sometimes supplemented by demonstrations on wooden models. Even in the early twentieth century, many medical students graduated without having performed a delivery. Most physician-assisted deliveries were done by general practitioners.

Many of Colorado's women lived on farms or ranches or in mining camps at some distance from medical care. Harriet Fish Backus was the wife of a mining engineer at the Tomboy mine above Telluride.[56] When her labor pains came, she walked down to the Miner's Hospital in town. It was more difficult for Harriet's friend, Amy. Amy's cabin was at the Liberty Bell, well above the Tomboy among 13,000-foot peaks. When her time came, at two o'clock in the morning, she was led by lantern, on horseback, down a twisting and narrow mountain trail. After "two agonizing hours . . . jolted beyond endurance . . . she arrived at the hospital only minutes" before delivering.

Usually the doctor was able to get to the patient. Dr. Charles Gardiner was called, one evening, to a distant ranch. After the long horseback ride and a prolonged and difficult delivery, the exhausted doctor fell asleep. The rancher, who had been away for the proceedings, returned home to find the three—wife, baby, and doctor—asleep in the same bed. The joke was on him, said the happy new father—paying Doc to

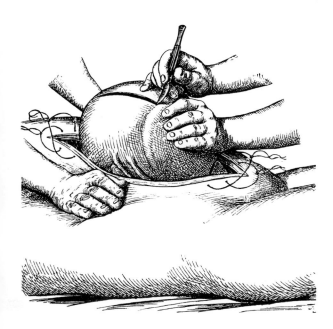

sleep with his wife![57] Dr. B. A. Peden of Man-zanola spent not one, but three nights at the ranch home of a woman with placenta previa, awaiting the hemorrhage which would gush from the misplaced placenta. Finally, it hap-pened and she went into shock. The doctor worked all day—the placenta had been ex-tracted, the dead baby delivered, and the bleed-ing stopped. The exhausted physician fell asleep at the house, awaking the next morning to find his patient better. Soon after, he reported, she was doing nicely, "taking iron, quinine, and whisky, and eating corn bread, butter, fat meat, potatoes and the like."[58]

Many women gave birth without the assis-tance of a physician. Some could not afford the fee (generally about twenty-five dollars) but were not about to accept charity or go to a county hospital. Among the German-speaking Russian immigrants who lived on the eastern Colorado plains, a pregnant woman expected, and re-ceived, little help.[59] She delivered in the tradi-tional way—kneeling and holding on to a piece of furniture, perhaps a chair, thereby avoiding soiling the family bedclothes. Unless there were complications, she probably returned to her farmwork in a day or two. Often, rural neighbors helped each other. One early Moffat County resident recalled how her mother was assisted in her delivery by a woman from a neighboring ranch; when the neighbor woman's turn came a few years later, the "compliment" was re-turned.[60]

In Colorado, as elsewhere, midwives were a popular alternative to physicians or to friends and neighbors. In some areas of the country, midwives were hospital- or medical school-trained, and their obstetric experience was often more extensive than that of many medical stu-dents and physicians. In some states midwives were licensed, or at least, as in Colorado, regis-tered. In other instances, however, the only edu-cation a midwife might have had was "on the job" and some were ignorant and steeped in superstition and mysticism. In the cities, mid-wives were especially popular among blacks and the foreign born. One Russian Jewish midwife of the 1880s was recalled as a respected figure in the community, often seen hurrying down the street in her "newly washed apron, swinging a black bag from her arm . . . on her urgent er-rands."[61] In addition to respect, the midwife might also receive a substantial reward, perhaps even a five-dollar gold piece.

Some physicians accused midwives of being indifferent to cleanliness. In fact, it was only in the late nineteenth century that aseptic and anti-septic procedures were introduced to obstetrics in order to prevent the dreaded and frequently lethal post-partum complication, puerperal, or "childbed" fever. A typical case of puerperal fever was described by a Colorado physician at a medical meeting:

> Who of us present here tonight cannot call to mind a case, after labor seemingly the most satisfactory which, from the second to the fourth day . . . was unexpectedly changed into one of the gravest and most alarming, by a sudden and extreme rise of pulse and temperature, distention of the abdo-men, tenderness in one or both iliac regions, ces-sation of the lochia and oncoming delirium? Our patient, who but a few days ago was full of hope and promise, now lies prostrate under a cloud of complications.[62]

There were innumerable therapeutic regimes available for puerperal fever—all of them equally ineffective for what we now know to be a particularly invidious bacterial sepsis, usually

13.14 Caesarian section was a very risky proce-dure and rarely done in the nineteenth century. When a baby was too large for its mother's pelvis, the result was fatal for the baby and some-times for the mother.

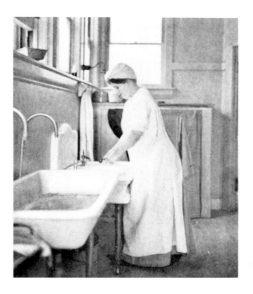

13.15 By the simple expedient of cleanli-ness—especially the washing of their hands by doctors, nurses, and midwives—the incidence of the dreaded postpar-tum killer, puerperal fever, was markedly reduced.

due to Group A beta-hemolytic streptococcus. This organism is the same one which causes "strep" throat and is part of the normal pharyngeal flora in asymptomatic carriers. The infectious basis of puerperal sepsis was suggested in 1844 by Oliver Wendell Holmes and demonstrated, a few years later, by Vienna's Ignaz Semmelweiss. The latter had pointed to the unwashed hands of medical students and physicians as the means by which puerperal fever was spread. Unfortunately, this was several decades before the emergence of clinical microbiology, and most physicians were unwilling to regard themselves as vectors of disease. The ideas of Holmes and Semmelweiss were ridiculed, physicians' hands remained unwashed, and thousands of women continued to die.

Eventually, the microbiologic basis of infectious disease was accepted, and by 1890 in Denver, Dr. Hawkins's Women's Hospital had instituted a rigorous regime of obstetric cleanliness.[63] In addition to hot soap baths, rectal enemas, and the like, Hawkins used vaginal douches with a hot solution of the antiseptic, bichloride of mercury, before delivery and for ten days thereafter. A variety of other precautions were taken. For example, after each delivery the room was "fumigated with sulphur and the floor scrubbed with a strong solution of corrosive sublimate . . ." The results of the Hawkins technique were said to "have been most remarkable."

In addition to Dr. Hawkins's maternity hospital, there were several "homes" for "unfortunate" women in Denver. Generally "unfortunate" meant pregnant, unmarried, and poor. Denver's Colorado Cottage Home was a private, non-sectarian institution established in 1888 as an "open refuge . . . for unfortunate girls and married women before and during confinement."[64] Several years later, the Florence Crittenden Home was opened—one of a national "chain" of such institutions.[65]

It was frequently pointed out that not all "unfortunate" women were poor or promiscuous; many were from "good" families and were simply ignorant of the biology of reproduction. While such ignorance might lead to an inappropriate and unwanted pregnancy, it also led to other problems as well. Dr. Jesse Hawes, emphasizing that he was not writing for "the purpose of tickling prurient ears," cited an example:

> One charming young lady of my acquaintance arose from her bridal couch and rushed, half clothed, to her mother's chamber, crying that her husband had offered her a gross, unpardonable insult . . .[66]

The young lady, he suggested, had probably been taught by a "shrew mother or by prudish, soured old maids that man's marital love is only legalized lust." She had obviously been uninformed that "a congestion of the reproductive organs of both sexes is normal and chaste under certain marital circumstances." Dr. Hawes felt that sex education was important and that the physician should play an important role in it.

Birth control became increasingly popular among middle and upper class Americans towards the end of the nineteenth century. A variety of techniques was used, ranging from coitus interruptus to rhythm methods to various prophylactic devices (condoms, tampons, womb veils or tents, cotton pledgets attached to a string) and douches (carbolic acid, bichloride of mercury, vinegar, and other chemicals). These methods varied in their degree of reliability. Others, such as the use of post-coital exercise, were predictably unreliable. Birth control, although it must have been a topic of medical discussion in early Colorado, was apparently considered an unsuitable one for publication. In 1899 one of the infrequent medical allusions to prophylaxis reported: "In Denver a small instrument is being placed in the os uteri of willing subjects for the purpose of preventing pregnancy." The brief note added that it was difficult to evaluate the results "on account of the secrecy observed by both parties . . ."[67]

There was one form of birth control about which Colorado's early doctors had definite opinions and which they did not hesitate to express publicly. They were virtually unanimous in their condemnation of abortion, even when it was considered necessary to save the life of the mother. Colorado's statutes relating to abortion were described by a turn-of-the-century lawyer as "exceedingly simple."[68] The law provided that any person convicted of attempting to "procure the miscarriage of any woman then being with child," could be sentenced to "a term not exceeding three years." If such an attempted abortion resulted in the death of the mother, the crime was deemed manslaughter "unless it appear that such miscarriage was procured or attempted by or under the advice of a physician or surgeon, with intent to save the life of such woman, or to prevent serious and permanent bodily injury to her."[69]

Colorado's physicians consistently pointed out that abortion was common. Supposedly, most M.D.s did not perform illegal abortions, but most acknowledged that they received inquiries from pregnant women, knew colleagues who were less fastidious than they, and were aware of professional and "criminal" abortionists. They were appalled at the "startling . . . frequency with which [illegal abortion's] serious consequences . . . come to our attention."[70] In 1899 it was said that in Denver "there must be a vast deal of this criminal business going on," and this was probably true, although less overtly, in Colorado's smaller communities as well. Furthermore, it wasn't just "unfortunate girls and degraded women" who were seeking abortions. In the words of one Denver physician: "The church-going woman and the dance-hall girl alike resort to the hair-pin and the catheter, jump down stairs, and fall from ladders."[71] Indeed, there were indications that most abortions were being requested by married, middle and upper class women. According to one physician:

> Among married people [abortion is done] simply because the people either want no children at all, or having one or two, want no more . . . People of moderate means think their rise in the world, either financially or socially, or both, will be hindered by even a small family of children . . .[72]

The woman who wanted an abortion had several choices. She could use any one of the many traditional methods, household chemicals, or an improvised instrument to induce an abortion herself or with the help of a friend. She could select one of many abortifacients advertised in newspapers and magazines, or she could seek the advice of a helpful druggist. Sometimes the attempt was successful, as was probably the case in 1903 in a Denver Coroner's report which described a "white, stillborn, male . . . found under the Colorado and Southern Railroad bridge at the edge of the Platte River . . ."[73] Often the attempt was unsuccessful and resulted in maternal hemorrage, infection, or other serious complications necessitating emergency medical attention.

Many women resorted to "criminal abortionists"—physicians, nurses, midwives, or non-medical quacks who were willing to perform an abortion outside of the statutory requirements. Done in secrecy, in basements and back rooms, often under the most unsanitary and primitive conditions, such abortions were also at high risk for serious complications. Periodically, abortions, whether self-induced or the work of a criminal abortionist, resulted in the death of the mother as well as the fetus. Finally, it was not unknown for a legitimate physician, sympathetic to the pleas of an "unfortunate"—perhaps a young woman whose physician he had been since she was a baby and whose family he knew—to perform an abortion outside of the law. In such a situation, Miss J---- might be reported as under Dr. S----'s care for some socially acceptable contagious disease requiring isolation from the prying eyes of friends and neighbors.

A symposium on abortion was held in Denver in 1903. At that time, according to the *Denver Medical Times*, "it was conclusively shown that the attitude of the regular medical profession is a unit against this common form of murder."[74] Dr. Hawkins considered the mother, and "oftentimes, the father," as accessories to "the heinous crime of abortion, a crime which is greater, more monstrous and horrible than that of murder in the first degree."[75] As to the abortionists themselves, they were "hell hounds," "sharks [and] fiends in human shape," "human vermin," and among "the most contemptible creatures on the face of the earth."[76] Abortionists, said Dr. Hawkins, should either "seek some other clime, or become the principal participant at a neck-tie party."[77]

Despite such strong feelings, there were few arrests for criminal abortion and convictions were rare. The infrequent examples were often cited in Colorado's medical journals. The first such conviction was apparently that of one Dan Dougherty of Gilpin County in 1871; he was sentenced to one year of imprisonment following the death "of the girl on whom the abortion was committed."[78] In searching the records of the state penitentiary, a Denver lawyer was able to find only four additional examples of incarcerations for criminal abortion—one of them for twenty-four hours.[78] In Denver, over the thirty-year period ending in 1902, a total of eighteen persons were charged with criminal abortion; three were convicted, thirteen were released without trial (two after admitting their guilt), and two were acquitted. "No wonder," said the lawyer, "that Denver is known as the Mecca of abortionists."

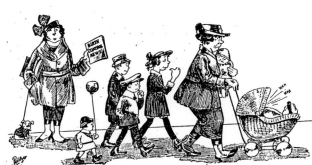

MAMMA, WHAT KINDA BOOK IS THAT LADY SELLIN'?

13.16 Even in the 1920s, the topic of birth control was not discussed publicly by most physicians.

Fetus and Newborn

Other than the ongoing denunciations of criminal abortion, little attention was paid in Colorado's medical literature to the fetus. Fetal anatomy had been described centuries before, but virtually nothing was known of fetal-placental-maternal biology and disease. Isolated examples of "monsters" and malformations were presented at medical society meetings. The ancient concept of "fetal impressions"—the idea that maternal experiences could result in a corresponding fetal malformation—was widely held. A number of instances were cited by one prominent Colorado physician, for example: "Case No. 16, a woman who had seen "her enraged husband cut three toes from a chicken had a baby with 'three stubs of fingers on one hand.'"[79]

Prematurity had a high mortality rate. The survival of a markedly premature baby was infrequent enough to warrant a report in Colorado's medical literature:

> Miss Lula Frey, who was born January 15, 1902 [in Denver] weighing but two pounds . . . now weighs twenty-five and a quarter pounds and is a healthy child.[80]

In 1913, the most popular exhibit at Denver's Lakeside Amusement Park was provided by a French physician, Dr. Martin Couney.[81] For a small admission fee, the fairgoer could examine a row of metal baskets, each containing a newborn baby. The baskets were the equivalent of incubators used for chicks, and the idea was that Dr. Couney's contraptions could be used to provide a controlled environment for newborns and, especially, prematurely born babies. Most physicians regarded the whole thing as just another example of medical quackery.

Infant feeding was one of the most controversial topics in medicine at the turn of the century. Most physicians agreed with Grand Junction's Dr. A. G. Taylor that mother's milk was "the only safe, perfect food for the baby."[82] The mother was expected to do everything she could to support lactation. In his paper entitled, "The incompatibility of higher education with the duties of motherhood." Trinidad's Dr. Henry Palmer warned:

> Look through our boarding schools and compare the glandless bust of the . . . young woman who spends half her nights over her mathematics or essays, with the plump rosy girl, with breasts like Venus, who goes to bed at dark, and would sleep over the most exciting novel Dumas ever wrote.[83]

As for those situations in which breast feeding was not possible, there was much discussion over the merits of cow's milk and of proper dilutions, methods of enrichment, the addition of sugars, etc. The calculations involved in the preparation of such formulae became so complex that one physician complained: "It is a little bit trying to go back to our schooldays and begin again to introduce algebra into our daily work."[84] The rapt attention of physicians to formulae and calculations offended Boulder's Dr. Kate Lindsay. "Here we have gone into the minutest details of taking care of the milk . . . the combinations, the percentages and calories . . . [yet] we have left out the main element. Everything is discussed but the mother herself, and the need for her cooperation."[85]

An interesting sidelight to early twentieth-century infant care was the "baby-show" held in conjunction with the National Western Stock show in Denver in 1913. Dr. Agnes Ditson described the event:

> Infants competed for prizes on a basis of mental and physical development, as determined by tests and examinations conducted by physicians . . . The human stock show bears the same relation to race improvement that the live stock show bears to stock breeding . . . It bridges the gap between scientific and practical eugenics . . .[86]

The hordes of naked babies, one to three years old, were judged on the basis of a long list of physical and psychological features. The best girl baby was awarded $100 in twenty-dollar gold pieces and a horseback ride around the arena with Buffalo Bill.[87]

13.17 Although introduced as early as 1881 in Europe, the incubator for prematurely born babies was a sensation when it was demonstrated at Denver's Lakeside Amusement Park in 1913.

13.18 Proper infant feeding was felt to be crucial in producing a healthy child.

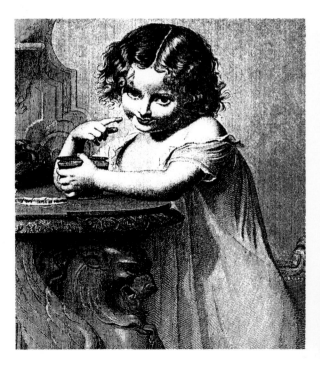

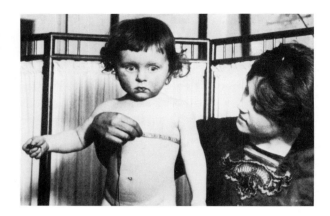

Pediatrics and Diphtheria

Childhood mortality was terribly high in the nineteenth and early twentieth centuries, and most of these deaths were due to infectious diseases. Among infants, the widely feared cholera infantum, or "summer diarrhea," was due to several bacterial, and probably viral, forms of gastroenteritis. Croup, whooping cough, pneumonia and other respiratory tract infections, as well as scarlet fever, measles, erysipelas, meningitis, smallpox, and tuberculosis, all contributed to the fact that one-third of all deaths in the U.S.A. occurred in the pediatric population. The most dramatic and the most devastating of the childhood infections was diphtheria.

By 1886 Denver's pioneer Dr. John Elsner had treated 400 cases of diphtheria.[88] Typically, as Elsner described it, fever, headache, and malaise were soon followed by a progressively severe sore throat. Examination of the child's throat revealed the characteristic "false membrane." The membrane was often black

> [and] the odor of the breath becomes fetid or even gangrenous. The breathing becomes greatly oppressed . . . [and] the patient passes into a semi-asphyxiated state, face livid, look anxious and frightened, eyes stare wildly, forehead clammy, and extremities cold. At each recurrence of the dyspnea the attack is more severe.[88]

Although some cases were milder, Elsner warned that the prognosis "must always be guarded . . . It is best not to express an opinion." Diphtheria usually occurred in outbreaks—Georgetown in 1879 ("the disease was of a mild type, there having been but 7 or 8 deaths among ten times that number of cases") and Globeville in 1900 ("the schools are closed . . . four deaths on October 20").[89] Sometimes multiple deaths occurred in the same family, as when the four children of Willard and Christie Head died within one week during an outbreak in southwestern Jefferson County.[90] The coming of

diphtheria to a town was treated as a major calamity. An Aspen newspaper headline of 1892 reads: "School Board and City Physician Hold Council of War—Close Schools, Rigid enforcement of Quarantine."[91] The board appointed a special health officer, Dr. Mollin, to "patrol the city and camp on the heels of the contagion, seeing that the [quarantine] signs are posted . . . and not lowered until such time as the building has been disinfected and every germ destroyed."

The problem in diphtheria was the membrane which gradually expanded and obstructed the victim's airway, slowly asphyxiating him. In 1885 a Chicago physician, Dr. Frank Waxham, dedicated himself to learning the newly introduced technique of intubation—the insertion of a metal tube through the mouth and down into the patient's trachea.[92] Waxham practiced the procedure for five months on cadavers, then on

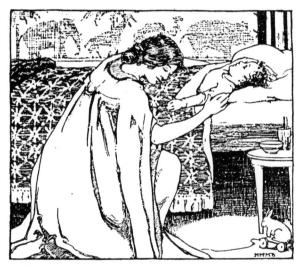

"steet urchins whom he hired for the purpose," and then on his own children. Finally, he began to use it in patients with diphtheria. Many of his patients had advanced disease and, not unexpectedly, some of them died. Unfortunately, "in the crowded districts of Chicago" where he worked, the deaths were attributed to intubation:

> This ignorant prejudice was often vented on Dr. Waxham and, more than once, he had to flee for his life from irate parents, who followed him with volleys of bricks, stones, or with knife or revolver. He did not dare to venture unarmed into the poorer districts of Chicago. Many times he had to beg or even pay parents for the privilege of saving the lives of their little ones through intubation.[92]

Waxham met similar, if less violent opposition, from some of his colleagues, and the A.M.A. appointed a committee to investigate his results. Its report enthusiastically supported Waxham's work. In 1893 the doctor and his wife came to

13.19 Dr. Agnes Ditson, seen here providing measurements for the Denver "baby show" of 1913. The baby show was held in conjunction with the Denver Western Stock Show.

13.20 Infant and childhood mortality was terribly high well into the twentieth century.

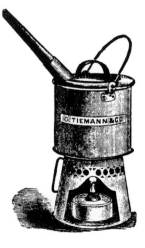

13.21 In the days preceding antibiotics and immunizations, the croup-kettle did little for the child with whooping cough, diphtheria, or pneumonia.

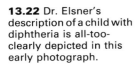

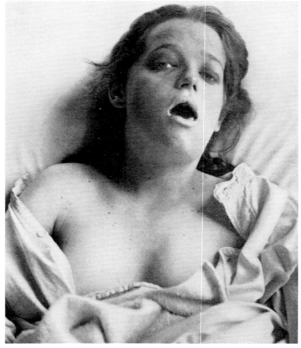

13.22 Dr. Elsner's description of a child with diphtheria is all-too-clearly depicted in this early photograph.

Denver to seek relief for her tuberculosis. The following year he reviewed for the Colorado Medical Society his experience with more than 500 cases of intubation.[93] He was appointed to a professorship at the University of Colorado School of Medicine and, until his death in 1911, instructed many Colorado physicians in this life-saving procedure.

The same year that Waxham performed his first intubation, Friedrich Loeffler demonstrated the bacterial agent which caused diphtheria, and a few years later, an antitoxin was developed. It was soon introduced to Colorado. The results were demonstrated quickly. In those patients in whom the antitoxin was used in Denver in 1895, the expected mortality of thirty percent was reduced to nine deaths in 140 cases.[94] Among twenty-nine of Dr. Waxham's patients who had received antitoxin, but were still sick enough to require intubation, twenty-seven survived.[95] Diphtheria did not disappear, however, and in 1906 it made a startling comeback. That year there were 122 diphtheria deaths in Colorado, and in the first three months of 1907, there were forty-eight more. The problem, said Dr. Waxham, was that the antitoxin was not always available, especially to the poor.[96] Massachusetts, he pointed out, had allocated $15,000 a year to Harvard Medical School to manufacture antitoxin, and it was provided, at no cost, to anyone who needed it. "Is it not time for Colorado to join the procession?" he asked. A state which could afford to gild its capitol's dome and spent $65,000 to "preserve game animals," could surely spend an estimated $5,000 a year to save the lives of its children. The legis-

13.23 Dr. Waxham demonstrating the use of endotracheal intubation for diphtheria.

lature agreed, but Governor Shafroth did not and he "pocketed" the bill.[97] His explanation to the Medical Society's Antitoxin Committee was that, "He could not see why the State of Colorado should furnish free antitoxin to the people any more than free horses and carriages to physicians." It was clear, many doctors responded, that the governor placed the lives of "fish and wild animals" above the lives of the people. Diphtheria continued to kill children and remained a significant problem until the introduction of toxoid and active immunization in the 1920s, and their subsequent incorporation into the childhood immunizations of later years.

When outbreaks of diphtheria and other contagious diseases occurred, one of the first acts was generally to close the public schools—usually on the advice of a local physician. Colorado's doctors played a significant role in the public schools from their very inception—as board members, sanitary inspectors, and school physicians. In 1909 the legislature passed an "Act Providing for the Examination and Care of Children in the Public Schools."[98] Written by Dr. Mary E. Bates and sponsored by Alma V. Lafferty, the only woman in the legislature, the law made Colorado the third state in the nation with a compulsory health inspection law for its public school children. It resulted in the discovery of undiagnosed medical problems in thousands of children and, in many instances, provided for their correction.

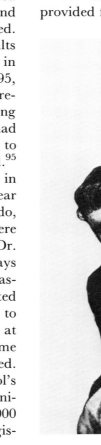

Hospitals

There are other specialties and many other outstanding physicians whom we cannot cover in this book.[99] The rise of medical specialization coincided with the emergence of the hospital as the focus of medical care in the late nineteenth and early twentieth centuries. We have mentioned some of them, and they ranged from Denver's large facilities to Rocky Ford's Pollack Hospital (twelve beds) and Paonia's Private Hospital (five beds). Despite such differences, there were were similarities. The "By-laws and House Rules" of Aspen's Citizen's Hospital (1892) provide a representative description of the day-to-day aspects of a late nineteenth-century hospital.[100]

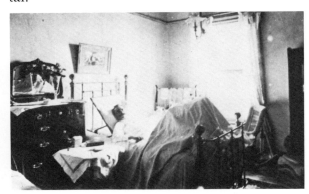

St. Joseph's Hospital
DENVER, COLORADO
Maternity Department
RATES

Private Rooms, per week $16.00, $18.00, $20.00 $25.00.
Private Rooms, with bath, per week $35.00; Suite $60.00.
Ward, per week $14.00.
Care of Infant $5.00.
Medicine and supplies at reasonable rates.
BILLS MUST BE PAID WEEKLY IN ADVANCE
FOR FURTHER INFORMATIONS WRITE TO THE SUPERINTENDENT

The Aspen Citizen's Hospital's corporate entity, or association, was governed by a board of directors. The board appointed various committees and approved staff appointments. The medical staff (i.e. the hospital's physicians) advised the board, controlled the professional aspects of the hospital, and admitted and discharged patients. A "resident physician," i.e. a doctor who actually lived in the hospital, "carried out the

instructions of the visiting physicians," made daily rounds, kept the medical records, and conducted the professional business of the hospital. The "matron" supervised "all the households of the hospital"—the wards and operating room, kitchens and dining room, laundry and supplies. She also supervised the nurses and "other female" employees. The nurses worked twelve-hour shifts, with half-days off Sunday and one weekday. They also had rooms in the hospital and were subject to a 10 P.M. curfew and to emergency call day or night. Their uniforms consisted of "blue and white seersuckers, simply made, with white apron and cap and linen collar and cuffs."

Patients could be admitted by any member of the staff or, "having applied in person," by the resident physician. Members of the hospital association who had paid their monthly fee of one dollar were entitled to bed, board, nursing, and medical care. Any other "reputable" citizen of the county could be admitted "upon payment, in advance, of the weekly rate." Patients with venereal or other contagious diseases were not eligible for admission. The opinion of a second physician was required before major elective surgery was done. Once admitted, a patient was forbidden to

use any profane or indecent language, to express immoral sentiments, to play at any game for money, to [use] intoxicating liquors, to have any [literature] of immoral or indecent nature, to use tobacco, [or to] spit upon the floor of the wards, hall, or stairways, nor out of the windows.[100]

Similar rules pertained to visitors, and the rules were rigidly enforced.[101]

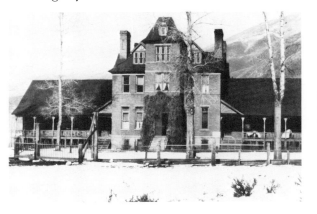

13.24 A private room in Denver's St. Joseph's Hospital.

13.25 Although undated, these rates suggest that this price list is not of recent vintage. Reasonable though they seem, they were to be paid in advance!

13.26 Aspen Citizen's Hospital. A one dollar a month subscription entitled the "policy holder" to hospitalization and care.

14 CLIMATOLOGY

Why, Coloradans are the most disappointed people I ever saw. Two-thirds of them came here to die, and they can't do it. This wonderful air brings them back from the very edge of the tomb, and they are naturally exceedingly disappointed.

P. T. Barnum, ca. 1872[1]

One has but to go onto our streets and meet the hale and vigorous men and women, many of whom came here as invalids, to be convinced that the climate we enjoy is one of our greatest treasures, to be valued more highly . . . than the stores of silver and gold locked up in the mountains . . .

First Annual Report of the Denver Chamber of Commerce, 1883[2]

FROM ITS EARLIEST DAYS, glowing reports of Colorado's climate attracted tourists and health-seekers. At first there were just a few hardy souls who were willing to make the difficult journey and endure primitive accommodations and food. With the coming of the railroads, the encouragement of physicians, and the advertising of entrepreneurs, Colorado's sunshine, altitude, dryness, and mineral springs evolved into a major industry. Concomitantly, there developed, in the late nineteenth century, the medical specialty of "climatology"—a forerunner of what is now called "environmental medicine." Colorado and Colorado physicians played a major role in this new area of medicine.

Within a year of the discovery of gold at Cherry Creek, the healthful effects of Colorado's climate were being touted. In 1859 the area's first business directory reported:

The salubrity of this vicinity is unquestionable. Indigenous maladies are entirely unknown . . . The air is dry, pure and extremely invigorating. Wet lands are nowhere and steadiness of temperature is one of the characteristics of the climate. In the summer, the heat of the day is never oppres-

sive and the nights are invariably cool and pleasant. The winters are mild . . .[3]

The impression of "salubrity" was not limited to Colorado's professional boosters. That same year, a pioneer wrote to his sister in Wisconsin:

I am sorry your health has been so poor . . . Why don't you leave that sickly place and come to this salubrious clime where sickness is almost unknown. You remember how miserable I was when I left your place. A few weeks of mountain air fully restored me to health and strength.[4]

By the 1870s such testimonials were appearing in eastern newspapers and national periodicals. World travelers such as Isabella Bird wrote, "The curative effect of the climate of Colorado can hardly be exaggerated . . . Colorado is the most remarkable sanitorium in the world."[5]

Eastern medical journals began to print articles with titles such as, "Colorado for Invalids."[6] Colorado's physicians added their own encomiums. In 1872 the *Report of the Territorial Board of Immigration* quoted the first president of the Colorado Medical Society, Dr. R. G. Buckingham:

That Colorado possesses a pure and healthful atmosphere, no one can deny . . . It has been my good fortune to have observed that in every case of chronic disease to which my attention has been called, none have failed to receive benefit, sooner or later, by a sojourn in Colorado . . .[7]

The word was spread and health-seekers came from all over the country to benefit from Colorado's healing climes. Isabella Bird found

consumptives, asthmatics, dyspeptics, and sufferers from nervous diseases, . . . here in hundreds and thousands, either trying the "camp cure" for three or four months or settling here permanently. All have come for health, and most have found or are finding it . . .[8]

One such health-seeker was young Howard Kelly.[9] A nineteen-year-old medical student at the University of Pennsylvania, Kelly had begun to suffer from various health problems, including "insomnia." He was advised to postpone his studies and come West. After several months building up his strength in Colorado Springs, the young man worked as a cowboy on a cattle ranch in Elbert County. Within a year he was sufficiently improved to return to his medical studies. Kelly subsequently became Professor of Gynecology at Johns Hopkins and one of the leaders of American medicine.

The advantages of Colorado's environment were enumerated everywhere. In addition to the benfits of its high altitude and mineral springs (discussed later in this chapter), boosters cited the number of "sunshine" days. Sunshine, it was said, and in particular, the "photo-therapy" of ultra-violet and other non-visible rays, were "of no inconsiderable importance in bringing about the cures of Colorado."[10] It was the "diathermancy" of Colorado's air, "its rarefication due to altitude . . . which enables it to readily allow the passage of the sun's rays without interposing resistance."[11] In addition, the dryness of the air tended to "abstract moisture from the tissues of the lungs and thus . . . promote their ready opening to atmospheric pressure . . ." The air was so pure, in fact, that pioneer Dr. W. F. McClelland told how, in the early days, a "quarter of beef, or the saddle of a black-tailed deer or antelope" could be hung outside for a week or ten days and yet provide "a steak which looked as new and fresh . . . as new-cut chops from a first-class meat market."[12] Rather than putrify, dead animals simply dried up:

I have seen the body of a dead horse keep its shape, with hide on most of its body, for over two years—which I used as a landmark in my professional visits in the night up and down Bear Creek

. . . Go through the streets, alleys and vacant lots of our city [Denver] and take a look at the dead dogs, cats, rats, and chickens which dry up with the hair and feathers on, and rattle if you stir them.[12]

The dryness of Colorado's air was cited as the reason for the rarity of malaria, so common in the eastern and southern parts of the country. An occasional Colorado case was reported, more as an example of the exception that proved the rule. Jokingly, Dr. McClelland cited the sergeant-at-arms at the state legislature, blaming his malaria on the man's workplace, with its "foul air . . . contaminated with the political legerdemain of his surroundings."[13] Actually, Greeley's Dr. Jesse Hawes concluded that malaria could be acquired in certain parts of Colorado, and years later, malaria's vector, the Anopheles mosquito, was demonstrated in southern Colorado.[14]

There were a few dissenters. After spending two months in Denver in 1872, Dr. H. Norton wrote of freezing cold, long winters, sand storms, and other meteorological horrors.[15] He found the bright sunshine to be "disagreeable," necessitating sunglasses, and his overall impression of Colorado's climate was that it was "prostrating instead of tonic." In another medical article, one

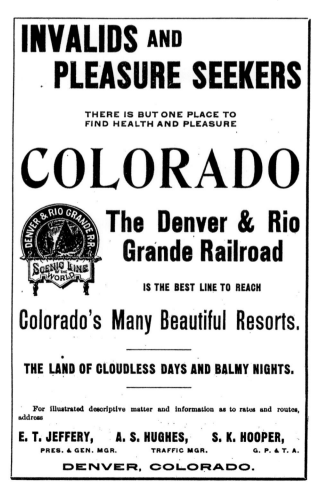

14.1 The railroads were among the most enthusiastic boosters of Colorado's healthful climate.

"not calculated to improve the reputation of Colorado as a health resort, it was said

> that the high altitudes there . . . often destroy all sexual desire and power in men and, what is yet more curious, that the altitude or climate has the reverse effect on women.[16]

Even some of Colorado's own physicians counseled their colleagues to show a little more restraint in their panegyrics to the healthful effects of Colorado's climate. Dr. Thomas Massey, Chairman of the Territorial Medical Society's Committee on Climatology, warned:

> It may be true, and doubtless is true, that to healthy men and women the climate of Colorado contributes nothing, save passing variety and exhilaration. That it is promotive of . . . longevity is more than questionable.[17]

Colorado Springs

Denver had been Colorado's original health resort, but the growing city was being transformed into a commercial and industrial center. Soon, Denver was replaced by Colorado Springs as Colorado's premier health resort. The town had been founded by General William Jackson Palmer as a health spa to which people would come on his Denver and Rio Grande Railroad.

14.2 In Colorado Springs's early years, even the elegant Antlers Hotel welcomed invalids. That changed.

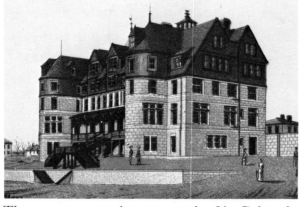

There were no springs to speak of in Colorado Springs, but nearby Manitou, a few miles away in the shadow of Pike's Peak, had more than its share. Palmer, along with his English friend, Dr. William Bell, and other American and English investors, built the area into a mecca for health-seekers. In late nineteenth-century America, these were were mainly "consumptives," i.e. people with pulmonary tuberculosis. Palmer and his partners were, in addition, seeking a particular class of health-seekers, specifically the upper and and middle class. The "Springs" was the place for sick people who were well off, the genteel and socially inclined, the educated and cultured, and the sports- and

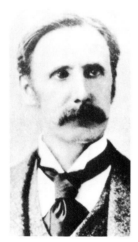

14.3 Dr. S. Edwin Solly was Colorado Springs's best known medical booster.

outdoors-minded. They rode horseback, played golf, and camped in comfortable quarters. In fact, Colorado Springs was compared favorably to Switzerland's grand health resort, Davos-Platz.[18] The hotels of Colorado Springs and the spas at Manitou Springs were never meant to cater to arthritic miners or tubercular immigrants from eastern Europe.

The area found an effective booster in Dr. S. Edwin Solly, himself a health-seeker from England. Dr. Solly's booklet, *The Health Resorts of Colorado Springs and Manitou*, praised the healthy climate of the area.[19] Solly gave detailed reports of the meteorological data collected by the U.S. Signal Service and compared Colorado Springs's weather with that of other cities. He described the climate's beneficial effects on nutrition and skin, the circulatory, renal, respiratory, nervous, and muscular systems, and on such ailments as anemia, renal disease, asthma, tuberculosis, dyspepsia, and so on. Unlike some of his more prejudiced colleagues, Solly did not claim that the area's climate would improve all diseases. In the matter of hemorrhoids, for example, he noted that the incidence of this "plague" was as "high in Colorado as elsewhere."

Dr. Denison and Climatology

Colorado's best known "climatologist" was Dr. Charles Denison. Denison had just begun his practice in Connecticut when he contracted tuberculosis. After traveling through the South, the twenty-eight-year-old doctor came to Denver in 1873. His health soon improved, and convinced that it was Colorado's environment that had cured him, Denison devoted the rest of his life to climatology—the study of the effects of climate on health and disease, especially tuberculosis. Denison's views were summarized in his book, *Rocky Mountain Health Resorts*, published in 1880.[20] In it he extols the climatic advantages of the state and the benefits of exercise and outdoor life. In addition, this was the era of Edison, and Denison was especially impressed with the medical potentials of atmospheric electricity. His investigations had demonstrated increased amounts of the oxygen derivative, ozone, in Colorado's "electrified" mountain air. Denison felt that the fact that ozone was an "oxidizing disinfectant" partially explained the salubrious effects of Colorado's climate on tuberculosis and other infectious diseases. Denison's book was a great success and he went on to write many papers on these and similar topics.[21]

In 1884 Denison and several colleagues founded the American Climatological Association. The following year, Denison established climatology as a science with his book, *The Annual and Seasonal Climatic Maps of the United States.*[22] The work was essentially an atlas of weather maps of the United States, presenting a huge compendium of meteorologic data in a clear and concise form. In reviewing the book, the *Journal of the American Medical Association* cited the "large number of people who are annually borne home in their coffins from the so-called 'Health Resorts' as solemn and silent testimonial to the ignorance of [most] physicians of the climate of various portions of their own country."[23] Denison's atlas provided a valuable source of medical information, and in commenting on the "perfection" of his maps, or "weather calendars," JAMA added:

> The profession [and] the people . . . owe Dr. Denison a debt of gratitude for his painstaking care and accurate work. [He] has commenced work in a mine which is far more valuable than any of those subterrestrial ones which have been opened in his native state.[23]

Denison's interests in climatology extended to what are now designated as ecological concerns. He deplored, for example, the "unreasonable and wanton destruction" of trees by the mining, railroad, and timber industries, and called for "forest conservation" by the state and federal governments.[24] His concerns were based on the his belief that forests exerted climatic effects and that deforestation would, through such alterations on Colorado's climate, adversely affect the health of its people.

Colorado's climate was publicized by a variety of spokesmen—not just physicians, but journalists and politicians, resort owners and developers, railroads and chambers of commerce. In 1879 Governor Frederick W. Pitkin recommended that the legislature appropriate funds to publish literature "setting forth the advantages which this climate affords . . . the afflicted."[25] Local boosters were also active. The town of Salida, for example, advertised that a few weeks in that community "will give new life and vigor to worn out and overworked businessmen."[26] The physicians of Colorado Springs donated funds to their chamber of commerce for the purpose of "advertising the climatic advantages" of their city.[27] All worked together to bring the health-seeker and, incidentally, his dollars to Colorado's "salubrious" climate. There may have been mixed feelings among physicians about the propriety of such

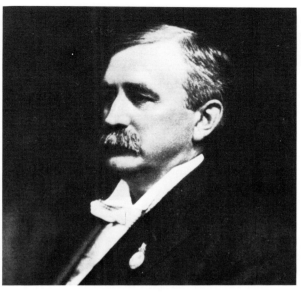

14.4 Dr. Charles Denison was a founder of medical climatology.

advertising and about the effectiveness of Colorado's climate in treating certain diseases, but there was little doubt that Colorado was the place to come if you had tuberculosis or asthma.

Asthma

The asthmatic no sooner reaches our magical land than he dispenses with physicians . . .
  D.H. Dougan, M.D. (Leadville), 1881[28]

Asthma is due to bronchospasm, a muscular contraction of the airways. This impedes the passage of air into and, especially, out of the lungs. The latter situation is characterized by expiratory wheezing, and during an attack, the patient may be in severe respiratory distress. The disease results from allergic phenomena but is influenced by a number of other factors.

Leadville's Dr. D. H. Dougan, who himself suffered from the disease, described the asthmatic as "an anxious, care-worn haggard sufferer, spending days and nights of unutterable torment, a constant care to family and friends, a source of solicitude and anxiety to his physician . . ."[28] Another asthmatic, author and Colorado health-seeker, Grace Greenwood, was even more dramatic:

> Asthmatics [are unhappy] men and women who, like shipwrecked mariners perishing of thirst, with water, water everywhere, gasp and fight for their scanty breath in a world of air. They find it not difficult to realize the sufferings of men suffocated in the mines, or the horrors of the Black Hole of Calcutta.[29]

All sorts of remedies were used to treat asthma, including the inhalation of chloroform or ether, the injection of morphine, and the ingestion of arsenicum or ipecacuanha. Newspaper advertisements offered all sorts of "irregular" and quack remedies. An 1871 issue of the *Rocky Mountain News* contained this example:

TO THOSE AFFLICTED WITH ASTHMA
Dr. M.M. Mitivier's Asthmatic Cigars Are An
Infallible Remedy for the Asthma
For sale at Steinhauer and Walbrach's Drug Store,
Larimer Street, near the Post Office[30]

Colorado's early settlers included a number of asthmatics who had come to the territory as prospectors, businessmen, and health-seekers. Many of them enjoyed remarkable relief from their disease. One of them, Mr. F.J.B. Crane, convened a meeting of asthmatics in Denver in December 1873. The results of their discussions were published in a little pamphlet, *Colorado and Asthma*.[31] The 117 participants had come from all over the country and lived in different parts of the state. Of these, sixty-two percent reported that their asthma had been cured since moving to Colorado, and an additional twenty-eight percent found that their symptoms had been "decidedly relieved." Even the remaining ten percent had noted some improvement.

Several popular travel books helped spread the word. The best known was Miss Greenwood's narrative of her western travels, *New Life in New Lands*. She had found, on visiting Colorado in 1871, that the air

> . . . is buoyant and delicious. It has all the ethereal properties of champagne. I drink it in long, deep draughts . . . [For asthmatics] I have to say that I do not believe there is out of Heaven such a place as the mountain land of Colorado.[32]

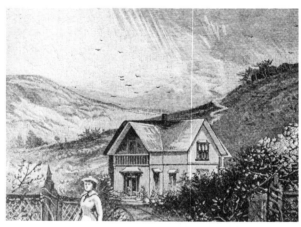

14.5 Author Grace Greenwood found Colorado's climate so beneficial to her asthma that she moved to this cottage in Manitou Springs.

Miss Greenwood was so impressed that she moved to Manitou Springs the following year. Denver's doctors were also impressed. In 1873 the Denver Medical Association passed the following resolution:

> The climate of Colorado . . . has a wonderfully curative power over Asthma. Nearly all such patients coming into this climate are relieved—at least so long as they remain here.[33]

The most exhuberant claims, however, were made by the state's non-medical boosters. From the Denver Chamber of Commerce in 1885: "Asthmatics as a rule are not only benefited but completely cured from the moment they reach our borders. The results in these cases are magical."[34]

Dr. Dougan had complained that is was impossible to estimate the number of asthmatics who had come to Colorado since, having been exposed to her curative climate, they never bothered to seek medical attention. In light of the many glowing reports from doctors, patients, travelers, and publicists, the brief comment of a later-day internist, Denver's Dr. James Arneill, provides an interesting insight. "Most of us have grown body weary, heart sore and mind mind distraught in our efforts to relieve and cure many of our stubborn cases of asthma."[35] Dr. Arneill's remark suggests that the effects of Colorado's climate on asthma were not uniformly miraculous.

Two aspects of Colorado's environment and their effects on health were studied with special intensity—altitude and mineral springs.

Altitude

This altitude is much too high for you . . . It makes a terrific pressure on your head and blood vessels . . . It would be too great a strain on your capacities.

S. Leach, Park County, Colorado
Letter to his "sickly" brother back East, 1864[36]

Colorado's early doctors agreed that the moderately elevated altitude of its Front Range and foothills communities was beneficial to health. Dr. Denison listed the salutory benefits "of a rightly chosen altitude," including "diathermancy and a heightened electrical state, . . . increased heart action, . . . and easy transpiration of vapor from the body . . ."[37] Altitudes of four to six thousand feet, and even a little higher in the foothills, were felt to play a major role in the climatologic effectiveness of Colorado's en-

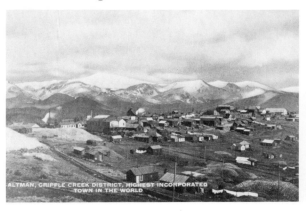

14.6 The medical effects of high altitude were reported by many of Colorado's physicians. Some of the mining camps were located above 10,000 feet, and many of the mines were much higher.

vironment. In 1902 Colorado Springs's Dr. Will Swan attempted to evaluate the effects of altitude on a variety of medical conditions.[38] In his survey, he asked physicians in the region to compare their present "high altitude" practice with their previous "low altitude" practice in other areas. The responses were inconclusive. For example:

> Fifty-one physicians saw more 'acute rheumatism' in their present 'high altitude' practice, while forty-five saw less. Nineteen physicians saw more 'acute lobar pneumonia' . . . while fifteen saw less. Fifty-two saw more 'billiousness, or other digestive diseases,' while ninety-six saw less.

These mixed results may have reflected the fact that "high altitude" in Dr. Swan's study referred to any site over 4,000 feet. Although most physicians felt that moderate altitude was beneficial, they generally agreed that truly high altitudes had some detrimental effects. To most Coloradans, high altitude began at 8,000 or even 10,000 feet. Many mining communities, including Leadville, were located at such altitudes. There were mines at 12,000 feet or higher, and for those who liked to ascend the peaks, there were more than fifty above 14,000 feet. In his 1864 guidebook to Colorado's mines, O.J. Hollister warned new arrivals to exercise caution:

> Doubtless you will experience the effects of a rarefied air. Upon moving about you will be filled plumb full of short wind. [If you] persist in violent exercise bleeding at the nose will result. You will observe an involuntary tendency to prolonged inspiration and forcible expansion of the chest.[39]

In 1879 Dr. W. Edmondson might have been describing today's tourist emerging from his car to admire the glorious scenery on 12,000-foot Independence Pass. Exhilarated after the long drive from Houston, and

> feeling fresh and buoyant, he starts to walk up an inclined plane with the same rapidity . . . to which he has always been accustomed. He becomes suddenly aware that there is something wrong with him. He pants for breath, his heart beats with painful violence, and he is . . . completely exhausted. He now realizes . . . that he is a stranger in a strange land.[40]

The most profound effects of high altitude were seen in the non-acclimated visitor who decided to take the burro ride or the cog railway to the top of Pike's Peak or to scramble up the trails on Long's Peak—both over 14,000 feet high. The cog railroad carried hundreds of tourists to the top of Pike's Peak daily. Typically, according to one observer, ten to fifteen per cent

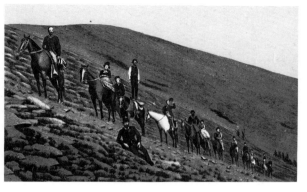

14.7 Altitude sickness was common among the tourists at the top of Pike's Peak.

were "slightly affected by the altitude. Most of them had nausea and a great deal of headache. Some went into a dead faint when they reached the top . . ."[41] A typical scene at the summit was described:

> The floor of the lunchroom [was] covered with people vomiting, some practically unconscious, others who could not take any food . . . One case in particular [was] an individual scarcely off the train [whose] lips became blue . . . with [the] ill-effects of the high altitude. He was given oxygen, and the lips soon became pink and [he] felt nicely. However, within ten minutes he grabbed a bag of oxygen as if it were a whiskey bottle, and ran for his train.[41]

The observer was describing some of the features of what is called "acute mountain sickness," a disorder which, in its extreme form, can result in cerebral and/or pulmonary edema—either of which can be fatal. Of greater import to Colorado's physicians than the acute effects of mountain sickness on the casual visitor were the possible long-term consequences of living at high altitude. One major concern was the effect of "rarefied air" on the cardiovascular system. Dr. J. N. Hall found that "the robust miners who work at 10,000 or 12,000 ft. elevation" tended to have enlarged hearts, their "cardiac area extending to the nipple line . . ."[42] Women were said to suffer from a variety of supposed altitude-related disorders. After nearly a decade of practice at altitudes of up to 10,000 feet, Dr. W. A. Jayne described a number of such problems, including:

> Nervousness, . . . undefined discomfort, unwonted irritability of temper, sleeplessness, . . . palpitation, headache, fullness of the head, neuralgia, gastric disturbance and, . . . in those of neurotic temperament, moderate loss of flesh and color. [Also] functional uterine derangements, . . . dysmenorrhea of the neuralgic and ovarian types, . . . and menorrhagia.[43]

A number of attempts were made to study the physiologic effects of high altitude. The most ambitious were those conducted by the famous

Oxford physiologist, J.B.S. Haldane on the summit of Pike's Peak in 1911.[44] With four trainloads of equipment, the group spent five weeks doing red blood cell counts, pulmonary function tests, and other analyses. If climatology was a prelude to environmental medicine, then the Pike's Peak experiments can be considered the forerunner of aerospace medicine.

Natural Springs and Mineral Waters

The inquisitive may want to know what are the medical properties of . . . springs. It would take a small volume to describe them. They range over the whole gamut of medical lexicography, and include, as the miners say, all the known "stinks." There are [about] a thousand of them in the state and the invalid who cannot be suited somewhere in Colorado need not look anywhere else for what he wants.
History of the Arkansas Valley, Colorado, 1881[45]

Water, emerging mysteriously and perpetually from the ground, has always had a mystical attraction for humanity. Sometimes crystal clear, fresh, and cold, sometimes murky, stinking, and hot, spring water has been used for medicinal purposes throughout history. Even after its geologic basis has been explained, its chemical composition analyzed, and its medicinal properties challenged, the supposed "healing" attributes of spring water have continued to be accepted by many people.

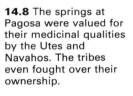

14.8 The springs at Pagosa were valued for their medicinal qualities by the Utes and Navahos. The tribes even fought over their ownership.

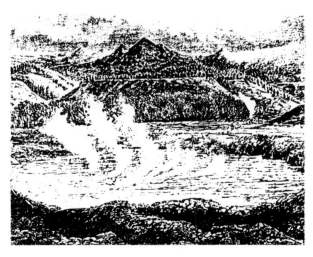

There are thousands of springs in Colorado's mountains. The Utes and other Indians had used the springs at Manitou, Glenwood, Pagosa, and other sites for as long as anyone could remember (Chapter 3). One of Colorado's earliest American visitors, Dr. Edwin James, described what he called the "Boiling Spring" near Pike's Peak as "a large and beautiful fountain of water,

cool and transparent, highly aerated with carbonic acid . . . [with] the grateful taste and exhilarating effects of the most strongly aerated artificial mineral waters."[46] Another spring was described as "sulfurous . . . impregnated with muriate of soda and other salts [and] may possess some active medicinal properties." In examining the springs, Dr. James carried out what may have been Colorado's first scientific experiment:

> [Nearby is a spring] which discharges no water, its basin remaining constantly full, and air only escaping from it. We collected some of the air . . . in a box, but could not perceive it to have the least smell, or the power of extinguishing flame, which was tested by plunging into it lighted splinters of dry cedar.[47]

Colorado's springs were described in the writings of many later explorers and mountain men. George Ruxton, for example, recalled relieving his thirst at a mountain spring:

> I dipped the cup into the midst of the bubbles, and raised it hissing and sparkling to my lips. Such a draught! Three times, without drawing a breath, was it replenished and emptied, almost blowing up the roof of my mouth with its effervescence. It was equal to the best soda-water, but possesses that fresh natural flavor which manufactured water cannot impart.[48]

By the 1860s entrepreneurs were developing some of the springs in the mining districts, building bath houses and primitive spas where the miner and the weary traveler could relieve their aching joints and muscles. One of the earliest was at Idaho Springs, near the Clear Creek and Central City diggings. Here, in 1863, Dr. E. S. Cummings built a small bath house.[49] Within a few years, the operation had been expanded. As described by a reporter for the *New York Tribune*:

> The soda springs are already turned to service. Two bath houses have been built . . . In one of these the water is so regulated that the bather may choose whatever temperature he prefers [and] the hot and cold springs come up so close together, that one may dip a hand in either at the same time.[50]

Natural springs were being developed in other locations. The emphasis had shifted from miners to tourists and health-seekers, and to combining the comforts of a resort with the health features of a sanitarium. William Byers, publisher-editor of the *Rocky Mountain News*, had a stake in the Hot Sulfur Springs in Middle Park.[51] The newspaper man solicited testimonials from patients

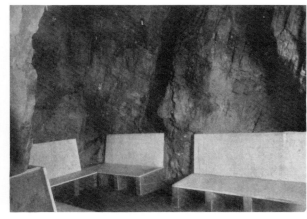

14.9 The vapor caves at Glenwood had been used by generations of Utes prior to their eviction.

and doctors alike. Mr. A. Sagendorf praised the Springs as having cured his severe dermatitis and Denver's Dr. Stedman referred to its waters as "an effective auxiliary to medical treatment." Poncha Springs's owner "spared no expense in making everything in and around these valuable springs attractive and comfortable," and Dr. J. L. Prentiss spent several thousand dollars developing his Royal Gorge Hot Springs at Canon City.[52] He promised to cure "rheumatics in three days to two weeks." A few of the springs were developed into large scale enterprises. Glenwood's Yampah Spring spewed three million gallons of steaming hot water into a pool (the "Natatorium") six hundred feet long.[53] By the 1890s the complex included an elegant bathhouse staffed by a resident physician, an "Inhalatorium," vapor caves, and a bottling plant. The sick were brought to Glenwood by rail from Denver; once there, they could stay at the eleg-

ant Hotel Colorado or any one of a number of lesser hotels and boarding houses.

The most famous, extensive, and accessible springs in Colorado were in Manitou. Just a few miles from Colorado Springs, Manitou was the crown jewel in General Palmer's plan to make the area into one of America's major resorts. He had a willing ally in Dr. Solly, who praised the salutory benefits of Manitou's springs in lectures, articles, and a monograph published in 1875, *Manitou, Colorado, U.S.A.: Its Mineral Waters and Climate*.[54] The monograph opened with a chemical analysis of the waters by Professor O. Loew.[55] The professor extolled the water's mineral composition, comparing it favorably with some of the best known spas in Europe. Next, after reviewing the medicinal use of mineral waters by the ancients, Dr. Solly pointed out that their "reviving and increasing popularity" demanded that physicians be aware of their value. Solly reviewed the Manitou's major springs—Navajo, Ute Soda, Iron Ute, Little Chief—listing each according to its mineral content, temperature, and other properties. Finally, the doctor presented his concept of human disease. Many diseases, he felt, were due to "increased venosity—a state [in which] the venous blood is in excess and circulates so feebly as to give rise to chronic congestions or stases of various organs, chiefly the abdominal organs . . . and causes the functions of these organs to be sluggishly or irregularly performed." This led to "catarrhs" of various mucous membranes

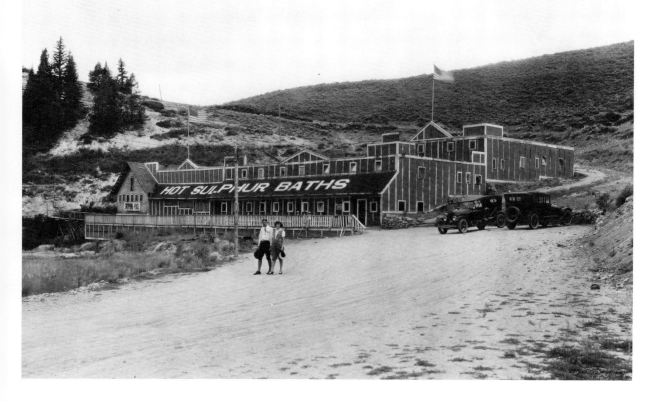

14.10 Hot Sulphur Springs was originally developed by Denver newspaperman and entrepreneur William Byers in the 1870s.

which, in turn, could result in various diseases of the liver, kidney and spleen, gout, dyspepsia and ulcer, and even tuberculosis and cancer. Certain of the waters at Manitou, whether imbibed, bathed in, or inhaled as vapors, could be expected to improve the increased venosity and catarrhs which resulted in these diseases. Other waters from other springs at Manitou had different compositions and properties and, therefore, different medicinal values. They would be effective in other diseases.

What sounds today like quackery, was actually well within the mainstream of nineteenth-century medical theory, and Solly's treatise was accepted as a learned and scholarly contribution. It was also received, with gratitude and reverence, by the Chamber of Commerce, the railroad, and the land developers and entrepreneurs. The sick, the lame, the elderly, and the just plain "run down," packed the Denver and Rio Grande's coaches and filled the growing number of hotels, inns, spas, bath-houses, and doctors' waiting rooms in the area.[56]

The public and the medical profession were bombarded with flyers, brochures, and promotionals attesting to the value of Colorado's medicinal springs. Some of the claims were reasonable, some borderline, and some outright quackery. A pamphlet touting Pueblo's Clark

Magnetic Mineral Spring is typical. Some excerpts:

> In Secondary and Tertiary Syphilis, Scrofula, . . . Cancerous and Ovarian Tumors, Eczema and Skin Diseases of all kinds . . . hundreds of patients come here, and in a few weeks return home entirely cured, after having tried all other means of cure.

> In Leucorrhea, Gonorrhea, Gleet, Female Weakness and Womb Troubles, the tonic effects of the water are at once apparent. All diseases of the Urinary or Sexual organs yield readily to treatment. Many cases of Impotency have been cured . . .[57]

Mr. Clark provided his patrons with "a large and elegant bath house and sanitarium and . . . a laboratory for the analysis of urine." They were advised to drink between twelve to sixteen glasses of warm spring water a day and to use the various tub, sitz, and vapor baths, massages, douches, etc. A list of prominent references included Colorado's Governor Alva Adams. Room and board was twenty dollars a week.

A few of the springs contained measurable amounts of radiation. They were advertised as "radium hot springs," and it was pointed out that for one fee, their patrons would benefit from two wonder drugs—mineral water and radium.[58]

Those who could not make the trip to Colorado's natural springs could still imbibe their waters. Beginning in the 1870s, Colorado's bottling industry provided the public with the benefits of it mineral waters. Manitou Table Water ("recharged with none but its own natural gas"), Manitou Ginger Champagne (prepared from a secret recipe containing ginger root), and Ute Chief Mineral Water were manufactured in Manitou Springs.[59] There was intense competition among the bottlers. The Manitou Mineral Water Company, for example, warned its public to "beware of imposition, counterfeits and false representations . . . Scrutinize every bottle closely . . . Accept none unless the neck label contains a facsimile of the word 'Manitou' in script . . ."[60] Regardless of the company, the promises were virtually identical—benefits similar to those which were offered at the springs themselves. By 1911 there were at least fourteen companies producing mineral water in Colorado, not only in Manitou, but in Denver, Boulder, and other communities.[61] Together, they bottled nearly one and a half million gallons valued at $104,000. This was just a drop in the national mineral water bucket, however, representing about two and a half percent of the country's annual output.[62]

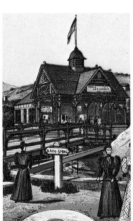

14.11 Manitou Springs was the creation of William Jackson Palmer and his friends. It was Colorado's most elegant and successful "watering hole" and attracted health seekers from across the nation.

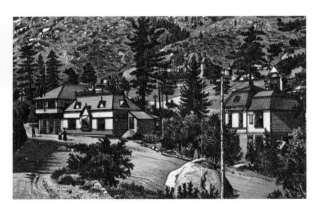

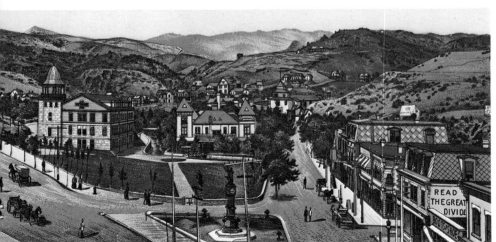

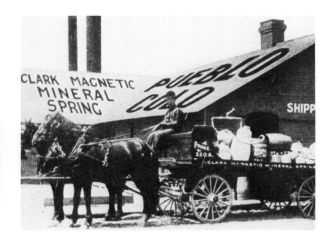

Finally, it should be noted that there was at least one published example of skepticism regarding the medical value of mineral springs and water among Colorado's early physicians. This is an article written by by Dr. E. C. Hill, Professor of Chemistry and Urinalysis at Denver's Gross Medical College, entitled, "The Mineral Water Fad."[63] Dr. Hill began by stating that "one of the most ancient of antique [medical] errors is the general belief in the universal efficacy of 'natural healing springs.'" Given the fact that there was some use for hot baths, that water is important, and that resorts are pleasant, Dr. Hill continued:

> Every thoughtful and unprejudiced practitioner of medicine must feel at times that the mineral water industry is considerably overdone and that the

BOULDER SPRINGS BOTTLING CO.,

SOLE AGENTS FOR

BOULDER - SPRINGS - MINERAL - WATER.

———o———

Recommended for
CONSTIPATION, DYSPEPSIA,
STOMACH, KIDNEY, LIVER
AND BLADDER COMPLAINTS.
GOUT AND RHEUMATISM.

ORIGINAL
"*Manitou*"
TABLE WATER
GINGER CHAMPAGNE

ABSOLUTELY pure and natural. Bottled recharged with NONE BUT ITS OWN NATURAL GAS. Unequaled as a table water or as a blend. Highly recommended by many physicians for stomach troubles, kidney or liver complaints. BEWARE OF SUBSTITUTES. See that each label carries our signature.
WRITE FOR LIST OF AGENTS AND LITERATURE.

The Manitou Mineral Springs Co.,   MANITOU, COLORADO.

general indiscriminate use of these waters does much more harm than good.[63]

Dr. Hill's comments were never heard by the public. They were submerged in a vast sea of mineral water marketing.

14.12 For those who couldn't come to Pueblo, the Clark Magnetic Mineral Spring provided bottled water for sale.

14.13 The Boulder Springs Bottling Company advertised its mineral water as effective in a variety of illnesses.

14.14 The Manitou Mineral Springs Company warned its customers to "beware of substitutes."

15 TUBERCULOSIS: THE WHITE PLAGUE

A dread disease, in which the struggle between soul and body is so gradual, quiet, and solemn, and the result to sure, that day by day, and grain by grain, the mortal part wastes and withers away . . . A disease which sometimes moves in giant strides, and sometimes at a tardy, sluggish pace . . .

Charles Dickens in *Nicholas Nickleby*, 1839

SOME OF THE INFECTIOUS diseases which were responsible for the high mortality rates of the nineteenth century were dramatic in their appearance—the gasping for air in diphtheria, the shaking chills of malaria, the horribly disfiguring lesions of smallpox. Tuberculosis struck quietly and insidiously, yet it was, by far, the greatest killer of them all. Because of the supposedly beneficial effects of its climate, many thousands of tuberculars, including a large proportion of its doctors and some who would become its most prominent citizens, made their way to Colorado. The disease accounted for a major portion of medical care in the state, led to the building of hospitals and sanitaria, and played an important role in the economic and social aspects of life in Colorado. For many years, as many as one out of every three Coloradans had active tuberculosis, one out of every four Coloradans died of the disease, and the state was known as much for "the white plague" as for its mountains and mines.

Tuberculosis is spread by droplet infection—the inhalation of aerosolized bacteria-laden droplets. The bacteria invade the lung, grow, and, although not toxic themselves, the infection results in host defense mechanisms which can destroy the affected pulmonary tissue. In some hosts, the process is self-limited—the infection is successfully contained and the bacteria enter a state of dormancy. A potential for reactivation continues to exist, however. In others, the primary infection is rapidly progressive and results in extra-pulmonary and even widespread lesions. In a few, the primary infection originates outside of the lungs, as in the disease which is caused by drinking milk containing the agent of bovine tuberculosis.

The onset of pulmonary tuberculosis is characterized by fever, night sweats, cough, malaise, and weight loss. The last feature led to the descriptive terms "phthisis" (i.e. wasting) and "consumption." The progressive destruction of lung tissue results in the formation of one or more cavities filled with white, cottage cheese-like material—hence, the term "White Plague." Small blood vessels are destroyed in the process, and the consumptive's chronic cough with its telltale traces of blood, eventually terminating in massive hemorrhage, is familiar as the tubercular's mode of exit in plays and operas, as well as in real life.

There is evidence for tuberculosis in prehistoric remains and many allusions to the disease in classical medical and non-medical literature.[1] The dissemination of tuberculosis is favored by poor nutrition and crowded living conditions, and with the Industrial Revolution and increasing urbanization, the White Plague became the leading cause of death in eighteenth and nineteenth century Europe and America. Most often associated with poverty and city dwelling, it did not spare the countryside or the more privileged classes. In England, for example, its victims included such literary lights as Shelley, Keats, the Bronte sisters, and Elizabeth Barrett Browning. The resorts of Italy, Switzerland, and France drew those who could afford the supposedly beneficial effects of their ambience and climate. Among Americans born around the turn of the century, at least eighty percent would be infected before they were twenty years of age. In Denver, where many tuberculars were drawn from other parts of the country, tuberculosis accounted for more deaths than the next three causes combined.[2]

In the early 1880s, medical textbooks were still pointing to such factors as heredity, climate, diet, mental status, and lifestyle as the key pathogenetic factors in tuberculosis. In 1882 the German microbiologist, Robert Koch, demonstrated that a bacterium, subsequently designated Mycobacterium tuberulosis, was the cause of the disease. With that discovery (and although there was continued resistance to the idea), the infectious—and contagious—nature of tuberculosis was established.

Although none was effective, innumerable medications were used in the treatment of tuberculosis. Alcohol and "tonics" such as strychnine were used as stimulants, heroin and opiates for cough, and various antipyretics for fever.[3] Dr. Darton Wright at the Navy Sanitarium at Fort Lyon, Colorado, advocated the use of mercury.[4] The Denver Medical Times reported on an anti-tuberculosis regime consisting of whiskey, kerosene, creosote, and guiacol, with "the dose of the kerosene and whiskey gradually increased from a teaspoon to a wineglassful of each . . . just before meals."[5] In order to counteract the wasting of consumption, many physicians urged "overfeeding"—diets containing huge quantities of milk, eggs, and other rich foods administered in multiple feedings throughout the day. The homeopaths preferred this approach. Dr. Julia Fitzhugh established a Milk Cure Sanitarium in Denver and Colorado's homeopathic journal urged "at least a gallon daily, gradually increased to two gallons . . . fairly hot in six feedings, drunk slowly . . ."[6] This approach, it claimed, would "add flesh faster than the ravages of the tubercle bacilli can waste it."

Colorado Springs's Dr. S. Edwin Solly concluded that "none of the specific forms of treatment . . . have been found encouraging to use."[7] Periodically, a new therapeutic breakthrough was reported. Denver's Dr. A. Zederbaum thought that koumyss, a mare's milk preparation used by the Tartars in Russia, might be useful. As for glandulin, "goat or calf lungs converted into a mush and worked up into tablets," the doctor stated, "I am not prepared to testify."[8] When Dr. Koch, the renowned discoverer of the tubercle bacillus, introduced a new wonder drug, "lymph," in 1890, the world rejoiced. Denver's Dr. Josef Meuer went immediately to Berlin to obtain some of the new material. The Denver Times hailed Koch's treatment as, "A phenomenal success . . . It has been demonstrated that the bacilli . . . yield to nothing but the lymph."[9] Immediately upon his return from Berlin, Meuer opened his Denver Sanitorium and began using the new therapy. Colorado's tuberculosis experts, including Dr. Charles Denison, were unenthusiastic about Koch's lymph. With the exception of Dr. Meuer and a few other physicians, lymph was never widely used by Colorado doctors, and as its ineffectiveness became apparent, it was discarded.

In some cases, medical therapy was supplemented by a surgical procedure, the induction of an artificial pneumothorax. Collapsing the

15.1 When Dr. Koch's "lymph" became available, Denver's Dr. Meuer quickly travelled to Berlin to obtain a supply. Like many other tuberculosis "cures," Koch's lymph was soon found to be ineffective and was discarded.

infected lung, thereby allowing it to rest, was thought to favor healing. In addition, it was was hoped that the bacteria, deprived of oxygen, would become inactivated. In 1901 Denver's Dr. C. B. Van Zant became the first to perform the procedure in Colorado, when he injected air into the pleural cavity of a young man who had suffered a massive pulmonary hemorrhage and become moribund.[10]

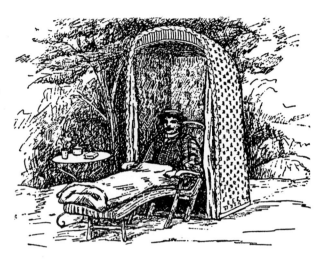

15.2 Consumptives were encouraged to spend as much time as possible out-of-doors. In the winter, they bundled up against the cold.

Mecca of Consumptives

Colorado is the Mecca of consumptives, and rightfully; for dry air, equable temperature and continuous sunshine are as yet the most reliable factors in the cure of that disease.

Denver Chamber of Commerce, 1887[11]

From its earliest days, Colorado's climate was being praised, not only for its beneficial effects on health in general, but for its special effects in tuberculosis. In 1860 a medical visitor wrote:

> To those laboring under a tubercular diathesis, no part of the globe promises more than this region . . . Here [consumptives] will find the long sought after elixir vitae.[12]

The same year, the *Rocky Mountain News* noted that "a hostel for invalids is to be opened at Wazee and G Streets in Denver."[13] The term "invalid" was a nineteenth-century euphemism for patients with tuberculosis, and if the hostel did indeed open, it was the first of many consumptive's rest homes, boarding houses, camps, and sanitaria to come. The state's doctors were truly convinced of the salubrious effects of Colorado's climate, and with an overabundance of physicians making it difficult to earn a living, they encouraged the tuberculous of the East, South, and mid-West to migrate to Colorado. Non-medical boosters and civic leaders viewed the medical immigrants as an important source of growth and capital.

Railroad brochures urged "invalids" to ride the rails to Colorado. The Union Pacific even provided specific medical references to document "the beneficial effect of Colorado's climate upon consumptives."[14] Denver's Chamber of Commerce pointed out that "incipient phthisis is generally cured and always benefited by permanent residence here." In particular, it urged tuberculous parents of "children who have possibly inherited the seeds of this insidious disease . . . to consider whether they do not owe it to these innocent ones to rear them in a climate where the assurances are so great."[15] As for Colorado Springs, a letter to the editor of the *New York Tribune* from a consumptive physician who had tried such celebrated European health resorts as Baden-Baden and Davos, proclaimed, "Colorado Springs is the best resort on the face of the globe for an invalid with lung disease."[16]

Colorado commercialism, the advent of climatology, and the ineffectiveness of regular medical therapy, coincided with the burgeoning theory that, since tuberculosis was characterized by progressive wasting, its treatment should be directed towards building up the consumptive's strength and, thereby, his ability to combat the disease. This could be accomplished, not only by eating large quantities of healthy foods, but by fresh air, sunshine, and exercise. What better place for this approach than Colorado and its vast outdoors?

Dr. Denison had expounded at length on the healthful effects of Colorado's sunshine and altitude. As for the air itself, Dr. Charles Gardiner recommended that, if fresh air was to benefit the consumptive, it should be "pure and free from dust and germs, dry and thin . . . cool—to act as a stimulant, and with an excess of ozone and electricity. In Colorado," he offered, "these climatic conditions do exist."[17] Furthermore, said Gardiner and his Colorado colleagues, if light and air were important, then:

> Five hours daily outdoors are not enough. We would aim at twenty-four hours . . . We cannot afford to waste a single hour in fighting . . . tuberculosis. Few people realize the vast difference that exists between a so-called well ventilated room and the open air—the former is enough to kill an Indian![17]

Tubercular cases, Colorado's physicians warned, "cannot expect to get well unless they come here determined to live out of doors."[18] Many health-seekers did not realize this. One doctor described a typical example, a young woman who had come 2,000 miles at great expense and inconvenience to try the effects of Colorado's climate. She spent her first four months sleeping in a dark, windowless room . . . As she did not improve . . . she decided to return home, convinced that she was as well off there as here.[19]

The doctor was called in to prepare her for the journey. He convinced her to stay, and after suitable exposure to Colorado's outdoors, a high calorie diet, and other measures, she showed marked improvement.

More common was the consumptive who, "chasing the cure in Colorado," was advised by his physician to immerse himself in open air therapy. One such invalid, young Thomas Galbreath, recalled:

> It is not unusual to see an invalid sitting on a covered porch, overcoated, furred, and blanketed, with hot bricks or a hot water bag at his feet. Meanwhile, snow is swirling and drifting over him, and the thermometer is not far above zero . . . When he reaches for the glass of water by his side . . . it is frozen hard.[20]

Dr. Gardiner introduced something of a compromise between the extremes of such outdoor exposure and indoor asphyxiation.[21] On a hunting trip in Colorado's mountains, the doctor was invited to spend the evening with a some old friends, a family of Utes whom he had treated in the past. The next morning, he was surprised to discover that:

> In spite of the very dirty humans around me and the dogs and the old elk meat, all smelling to heaven, the air inside that teepee was as fresh as if I were outdoors. I decided that this . . . was an ideal kind of structure for my tubercular patients, a place where they could be warm and comfortable and not loaded down with blankets and hot water bottles in cold weather, yet with a constant interchange of fresh out-of-doors air all the time . . .[21]

The basis for this effect was a central fire, a hole in the top of the teepee, and a gentle inflow of outside air through a slight opening at the bottom of the tent, around its circumference. The doctor's discovery soon evolved into the Gardiner Tent. Manufactured by the Colorado Springs Tent and Awning Company, it was constructed of "very heavy duck," was sixteen feet in diameter, and was heated by a wood or coal stove. The tent became very popular and, in many variant forms including wooden tent-like structures, became virtually synonymous with the open air therapy of tuberculosis.

Some consumptives devised other arrangements. Thomas Galbreath's landlady allowed him to build his own indoor-outdoor facility, a

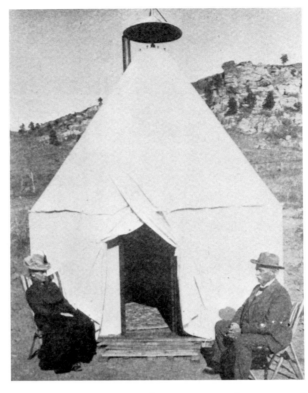

15.3 Dr. Gardiner's tent was a popular compromise between the extremes of the frozen outdoors and the warm, but unhealthy, indoors.

ten-foot square room in a corner of an unused stable. The young invalid nailed strips over the gaping boards and lined the walls with newspapers. The windows were kept open, and in the event of a storm, Galbreath had constructed a device which allowed him to close the windows without leaving his bed.[22]

Much more elegant arrangements were available for those who could afford them. One contraption was an "indoor-outdoor" bed. "Concealed under the seat of a davenport in the room," its dome-shaped top revolved and, "by

15.4 Some tents were more substantial than the Gardiner tent and others less.

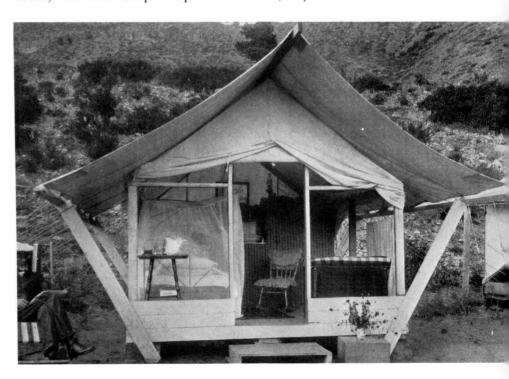

15.5 For those who preferred to stay indoors, there were a variety of indoors-outdoors contraptions available.

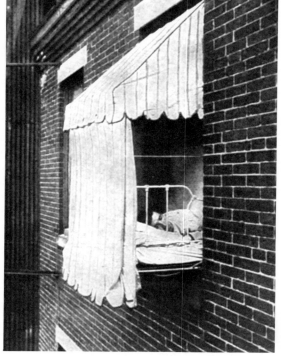

15.6 Sleeping porches were common and can still be seen on many older homes in Denver and other cities in Colorado.

15.7 City dwellers with access to a roof top could make other arrangements.

afternoon and rode from Colorado Springs to Manitou. There they refreshed themselves with mineral water and a meal before riding back. Gardiner recalled that, "Once or twice some one would cough up some blood, and then we would hunt up a hack and send him home." Years later, one of his recovered consumptives told him, "I owe my life to those rides . . ."[27]

Some young men were sent out to Colorado's ranches to build themselves up. One doctor recalled a young consumptive minister who was so sick that he could not even preach.[28] Years later, the doctor did not recognize him, "a typical looking cowboy . . . appearing entirely well [and] now back to preaching." Dr. Eugene Littlejohn came to Montrose where he spent time on a ranch for his tuberculosis. From his own experience, he wrote:

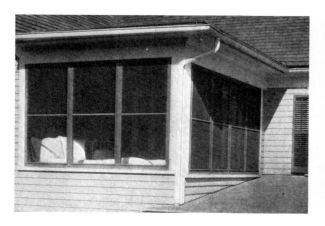

swinging it over to the inside, the occupant found himself out in the open, protected by a heavy wire screen . . ."[23] Another was Dr. Denison's "sleeping canopy." This consisted of a bed with an iron frame supporting heavy drapes; placed next to an open window, the bed provided both the "comforts of indoors [and] the same exhilaration on awakening in the morning as when arising from a cot in an open tent."[24]

The standard indoor-outdoor arrangement, however, was the "sleeping porch"—essentially a room which was open to the outside, screened or lined by windows.[25] Some were modest—wooden additions jutting out from the house on supports. Others were built with the house, and some houses, especially those used to board health-seekers, had as many as five or six sleeping porches. It was said that in Denver and Colorado Springs, perhaps one-third of the homes had at least one sleeping porch. They may still be seen in the older neighborhoods of those cities.

Exercise was considered an essential component of outdoor therapy. One doctor advised his eastern colleagues that, "in sending your patients to Colorado, you are putting them, as it were, in a gymnasium."[26] Another recalled that:

> In the '80s . . . it was not at all unusual to see patients take their 'daily dozens,' to see them use Indian clubs or dumbbells, or even to have them use pulley weights. Exercise was supposed to strengthen their lungs.[27]

Horseback riding was especially popular. Dr. Gardiner organized a group which met every

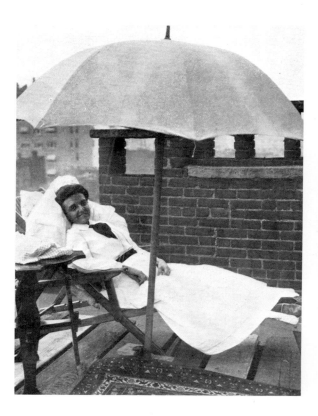

The best thing for the consumptive to do, as early as he can after arriving, is to . . . board at some nice ranch, take an interest in what is going on, help to attend to the poultry or horses, and, if he is able, assist in riding after the cows.[29]

Others were advised to "rough it in the mountains." One anonymous consumptive wrote the *Medical News* that he was living in a log cabin on the Eagle River, subsisting on game, and sleeping in a tent.[30] His "daily loss of phlegm" had been markedly reduced and he was "slowly but surely getting well without medicine of any kind." Whereas he had been contemplating certain death "with the utmost equanimity a few months ago," now he was thinking about the future and even considering taking out a mining claim. For more social health-seekers, the Rocky Mountain Tenting Tour Association offered group tours.[31] On one such jaunt, nine "consumptives" travelled 1,000 miles around the state, complete with tents, horses, wagons, attendants, a physician, and a physical culturist to supervise exercise.

Invalids

In Colorado, we point with pride to many of our most eminent physicians and say, 'He was once tubercular, and came into this state on a stretcher, now look at him, a perfect specimen of health.'

Colorado Medicine, 1911[32]

The consumptives came by the thousands. They had their disease in common, but they varied greatly in their backgrounds and in their means. Most were young adults, mainly men, but a significant number of women also came. Thomas Galbreath's experiences were typical. Five days after learning he had tuberculosis, he was on his way to Colorado:

What magic there was in that name. Colorado! To my mind it was truly Eldorado! No matter how much I suffered from the thought that the bottom had dropped out of all my years of planning, I never for one moment doubted that I was to be well . . .[33]

His doctor back home had told him to stay for three months and to exercise as much as possible. After six months, he was in worse shape than when he had arrived. The young man then consulted another doctor, who advised him to give up his exercise and to:

Sit down from morning until night. Force yourself to eat plenty of nourishing food—rare meat, milk, raw eggs. Keep in the open [air], and don't worry. You are to work your own cure. Under this advice I began truly to chase the cure.[33]

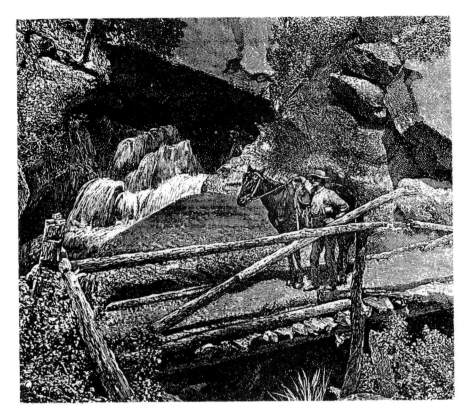

15.8 The incipient consumptive arriving in Colorado was encouraged to exercise. Horseback riding was especially popular, and this young man near Pike's Peak may have been a recently arrived consumptive following his doctor's advice.

Galbreath is known to us because of his little book of reminiscences. Otherwise, he would have been just one of the thousands of unremembered "lungers" who came, survived, and remained in Colorado, or returned home, or who died and were buried here or "back East." Some of the unfortunate ones are briefly memorialized in the records of Denver's coroner:

Thomas Brosnan, about 22 years old, unemployed, arrived from New York one week ago, residing in Mrs. Shaw's boarding house—"severe pulmonary hemorrhage during the night."

John Alexander, 26, bricklayer, recently arrived from Ohio, living in a tent—"violent pulmonary hemorrhage."

Charles Wilson, age unknown, cook, wife and family still in Ohio, living in a rooming house—"taken with a pulmonary hemorrhage while at work at Pell's Oyster House."

Beatrice Brown, 19, unemployed, living with her sister, arrived two months ago from Illinois—"tuberculosis."[34]

Others survived and are remembered for their accomplishments. Among Colorado's health-seekers were politicans such as Governor Frederick Pitkin and Denver's Mayor Robert Speer, poets such as Helen Hunt and Charles Kingsley, merchants such as J. Jay Joslin, railroad magnates such as J. J. Hagerman, and civic leaders such as Lawrence Phipps. As expressed in an 1890s book on "the great West":

Chasing the Cure in Colorado

Being Some Account of the Author's Experiences in Looking for Health in the West, with a Few Observations That Should be Helpful and Encouraging to the Tubercular Invalid, Who, Either from Choice or from Necessity, Remains in His Own Home to "Chase the Cure"

By
THOMAS CRAWFORD GALBREATH

With an Introductory Word by
M. BATES STEPHENS
Maryland State Superintendent of Education

Published by the Author
856 South Logan Avenue
DENVER, COLO.
1908

15.9 Young Thomas Galbreath, like thousands of other consumptives from the East, came to Colorado to "chase the cure." His reminiscences provide some valuable insights into the experiences of the consumptive immigrant.

The influence of the invalids is seen in all the greatness [of Denver and Colorado]. They are New Yorkers, Bostonians, Philadelphians, New Orleans men, Englishmen . . . the architects, doctors, lawyers, and every sort of professional man.[35]

Especially the doctors. An early twentieth-century survey found that one-third of Colorado's doctors had come to the state because of tuberculosis in themselves or a member of their family.[36] An unknown number died of their disease. Dr. Charles Manly, came to Colorado as a young man, managed to graduate from medical school in Denver, founded a medical journal, and wrote numerous papers on tuberculosis, before he succumbed at the age of twenty-nine.[37] The survey's respondents were, of course, the survivors. Of that group, sixty-seven percent considered themselves cured and fifteen percent had arrested disease. The remainder, presumably, still had active disease. Dr. Jacob Reed was thirty-five when he was told he had six weeks to live. He was brought out from Philadelphia on a mattress . . . and lived for many years, a specialist in tuberculosis in Colorado Springs.[38] Dr. A.C. Lusby was twenty-nine and practicing in Kentucky when he began to cough. He and his family came to Denver, where his consumptive brother had already moved. Working as a door-to-door salesman to support his family, Dr. Lusby was advised to try ranch life. He moved to the rural community of Brush, where he practiced for more than thirty years.[39] Colorado had many physicians who specialized in tuberculosis

and some of them were nationally recognized as authorities in the field. Nearly all had come to the state because they (e.g. Drs. S. Edwin Solly, Samuel Fisk) or their wives (e.g. Mrs. G. B. Webb, Mrs. S. G. Bonney) had the disease. Solly, Fisk, and Webb are discussed elsewhere and Bonney later wrote one of the standard textbooks on tuberculosis.[40] The dean of the state's tuberculosis specialists, Dr. Charles Denison, came to Colorado in 1873 because of his tuberculosis. Nearly three decades later, he pointed with pride to the fact that, during that time, he had cared for "some 4,000 lungers," most of them referred by other physicians.[41]

Results

It is a common saying in the East, "If you go to Colorado [for tuberculosis], you must live there forever after; you can never return East."

F. I. Knight, M.D. (Boston), 1890[42]

There was more substantial evidence to support the benefits of Colorado's climate in treating tuberculosis than just anecdotal observations. Three major studies, published between 1880 and 1890, showed remarkably similar results. Of Dr. Denison's original 202 cases, nearly seventy percent had shown clinical improvement.[43] Of Samuel Fisk's one hundred patients, sixty-seven percent were improved.[44] Many of the others, according to Fisk, did not do well because of their own "imprudence," such as excessive exercise or premature return to their homes in the East. Finally, sixty-seven percent of Dr. S. Edwin Solly's consumptives also showed improvement.[45] Again, the results would have been better, it was claimed, "had some [patients] exercised forbearance in delaying their return until their disease was more decidedly arrested."

Sanitaria

The past few years have witnessed a movement in favor of the sanitarium treatment of tuberculosis that has . . . amounted almost to a stampede.

W.T. Little (Canon City), 1904[46]

Prior to the 1900s, the thousands who came had to find non-medical accommodations. The hospitals didn't want them and most consumptives did not want to be confined to hospitals. A few went off to small towns around the state and fewer, still, to ranches or to cabins or tents in the mountains. The wealthy, at least in the earlier years, were allowed into the better hotels or rented apartments or houses. The great majority remained in Denver or Colorado

Springs and lodged in boarding houses, cheap hotels, private homes, or small establishments which "catered to invalids." At The Maples, for example, the proprietress, Mrs. Fleming, "spared no pains to provide her guests with all the comforts and conveniences."[47] Furthermore, Mrs. Fleming saw to it that there was no "plugging" for a particular doctor. Those who preferred the outdoors could board at Mrs. Lare's Tent Sanitarium for a dollar a day. Dr. William Beggs advertised his "Private Home for Early Tuberculosis," where "a limited number of cases . . . will be received for private treatment and supervision."[48]

The Oakes Home was Denver's largest establishment of this type. The Reverend Frederick W. Oakes, an Episcopalian priest, came to Denver from Leadville in 1894. He soon set about to establish a place "for that class of refined and cultured men and women [consumptives] . . . who find it not an easy thing to secure healthful and congenial surroundings . . . within their means."[49] He was quite successful and, over the years, the "Home" expanded to twenty-five buildings (including its main structure, "Hearts Ease") housing 150 patients.[50] It charged eight dollars a week and was always filled. It had no medical staff and each resident was cared for by his own private physician. The house rules were strict. For example: "If a man is seen to expectorate on the grass he is cautioned. If he commits the same offense again, he is ordered away from the place."[51]

To many physicians, it was clear that:

> In so serious and obstinate a disease as consumption, its successful treatment demands our attention to every detail of the patient's life . . . each and all of these matters should be supervised . . .[52]

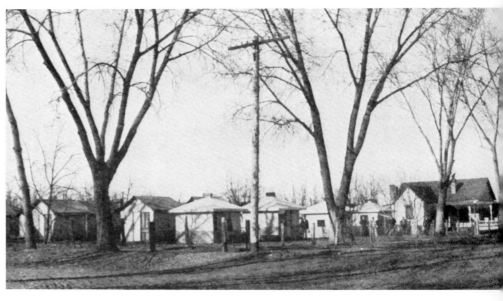

This could only be accomplished in a controlled environment under the control of physicians. In 1884 Dr. Edward Trudeau opened the nation's first tuberculosis sanitarium, at Saranac Lake in upstate New York. Here, selected patients were admitted and subjected to a strict, medically supervised regime which included diet, outdoor therapy, medication, sanitation, and education. It was not until 1899, however, with the opening of Denver's National Jewish Hospital, that the sanitarium movement appeared in Colorado.[53] Within a decade, more than a dozen major sanitaria and a number of smaller ones had opened in Colorado. A few were located in such smaller communities as Boulder and La Junta, but most were in Denver and Colorado Springs.

Denver's premier sanitarium was the Agnes Memorial Sanitarium, opened in 1904 and costing half a million dollars.[54] Located on forty

15.10 Many private homes, boarding houses, hotels, and "private tent sanitaria" provided lodging for consumptives who could afford them—not only in Denver, but in many small communities throughout the state.

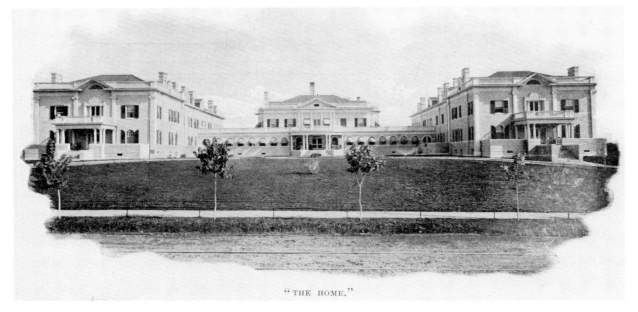

"THE HOME."

15.11 Reverend Oakes's "Home" in Denver was intended for "that class of refined and cultured men and women . . ." who could not afford other arrangements. Its rules were strict.

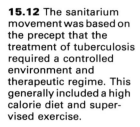

15.12 The sanitarium movement was based on the precept that the treatment of tuberculosis required a controlled environment and therapeutic regime. This generally included a high calorie diet and supervised exercise.

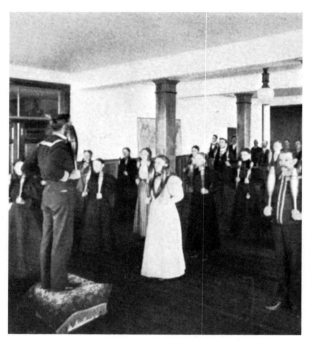

acres seven miles east of Denver, the institution was funded by Lawrence Phipps and named in honor of his mother. The purpose of the sanitarium was to provide "six months or so . . . of outdoor living, physical quiet, abundant nourishment, and medical oversight, at a small cost . . . for persons with early disease whose return to wage earning is urgent."[55] The facility was impressive: "in every detail the most thoroughly built and equipped institution possible . . . No expense was spared." Agnes had electricity and central heating, as well as X-ray facilities and clinical laboratories. The architecture was "Spanish mission" with roofs of red tile. The main building was connected by open cloisters to two patient pavilions and the total capacity was about 150. The cost for a room was twelve dollars a week (about a week's wages for a working man), but lower-cost open-air pavilions were subsequently built for those who could not afford that amount. Concerts and other "entertainments" and all sorts of activities were provided.[56]

15.13 Agnes Memorial Sanitarium, built by millionaire Lawrence Phipps, was the last word in institutionalized tuberculosis care.

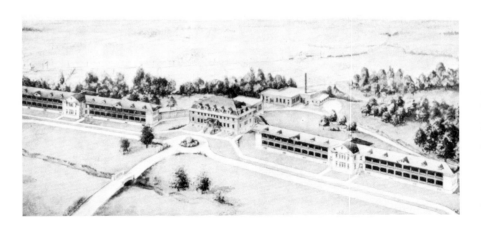

Other sanitaria were opened in metropolitan Denver by various church and philanthropic organizations. These included the Swedish National Sanitarium (1908, in Englewood), the Evangelical Lutheran Sanitarium (1905, in Wheatridge), and the Dutch Reformed and Christian Reformed Church's Bethesda Sanitarium (1914).[57] At the opposite end of the spectrum from the "Agnes" was the YMCA Health Farm.[58] Here, each of the forty-two patients had a "tent-cottage" containing an iron bed, stove, spare furniture, and "toilet apparatus." Built in 1903, the "co-operative colony" charged twenty-five dollars a month and was intended for "men of small means and any or no creed," mostly young white collar workers "whose contracted chests and round shoulders told of hours spent bending over desks or behind counters . . ." Now, they spent their time out of doors, caring for the sanitarium's gardens, orchard, and farm. Some plans for sanitaria never materialized—for example the huge National Sanitarium Hotel, a proposed "grand resort for those who are able to pay."[59]

Colorado Springs was the place for people who could afford to pay, and the ultimate in upscale sanitaria was Cragmor.[60] Conceived by Dr. Solly and built on land and with funds provided by William J. Palmer, Cragmor was based on Solly's vision of an "institution for the well-to-do."[61] The plan was to apply profits derived from one hundred paying patients to the costs of fifty patients who could not afford care. Solly died soon after the complex was opened, however, and under the guiding hands of Dr. Alexius Forster, the sanitarium evolved into something of a "country club" for consumptives. The emphasis at Cragmor was on relaxed gentility, good times, social graces, and the like. Colorado Springs invalid and latter-day historian, Marshall Sprague, compared Cragmor to an ocean liner, still ablaze with light and social activities at three o'clock in the morning.[62] The essence of Cragmor is found in *Ninety-Eight-Six*, a periodical consisting of chatty articles, literary fluff, and news items written by its patients and staff.[63] A typical newletter, written by patient-correspondent "Genevieve" to "Dear Louise," discussed prospects for next summer's flowers; described a call from a Colonel Sutphin, who would be spending the season at the Broadmoor; included other miscellaneous social patter and gentle gossip; and a told of a recent night's entertainments of "dramatics, songs, piano recitals, and dancing." With regard to the latter, the correspondent noted "it is a rare treat to be wheeled into the dining room in bed, and be

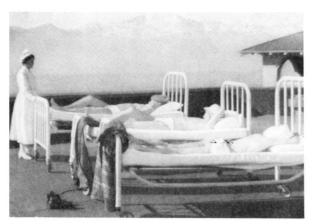

entertained better than you could ever be by going to the city . . ."[64] Elsewhere, Genevieve reminded Louise of the "Samoan dancers who entertained us one Monday a few months ago . . ."[65]

There were quite a few sanitaria in the Colorado Springs area. Like Cragmor, Nordrach Ranch was private, but the ambience was quite different. Nordrach's founder and director, Dr. John White, demanded rigorous adherence to a German-inspired therapeutic regimen of fresh air, overfeeding, and rest.[66] Some of the patients felt like prisoners and referred to White as "the warden."

The Glockner Sanitarium had an interesting history.[67] In 1881 two tuberculous teenagers from Ohio, a brother and sister, arrived in Colorado Springs with their nurse. The boy died soon after their arrival. The girl recovered and met and married another consumptive, Albert Glockner. Before his death in 1888, Albert had discussed the need for a sanitarium in Colorado

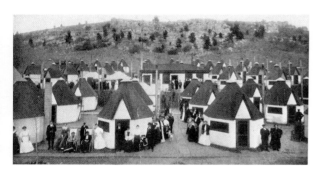

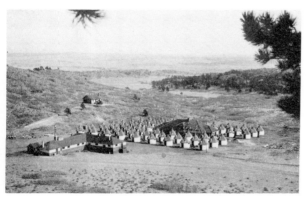

Springs. Now in her twenties, the young widow raised $25,000 and in 1890 opened the Albert Glockner Memorial Sanitarium, the first tuberculosis sanitarium in Colorado. The patients were charged one dollar a day, and Mrs. Glockner made up the deficits, but soon finding herself in financial jeopardy, she gave the sanitarium to the Sisters of Charity of Cincinnati and moved back to Ohio.[68]

There were a number of non-church, non-private sanitaria as well. The Union Printer's Home was founded in 1892, supported by a million dollar investment and fifteen cents a month from each of the International Typographical Union's 50,000 members.[69] The Woodmen Sanitorium was established by a fraternal-insurance society, the Modern Woodmen of America, on a ranch northwest of town. Opened in 1909, the sanitarium included rows and rows of neat wooden, octagonal variants of Dr. Gardiner's famous tent—each one painted white with a red roof.[70] Hospitalization was free to members, and new patients were advised to bring warm clothing with them, including "one cap with ear flaps," and "not less than six handkerchiefs."[71]

National Jewish Hospital, the JCRS, and Poor People

None who can pay can enter—None who enter pay.
Motto of National Jewish Hospital
for Consumptives

He who saves one life is considered as if he preserved the whole world.
Motto of the Jewish Consumptives' Relief
Society Sanitarium (from the Talmud)

It was bad to have tuberculosis, but it was worse to be poor and have tuberculosis. In Denver most private hospitals would not admit indigent tuberculous patients, and even the County Hospital provided only a few beds for the thousands of poor consumptives who were "on the street." In the 1890s there were no sanitaria, and the poor could not afford even the cheapest boarding houses which accepted paying invalids. This was true, not only in Denver, but in other cities across the country. It was particularly true of America's Jews, many of whom had come from the ghettoes of Europe to the ghettoes of New York, Chicago, and other cities and who, on either side of the Atlantic, living in crowded, unsanitary, poorly ventilated tenements and inadequately nourished and clothed, were especially susceptible to tuberculosis.

In November 1889, leading members of Denver's Jewish community met and determined to

15.14 Colorado Springs's Cragmor was the most socially upscale of Colorado's sanitaria.

15.15 Ninety-Eight-Six was a chatty magazine produced by Cragmor's patients and staff. Its name referred to normal body temperature—a goal of the consumptive.

15.16 Nordrach Ranch was based on a strict German therapeutic regime. The patients referred to the sanitarium's director as "the warden."

15.17 The Modern Woodmen Sanitarium was a large tent colony established by the fraternal organization.

build a tuberculosis hospital for poor people. Led by Rabbi William Friedman, they raised money, acquired land, and in 1892 constructed the first of National Jewish Hospital's buildings.[72] Unfortunately, no sooner was the building completed, than the nation entered the "recession" of 1893, and the hospital was not opened until 1899. At that time it became the first sanitarium in Denver. Furthermore, as was clearly stated, its goal was different from other sanitaria:

> It was erected and is maintained for the poor, irrespective of their creed, for those only, of whatever nationality or faith, who have not the means to procure in other institutions the care and treatment their condition requires.[73]

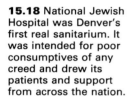

15.18 National Jewish Hospital was Denver's first real sanitarium. It was intended for poor consumptives of any creed and drew its patients and support from across the nation.

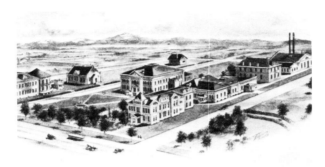

Thus, N.J.H. not only welcomed the poor consumptive to its doors, it specifically limited its facilities to this group of medical outcasts. "No patient who is able to pay can be admitted. It is exclusively for the indigent."[73] Obviously, Denver's small Jewish community could not, by themselves, bear the financial burden of this policy for long. National support was solicited, patients were drawn from across the country, and the hospital grew. Applicants for admission had to have a demonstrably "reasonable chance for recovery." The staff included some of Denver's best known physicians, all volunteering their services.[74]

Within a few years, some members of Denver's Jewish community saw the need for another tuberculosis hospital—one different from N.J.H. Large numbers of eastern European, mainly Russian Jewish immigrants were beginning to arrive in Denver. The newcomers differed from their Jewish predecessors, many of whom were of German origin, educated, and successful merchants or professionals. In addition to being poor, the new arrivals were very "foreign," unsophisticated, uneducated, and unskilled. They were religious, Yiddish-speaking, and sickly. Quite a few had tuberculosis, often to an advanced degree. National Jewish Hospital, with its funding and patients drawn nation-

15.19 The influx of large numbers of Russian Jews to Denver in the early 1900s, many of them with tuberculosis, led to the establishment of J.C.R.S.

ally, could not meet the needs of these people. Furthermore, N.J.H. would not admit consumptives with advanced disease. Thus, the need for a new hospital.[75] In 1903

> in a dingy room on West Colfax . . . a small group of people, most of whom had at one time harbored the tubercle bacilli in their lungs, met for the purpose of devising means of how to help destitute Jewish consumptives in Denver . . . A collection was made, and the magnificent sum of $1.10 was realized.[76]

That was how Dr. Charles Spivak, one of its founders, described the origin of the Jewish Consumptives' Relief Society, better known as the J.C.R.S.[77] Despite its inauspicious beginnings, within a year, the J.C.R.S. had acquired twenty acres of farmland in Edgewater, a mile from the end of the "car line" on the West Colfax Avenue. From its original six tents and seven patients, it had grown, within another year to a three-story brick building and twenty-six tents. Like National Jewish Hospital, the J.C.R.S did not charge its patients. Unlike N.J.H, the J.C.R.S was mainly for Denver's Jews and accepted patients in all stages of tuberculosis. Also, unlike N.J.H, its main support was derived from working class people and labor unions, and it identified more with the orthodox storefront congregations of Denver's West Side than with the establishment reformed Jews of Temple Emmanuel. The J.C.R.S.' *First Annual Report* proudly listed, among the donations received in 1905:

> B. Feldman—one box apples
> Mrs. Greenberg—one bedspread
> J. Laskowitz—one commode
> Mrs. Steinberg—one pillow and feathers[78]

In fact, there was friction between the two sanitaria and their respective supporters. N.J.H., as the senior institution, was concerned that the interloper would attract large numbers of destitute consumptive Jews to Denver. This, in turn, would have a negative impact on the city's non-Jewish majority. Furthermore, the two sanitaria would be competing for financial support from the same pool of donors. The N.J.H.'s publication, *The Outlook*, referred to the J.C.R.S as that "tent cottage sanitarium" and as "an impractical Utopian dream."[79] The J.C.R.S. complained that the N.J.H. interfered with its fund raising activities.[80] The dispute continued to simmer for years, but both institutions were successful and continued to expand. By 1926 the J.C.R.S. was a 300-bed hospital with excellent facilities for the care of tuberculous patients.[81]

Other than these two institutions, facilities for the care of Colorado's indigent consumptives were virtually non-existent. The state which claimed to be the nation's leader in tuberculosis therapy made virtually no provision for its own poor people with the disease. It was not until 1914 that Denver opened a Tuberculosis Dispensary for outpatients—the only such publicly supported clinic in the state.[82] In addition to a few charity beds at some of the private sanitaria, there were two small non-public facilities available for indigent tubercular men and women. In 1909 a consumptive young student from Ohio, Frank Craig, set up his tent on the western edge of Denver. He was joined by others, donations were solicited, and within a year, the Craig Colony, a tent sanitarium for fifty homeless, consumptive men had been incorporated.[82] In 1913 a poor tuberculous young woman knocked at the door of a Denver home and collapsed in the arms of the lady of the house. This incident eventually led to the founding, in 1915, of Sands House, a forty-bed home for destitute tuberculous women.

Tuberculophobia

Tuberculophobia—the unnecessary dread and fear of tuberculosis which has lately affected the public.
C. E. Cooper, M.D. (Denver), 1904[83]

Colorado is most glad to welcome the contents of the purse the invalid brings with him, but she would greatly prefer that the invalid should not accompany the purse.
T.C. Galbreath (Former "invalid"), 1908[84]

Although in the early days, consumptives were generally welcomed to Colorado, even then there were signs of growing callousness and hostility toward the "invalids." Isabella Bird, visiting Colorado in the late 1870s, commented on this attitude, citing one Colorado Springs landlady in particular. While one of her consumptive boarders was dying in the next room, the landlady and her other guests were in the parlor, talking, laughing, and playing backgammon. Mrs. Bird recalled: "No one laughed louder than the landlady . . . All this time I saw two white feet sticking up at the end of the bed."[85] The dying man's brother, himself sick with tuber-

culosis, came out of the invalid's room, groaning and sobbing.

> And still the landlady laughed . . . Afterwards, she said to me, 'It turns the house upside down when they just come here and die. We shall be half the night laying him out.' The corpse lay there the next day, without even a cover on its face.[85]

One problem was the misinformation that some Eastern physicians were giving to their consumptive patients. Many were told to get on the train, spend a few months in Colorado's healthful climate, and return home—cured. One doctor suggested that his patient needn't bother to consult a physician on his arrival in Colorado—just to:

> Walk a mile or two before breakfast and [adhere] to a diet [sufficient] for a smelter hand. The patient struggled on with this advice for two weeks, when complete exhaustion came to his rescue.[86]

Another was told that, once in Colorado, all he had to do was eat six raw eggs every day, and nature would do the rest.[87] Not only were eastern physicians providing their patients with misinformation, they were sending their sickest patients to Colorado. In the twelve years between 1908 and 1920, there were more than 23,000 deaths due to tuberculosis in Colorado. Of these nearly 10,000 died within a year of their arrival, and, of these, nearly half were dead within the first three months! Denver's Dr. H. G. Wetherill warned his eastern colleagues:

> Many tuberculous patients are hurried to the grave by a trip to Colorado . . . Patients who have not the strength or vitality to lead an out-of-door life in New Jersey will get little or no benefit in Colorado.[88]

Even worse than the misinformed consumptive, and the incurable case, was the tubercular who was misinformed, incurable, and indigent. In 1895 Denver's Dr. Charles Manly wrote: "No worse place exists than Denver for the penniless consumptive."[89] A Denver clergyman told an all too familiar story, that of a young man from New York, who, loathe to leave his home, waits until "the disease has got a fatal grip." Finally, his friends and family raise some funds to send him to Colorado. The trip takes all of his money and finally:

> He reaches his Mecca—Denver. He goes to some cheap lodging house, where the surroundings are anything but healthy, and begins the hopeless search for light work. In a few days the poor fellow is . . . sick, hungry, shelterless. This is the story of scores of young men in this city today. The

kindest thing is to send them back . . . that they may die with friends about them . . .[90]

Denver bore the brunt of this influx of indigent consumptives to Colorado. Sometimes they were carried off the train on stretchers:

Visitor: Was there an accident? I saw them carrying someone into the station on a litter.

Denverite: Oh, no. That was a lady suffering from consumption, brought here for benefit from our climate. Such scenes are not uncommon at the Union depot.[91]

From the depot they might be taken directly to the County Hospital. The hospital's director observed:

Nothing is more cruel, revolting, or inhuman, than to send a helpless tubercular . . . without means of subsistence . . . What chance do people situated like that have?[92]

Ironically, as we have seen, Denver, and Colorado, had fewer facilities for indigent consumptives than most cities and states. One reason was: "It was feared that should it become known that we take good care of our indigent consumptives, we would soon be overwhelmed . . ."[93]

In addition, like the landlady in Colorado Springs, and many Coloradans in general, young Thomas Galbreath commented:

The heart of the average Denverite has become hardened toward the tubercular patient ["lungers" they are everywhere called], and human sympathy is conspicuously absent.[94]

Most significant, however, in this change of attitude toward the consumptive, was the fear of acquiring the disease. This had not been a consideration in the early days, when many physicians believed that tuberculosis was not "indigenous" to Colorado and that all of Colorado's cases were in immigrants who had been infected elsewhere. It didn't take very long for this fallacy to be dispelled. As physicians began to emphasize the contagious nature of tuberculosis, there developed an "unreasoning fear as to the dangers of direct infection [and] a popular prejudice against association with the consumptive."[95]

Now, the once-courted tubercular had to disguise his illness in order to obtain lodging. After having been rejected by seven boarding houses, young Galbreath soon learned the secret to finding a place to stay. At the eighth establishment: "It was surprising the number of diseases I found represented, [yet] everyone coughed— dyspeptics, rheumatics, nervous wrecks, heart patients . . . all coughed."[96] Want ads specified,

"No invalids need apply." People crossed the street to avoid a consumptive. The legislature considered a bill which would require a "lunger" to wear a bell around his neck.[96] Hospitals announced that "owing to the prejudice against consumptives, they will no longer be received as patients . . ."[97] James J. Waring, then a medical student recovering from tuberculosis, was allowed to stay at Colorado Springs's Antlers Hotel—if he promised to use the freight elevator.[98] The *J.A.M.A.* printed a rumor that Colorado might be considering the exclusion of tuberculars from its borders.[99]

In a comment reminiscent of current concerns over AIDS, an anonymous "visitor from the East" wrote, in 1909:

The public attitude toward tuberculosis [in Colorado] . . . is made up of ignorance, selfish stupidity, and hypocrisy . . . There is a senseless panic . . . To an avowed patient, not a hotel, boarding-house, or rented home is open, not a job is available.[100]

The editor of the *Denver Medical Times* asked, "Is Denver destined to share the fate of Mentone?" This French town, because of its "ideal" climate, had attracted "all the unfortunate consumptives of Europe."

Today, Mentone . . . is bacillus ridden and a pest hole. The once strong, healthy inhabitants are today coughing, bleeding consumptives. The soil is contaminated . . . It is no longer a health resort.

Will this be the fate of Denver and Colorado Springs? It surely will be unless precautions are taken.[101]

Precautions

The phrase, "No expectoration, no tuberculosis," has become an axiom in phthisology.
        W.N. Beggs, M.D. (Denver), 1911[102]

In addition to discouraging the immigration of consumptives, such precautions included the institution of various public health measures. Some of these were rudimentary, such as urging consumptives to avoid kissing, or even handshaking. Yet, a visitor to Denver complained:

One may go to any drug store or ice cream parlor and drink a glass of Coca-cola or eat a plate of ice cream immediately after a person with active tuberculosis has done the same, the glasses and spoons not having been sterilized.[103]

To the average Coloradan, layman and physician alike, the most obvious, and obnoxious, means of spreading the tubercle bacillus was the consumptive's habit of expectorating his sputum. Denver's Health Commissioner summarized the situation: "The constant spitting upon our sidewalks, streets, houses, and public conveyences, has done much to disseminate the tubercular germs throughout our city."[104] The editor of the *Denver Medical Times* provided a more picturesque analysis:

> In neither [Denver nor Colorado Springs] can a woman walk down the street without gathering on her skirts a sickening mass of bacilli-laden sputa of all ages and stages quite sufficient . . . to sow a family harvest of death.[105]

Spitting was the trademark of the consumptive. Senior Denverites recall a popular children's ditty, sung to the tune of "For he's a jolly good fellow":

> We are the jolly consumptives.
> We are the jolly consumptives.
> Hoch! Chu! Ping!
> Hoch! Chu! Ping![106]

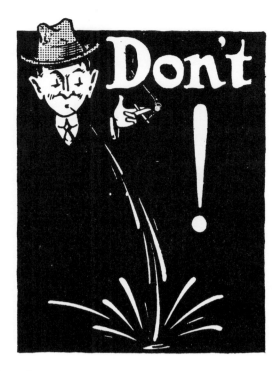

15.20 Signs such as this were posted all over Denver. Some found them offensive.

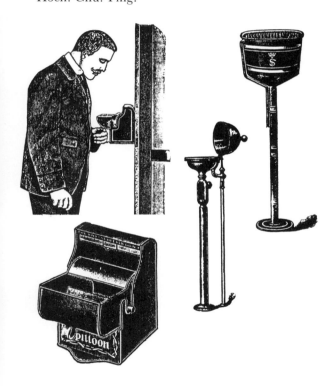

Indoors, in order to contain the flood of infectious sputum, the spittoon or cuspidor was recommended. "Unfortunately," it was pointed out, "not all spitters are good aimers."[107] Another observer commented that, although "a fair number of male patients may possess a certain dexterity in disposing of their sputum, I have yet to find a woman who knows how to hit the spittoon."[108]

Out of doors, a variety of means was available to dispose of the consumptive's sputum. One possiblity was "Japanese paper napkins [which could be] placed in a rubber tobacco pouch immediately after using, and later burned."[109]

Even better were the various "spit cups" which had become available—metal cups containing disposable paper receptacles. It was recommended that the paper be removed every twelve hours and burned and that the metal cup be boiled daily. One popular variety was "flanged—to make the closing of the cup noiseless." A package of fifty cost one dollar.

Anti-spitting campaigns were undertaken. In 1897, for example, the ladies of Denver's City Improvement Society placed "Do Not Spit" signs on telephone poles and in boarding houses, saloons, dairies, hotel lobbies, and even police headquarters.[110] A "smaller placard was placed in the public library—where a larger placard might have been objectionable."[111] A few citizens did object to the signs, including those merchants who denied that Denver even had a tuberculosis problem and some women who complained that "the signs turned their stomachs."[112] Others felt that they were "an effort to hound down and humiliate the poor consumptive."

Even as late as 1910, a national tuberculosis journal was pointing out that Colorado had never taken "any legislative or restrictive steps against the disease."[113] In 1913 the state finally passed a law requiring physicians to report their tuberculous patients to the appropriate health authorities.[114] Other public health measures were included in the law, such as a requirement that all premises vacated by consumptives be cleansed and disinfected. A number of private efforts were also beginning to be made to deal with what had come to be known as "Colorado's burden." In 1908 the organization subsequently

15.21 Indoors, the expectorating consumptive was encouraged to use a spittoon. Some spittoons were of the usual variety, while others were more elegant or exotic. The problem with spittoons was that "not all spitters are good aimers."

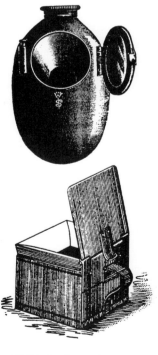

15.22 Outdoors, the consumptive was urged to use a sputum cup or flask.

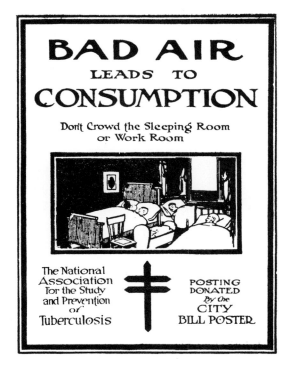

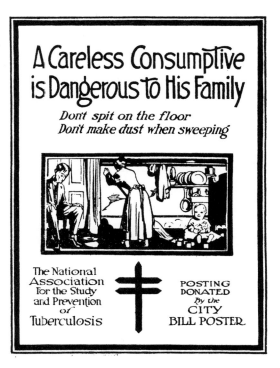

15.23 Finally, in the early twentieth century, active efforts were being made to educate the public about tuberculosis.

15.24 Tuberculosis prevention programs were intitiated among Denver's schoolchildren, especially in T.B.-prone neighborhoods. This is an open air rest period in west Denver's Chelthenham school in 1922.

known as the Colorado Tuberculosis Association was founded.[115] In addition to raising funds for free outpatient care and lobbying for public health measures, the association sponsored a variety of anti-tuberculosis educational programs.

One especially notable effort was the "open air school." Based on a study which showed that many of Denver's schoolchildren were underweight, anemic, or otherwise "defective," and the high incidence of tuberculosis among the parents of west Denver's Jewish children, a program was instituted in the neighborhood's Chelthenham public school.[116] The daily program, meant to build up the children's resistance to tuberculosis, included a shower, a hearty lunch accompanied by two glasses of milk, and rest periods. These were outdoors, on the school's roof, with the children bundled into "Eskimo costumes" during the winter months. Under this regimen, each child gained an average of two pounds a week, and "one little girl who was

apathetic and never smiled, became one of the happiest in the class and gained ten and a half pounds."

At last, by the 1920s, Colorado and Denver and other communities were beginning to deal with the White Plague in a systematic and modern fashion, approaching the disease from a variety of medical, public health, and sociologic aspects.

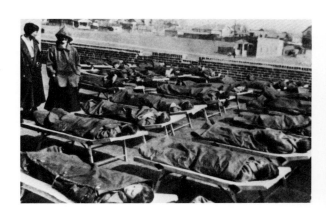

16 SMALLPOX: THE RED PLAGUE

One glance was enough! The swollen pustular face, the delirium, the fingers scratching at the face, and the smell . . . Confluent smallpox! I had seen many cases like it before. I did what I could, put lard on the scarred and bleeding face, and tied the hands to protect the eyes. I told the family what it was. No one spoke.[1]

C. F. Gardiner, M. D. (Meeker), 1890s

D R. CHARLES GARDINER described this as a typical case of smallpox. He had made a fifty-mile "housecall" to a remote cabin on Colorado's western slope. Holding a lantern to the face of his patient, a fifteen-year-old boy, the doctor had made the dreaded diagnosis.

Indeed, the Red Plague was probably the most dreaded of mankind's many afflictions. It was the same disease which had ravaged the features of an Egyptian pharoh in the fourteenth century B.C., wiped out three and a half million Mexicans early in the seventeenth century, and killed half of Iceland's population in 1707.[2] Well into the twentieth century, between 1920 and 1930, nearly half a million Americans would contract smallpox and 5,000 would die of the disease.[3]

Smallpox is due to a virus. Limited to the human species, it is spread by the inhalation of virus-containing droplets. The inhaled virus multiplies, and within a week or two, the host develops a "flu-like" illness. Several days later a rash appears, first on the face, then everywhere. Small red papules become blisters and then pustules. As in Dr. Gardiner's patient, they may become confluent and the patient's face swollen and unrecognizable. Scabs form in about ten days, and if the patient survives, they fall off in three or four weeks, leaving their characteristic pitted scars. Smallpox is one of the most contagious diseases known to man. The patient is infectious for about four weeks—from the appearance of the rash until the time that the scabs fall off. Since animals do not develop smallpox, the disease requires a continuous chain of infected human beings. Such an unbroken chain has persisted for at least three millennia. There has never been any effective treatment for smallpox, but survivors have lasting immunity to the disease.

In 1798 the publication of a little pamphlet by an English country doctor marked a medical milestone.[4] Dr. Edward Jenner had observed that previous infection with cowpox, a mild disease acquired from cattle, conferred immunity to smallpox. This fact, well-known to milkmaids and a part of country folklore, was taken a step further by Jenner when he used material ob-

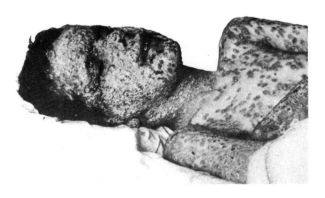

16.1 Dr. Gardiner's patient, a fifteen year old boy, had confluent smallpox, the type illustrated here. The outcome was all too obvious.

tained from a cowpox infection to infect individuals who had never been exposed to smallpox. The procedure, termed "vaccination" (after the medical term for cowpox), did indeed confer protection against smallpox. Vaccination was hailed by some and denounced by others, a situation which would continue well into the twentieth century. Jenner's accomplishment, it should be recalled, was made prior to any knowledge of the microbiologic nature of infectious disease or of the biologic basis of immunity. One year later an American physician, Dr. Benjamin Waterhouse, received a supply of vaccine from England. On July 8, 1800, he vaccinated his five-year-old son and others in his household.[5] Again there was opposition, even threats of violence, but Waterhouse received powerful support from Thomas Jefferson and, eventually, most physicians.

Nevertheless, arguments over vaccination continued in legislatures and churches, among school boards and city councils, and in newspapers and medical journals. Without a uniform policy of compulsory vaccination and until the need for re-vaccination was realized, devastating outbreaks continued throughout the nineteenth century. In 1871 smallpox killed 2,000 in Philadelphia; the next year 1,000 died in Boston. During the great pandemic of 1881-1883, with the spread of disease fostered by immigration and the railroads, tens of thousands died in the U.S.A.

In the West, the first outbreaks of smallpox occurred in the eighteenth century, in the settlements and pueblos of New Mexico. Vaccination having been accepted early in Spain, the Spanish government sent a flotilla in 1803 to vaccinate the population of her colonies.[6] This was done by the establishment of a "human chain" to maintain the cowpox infection during the long voyage to the New World. A group of orphan boys served this function. Every two weeks, a new pair of boys was inoculated with material from a previously infected pair, thereby maintaining the virus. From Mexico City to Chihuahua, and finally to Santa Fe and the pueblos, the procedure was continued, with the relentless determination so typical of Spanish colonialism. As elsewhere, there was resistance, notably in the pueblos of Zuni, Laguna, and Acoma, but by 1805 several thousand Indians and settlers had been vaccinated.

In 1837 an American Fur Company steamer, carrying supplies to the trappers on the upper Missouri, also brought smallpox and wiped out several tribes of Plains Indians. In the next few years, the Red Plague devastated tribes throughout the West.

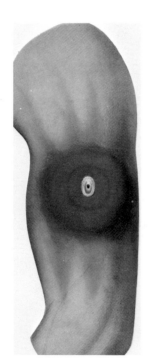

16.2 Vaccination was introduced by Jenner in 1798. Most Americans remained unvaccinated, however, and devastating outbreaks of smallpox continued throughout the nineteenth and early twentieth centuries. In Colorado, the disease struck down Indians, Hispanics, and Anglos indiscriminately.

The Pox in Colorado

In early nineteenth-century Colorado, vaccination could have been introduced by either of two routes. From Santa Fe, the "human chain" was said to have extended to a few New Mexican settlers along the upper Rio Grande in southern Colorado. Although this route may have been successful, the second was not. The Long expedition, entering Colorado from the east, had been ordered to vaccinate any Indians they met along the way. Unfortunately, as the expedition's physician and chronicler, Dr. Edwin James noted, the vaccine had been ruined when a keelboat overturned on the Missouri River, long before the group reached Colorado.[7]

Certainly, vaccine would have been useful at Bent's Fort where, in 1829, the first recorded outbreak of smallpox in Colorado occurred.[8] With the fort still under construction, the disease appeared among a newly arrived party of Mexican workers. It soon spread to the others, including William Bent and Kit Carson. Bent warned the Indians to stay away until the disease had run its course. How many neighboring Cheyennes and Arapahoes were infected by that particular outbreak is unknown. However, a particularly devastating epidemic occurred among the Arapahoes in 1855. That year the tribe was so decimated that they were unable to engage in their annual buffalo hunt. Instead they resorted to stealing sheep and cattle. The government, unimpressed with their excuse, canceled their annuity.

On a wagon train, an outbreak of smallpox was equivalent to its occurrence on board ship. In 1861 the Russell brothers, in five wagons, were returning to Georgia to join the Confederate army.[9] They were well on their way when Dr. Levi Russell diagnosed smallpox in one of the party. Unable to turn back, he quarantined those who had been exposed into one wagon, disinfected their clothing, and since few in the party had been vaccinated, awaited the inevitable. Ultimately, seventeen members of the party developed the disease. Four died, including a child.

The first recorded outbreak of smallpox in Denver occurred during the summer of 1860. Apparently a mild one, it was sufficiently threatening to inspire the appointment of a city physician, Dr. J. T. Hamilton.[10] The frontier town's fear of Indian attacks was compounded by an outbreak of smallpox among the Cheyennes in 1862. The *Rocky Mountain News* announced: "Dr. Feld has just received from the

East a lot of fresh and pure vaccine matter. He can be found at his office on 5th Street."[11]

In 1877 an epidemic swept through the southern part of Colorado. The population of that part of the state was mainly Hispanic, there were few physicians, and health care was poor. Father Pinto, the pastor of Las Animas county, described the outbreak:

> Supposedly brought from New Mexico, for nearly three months the disease was confined to . . . five or six miles around Trinidad. Then it spread all over the county. At least one thousand were attacked [out of a population of about 9,000], with a mortality of over four hundred. Cleanliness, proper care, vaccination, etc. could have saved, to say the least, two-thirds . . .[12]

The Hispanics of Las Animas county did receive some medical attention. Dr. Michael Beshoar travelled in a buggy throughout the county, vaccinating everyone he could find. Father Pinto served as his assistant, adding the church's authority in trying to pursuade the frightened and suspicious people to permit their children to be vaccinated.[13] Father Ussel at Walsenburg estimated that there were 320 deaths in neighboring Huerfano county, nearly all among the Hispanic population. The county clerk noted that he knew " . . . of but one Mexican case where a doctor was called." The State Board of Health calculated that in Huerfano County ten percent of the population died as a result of the epidemic.[14]

Fear gripped the state during such epidemics. Travelers were afraid to enter a new community, while townspeople regarded newcomers as possible sources of infection. The recollections of a visitor to Del Norte in 1877 are typical:

> Smallpox was raging . . . Mother was very much frightened. The hotel room had just been fumigated [and] mother was certain that someone had just died of smallpox in that bed . . . The next day as they started out by stage for Lake City, they were cautioned to put asafetida and camphor gum about their clothes, and to hold their handkerchiefs with carbolic acid over their noses if they met anyone, especially a Mexican.[15]

In 1880, Lieutenant B. J. Byrne, an army doctor on his way to Fort Lewis, found himself stranded in Mancos, Colorado, as a result of smallpox.[16] During a rest stop in that town, Byrne was asked by a local boy to examine his sister. He diagnosed smallpox. The stage driver, having heard of Byrne's brief contact with the dread disease, would not allow him to reboard, telling him that if he did, there would be a riot on their arrival in Durango. Stuck in Mancos and facing an epidemic, Byrne contacted the

surgeon at Fort Lewis, told him of his plight, and requested a supply of vaccine. Eventually he was able to vaccinate everyone, the epidemic was prevented, and Byrne received the grateful thanks of the townspeople. Ironically, Durango was unable to prevent a subsequent outbreak of smallpox. A few years later a passenger on the Durango train was found to have the disease.[17] He was brought to Mercy Hospital where, one by one, the sisters and others contracted the disease. The hospital had to be closed for five months.

Nor were the mining camps, isolated as they were, immune to the disease. Several legends tell of Silverheels, a beautiful saloon dancer who lived in Buckskin Joe, a camp near Fairplay.[18] During a smallpox outbreak, Silverheels, disregarding her own safety, was said to have nursed many of the afflicted miners. Coming down with the disease herself, her face now covered with the pox, she disappeared from the town. Years later, glimpses of a mysterious, heavily veiled lady were reported, periodically, by people in the area.

The mining camps were distressed by the bad publicity engendered by reports of smallpox epidemics in their communities, particularly when those reports appeared in the newspapers of rival towns. The *Lake City Times* resented what it considered exaggerated reports of an outbreak of smallpox in its community:

> The *Times* wishes to impress upon the minds of the pencil pushers employed on many newspapers . . . that a gross injustice is being done to the bussiness interests of this county by the publication of wild, exaggerated reports . . . Certain papers published in Grand Junction, Gunnison, and Salida deserve censure for the efforts they put forth to frighten people who have friends in Lake City . . . There have been some five cases of smallpox here [and] the authorities now have full control of the situation . . .[19]

Quarantine and Pesthouses

Since there was no specific treatment for smallpox, outbreaks were dealt with in three ways—the identification and reporting of cases, isolation of infected and exposed individuals, and vaccination of the rest of the population. In 1893 a state law required that all cases of smallpox be reported to the proper health authorities, not only by physicians, but by private citizens as well. Noncompliance was punishable by a fine of up to $100. Local governments were given the power to take whatever means necessary to prevent the spread of the disease, to establish suitable hospitals, and to provide vac-cination.[20] Unfortunately, the law was fre-quently ignored and variably enforced. In 1900 Denver's Health Commissioner was considering action against the superintendent of School Dis-trict No. 2 for failing to report cases of smallpox, and a few years later, a Denver physician was fined fifty dollars for a similar offense.[21] Quick action was needed when a case of smallpox was discovered. Such was the case when Dr. Jesse Hawes diagnosed the disease in a "tramp" re-cently arrived in Greeley. Dr. Hawes's actions were published as a model by the State Board of Health:

All persons who had come in contact with [the tramp] were immediately vaccinated . . . [His] room was thoroughly saturated with the fumes of burning sulfur. All bedclothing, clothing, etc. not carried with the patient to the pesthouse was burned. A vaccinated nurse remained with him until his death [and] no person except myself came in contact with him. When visiting him I wore a special suit that was removed immediately after visit and placed in an atmosphere of sulphurous acid, and my whole person was sponged with a 2% solution of carbolic acid. After his death, all clothing, bedding, etc.. was burned and the house was thoroughly fumigated.[22]

When a community faced the prospect of a smallpox epidemic, an officer of the State Board of Health was frequently called in. Such was the case in Cripple Creek in January 1901.[23] Twenty-five cases had already been identified when the consultant arrived from Denver. Within a day, he had arranged for a house-to-house inspection of the city, vaccination of the populace, estab-lishment of an isolation hospital, fumigation of infected houses, and—no small achievement in a mining camp—closing of the dance halls![24]

Unfortunately, many outbreaks were not handled with equal aplomb. On March 25, 1899, a worker named Charles Cain arrived at the Denver and Rio Grande railroad construction camp near La Veta in southern Colorado.[25] That night he became ill and developed a rash. Sometime later, several of the camp's thousand workers became ill and were "hospitalized" in the billiard hall in La Veta's hotel. They were soon joined by others. The men mingled with the hotel's guests and used the same washroom. When, at last, the diagnosis of smallpox was made, and with the threat of panic in the air, the board's Dr. Henry Sewall was asked to come and advise the town. At a hastily called town meeting, Sewall outlined a course of action—quarantine, vaccination, and so on. Unfortu-nately, "considerable feeling" existed among the

three key parties whose cooperation was neces-sary to effect such measures—La Veta's officials, the county authorities, and the bosses at the construction camp. Their efforts were less than ideal, and as a result, there were a large number of cases and a dozen deaths.

Sometimes, rather sophisticated epidemio-logic detective work was used to track down the source of an outbreak. *Colorado Medicine* re-ported:

On November 15, 1898, a sheep-herder from New Mexico suffering from the disease passed through the city [of Denver]. Ten days [later] two railway employees with whom he had come in contact developed smallpox; a week later the child of one of these men and a sister of the other were taken down . . . No further manifestations have been dis-covered due to this infection and we regard it as ended.[25]

At about the same time, other outbreaks were traced to a "negro from Pueblo, a Denver businessman returning from Texas, and an actor recently arrived from Mexico." In each instance "all persons whose exposure [was] great were removed to the [isolation] hospital or kept under surveillance for two weeks and vaccination done . . ."[25] A Denver ordinance required conductors on incoming trains to telegraph ahead if they suspected smallpox in any of their passengers. The following year, a Kansas Pacific passenger was found to have smallpox. In strict compliance with the law he was escorted directly to the mayor's office and from there quickly to the County Hospital.[26]

The same Denver ordinance required the quarantining of infected persons. This meant that an individual, or a family, might be isolated in their home for a few weeks, or sent to the dreaded smallpox hospital—the "pesthouse." For example:

On March 20 [1899] the police and one of the medical inspectors discovered at 1837 Wynkoop Street a family, one member of which had arrived in Denver from Victor [where there was an out-break of smallpox]. She had an eruption when she came to town . . . but no physician had been called. The whole family was removed to the quarantine hospital.[27]

In 1881 Denver's pesthouse consisted of a two-room building staffed by an attendant. In 1885 a new isolation facility, Sand Creek Hospital, was built nearly seven miles northeast of down-town. The hospital consisted of three buildings with sufficient space for fifty patients. There was also a "stable and a modern ambulance, for smallpox only, kept constantly in readiness."

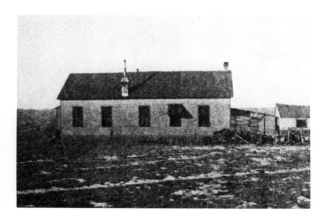

Nearly three decades later, in 1914, Sand Creek Hospital admitted 103 patients. To Denver's residents, the pesthouse had all of the allure of the Black Hole of Calcutta. Nevertheless, its superintendent noted that "not a single complaint was received from any of the patients . . ."[28] The Sand Creek "pesthouse" continued to be used until World War I.

Vaccination and Anti-Vaccinationists

As elsewhere, there was much opposition to vaccination in Colorado. Some of this was based on the fact that, in a small number of instances, the procedure was followed by complications. Edwina Fallis recalled being "scratched" by the doctor when she was seven years old. The vaccination "took" so well that it "nearly took my arm and my life too." For a week, she had to sit by the fire while her mother squeezed soap suds over the sore.[29] Such complications, and deaths, were stressed by those who were opposed to vaccination.

Dr. E. Stuver, a physician in Fort Collins, responded to

. . . the misguided anti-vaccinationist [who], allowing his imagination to run away with his judgement, holds up his hands in horror, and with bated breath, and a scared look, calls our attention to the horrible diseases and occasional deaths caused by vaccination.[30]

Such rare occurrences, said Dr.Stuver, are "but a tiny, trickling rill alongside the great river of beneficence which this grand discovery has brought to soothe and save suffering mankind."[30]

Sometimes physicians had to appeal to nonmedical motives in promoting vaccination. During an outbreak in Greeley, Dr. Jesse Hawes used what might be called "reverse psychology" to pursuade a rancher to have his children vaccinated.[31] Noting that if the family came down with the pox he would probably have to make

daily housecalls for about six weeks and that each housecall would probably net him fifteen dollars, Dr. Hawes told the rancher that he would, of course, prefer that the family not be vaccinated. The rancher, quickly taking into account the financial as well as the medical aspects of the matter, quickly responded, "Doc, I'll bring them in at nine o'clock in the morning."

The miners of Cripple Creek were not quite so easy to deal with. In 1901, during an outbreak of smallpox, the State Board of Health urged that all of the miners in the district be vaccinated.[32] When the manager of the Gold Coin mine made vaccination compulsory for his men, he "stirred up a regular hornet's nest." The Miner's Union resolved that its members would not subject themselves to still another outrageous action by a ruthless mine owner and "it seemed that a good deal of trouble might be occasioned." Fortunately, the union, perhaps feeling that other capitalist-worker issues were more worthy of battle, withdrew their opposition.

Compulsory vaccination was seen by some as an infringement on personal liberty. The *Colorado Medical Journal* responded to this argument by quoting the U.S. Supreme Court's decision supporting a state compulsory vaccination law:

Real liberty for all could not exist under the operation of a principle which recognizes the right of each individual to use his own [liberty] . . . regardless of the injury that may be done to others.[33]

Some opposed vaccination on religious grounds. The *Denver Medical Times* noted, sardonically:

There are quite a number of cases of smallpox in Idaho Springs. In every instance the persons had not previously been vaccinated. Then again Idaho Springs has quite a colony of 'eddyites,' so-called Christian Scientists.[34]

Battles between pro- and anti-vaccinationists, a national phenomenon, were fought well into the twentieth century in Colorado. The public schools were the most frequent battlefield. This letter was sent to a teacher by a parent in 1900:

Dear Madam:
I do not want my daughter vaccinated, as I am strongly opposed to that mode of Medical Practice. It is pure and simple a medical fake and delusion . . . When the virus is once injected . . . they are never as healthy as before . . . Do not insist upon Marguerite being POISONED by vaccination.[35]

The following year, Denver's Health Commissioner attempted to enforce a city ordinance

16.3 Sand Creek Hospital was Denver's facility for the isolation of smallpox patients. In 1914, 103 patients were admitted. Many other Colorado communities had their own smallpox "pesthouses."

which required the vaccination of all public school children. Hundreds of unvaccinated children were expelled from school, and the matter was brought to the district court. In a test case, the judge directed the principal of one school to admit a brother and sister despite their failure to produce certificates of vaccination, a temporary victory for the anti-vaccinationists.[36]

16.4 Although opposed by the anti-vaccinationists, some school districts required evidence of vaccination before a student could be enrolled. The issue was fought in the courts.

Central City, Colorado, *Dec. 6* 190 *1*

This is to Certify

That *Gertrude Barber*

has been vaccinated by me this 6 day of

Dec 190 *1*

A. Ashbaugh

Within each school district there was a constant shuffling of responsibility for making decisions regarding vaccination, with the community, physicians, newspapers, churches, and individuals often polarized and school boards and county health officials caught in the middle. In 1904 the State Board of Health recommended to the Superintendent of Public Instruction "that all pupils must show signs of recent successful vaccination before being allowed to attend school."[37] Unfortunately, there was no law by which the board could enforce this regulation. Finally, an outbreak of smallpox in the Cripple Creek District brought things to a head in 1906.[38] After twenty-nine cases had occurred, the Victor School Board issued a compulsory vaccination order. This time the court found the order to be lawful, a precedent which was used by officials in other communities to compel the vaccination of Colorado's public school students.

The anti-vaccinationists continued their fight, however—a fight which would culminate in the worst outbreaks of smallpox in Colorado's history. In 1911 a state senator introduced legislation to repeal the compulsory vaccination law.[39] The same year there were 472 cases of smallpox in Denver. In 1914 New York, a city with a compulsory vaccination law and a population more than twenty times that of Denver, had one-fifth as many cases of smallpox.[40] In 1920 an anti-physician organization called the Colorado Medical Liberty League (Chapter 21), focused its attention on the compulsory vaccination law.[41] The following year, the mortality rate for smallpox in Denver was fifty percent, virtu-

16.5 The successful opposition to compulsory vaccination culminated in a devastating outbreak of smallpox in Denver in 1922. There were nearly 500 cases and 144 deaths. This child is being vaccinated at Denver's city hall during an earlier epidemic.

ally all in people who had never been vaccinated. The city physician noted that:[42]

As soon as the death record appeared in the newspapers the people began to flock to the Health Department and demand to be vaccinated. There was no compulsion and no arguments . . . 3,309 people were vaccinated in one day and [about] 50,000 in the city.[42]

With obvious satisfaction, he added:

I think it is the first time that such a thing has occurred, and for the medical fraternity, who for years have been insisting on vaccination, it was a great victory.[42]

Although vaccination was now compulsory for public school students, it was still not required of anyone else, and during the five years between 1918 and 1923 there were thousands of cases of smallpox in Colorado and more than 300 deaths.[43] In one ten-week period in 1922, from mid-October until the end of the year, there were nearly 500 cases in Denver, with 144 deaths.[44] Nationally, smallpox was enjoying its "last hurrah," with more than 200,000 cases in the outbreaks of 1920-1921 and 1924-1925. The anti-vaccinationists had succeeded in placing the U.S.A. second only to India in the incidence of this preventable and devastating disease.[45] Future years would see the increased use of vaccination (though not without continued opposition) and the decreasing frequency of smallpox. Although the appearance of a case nearly forced the postponement of the opening of the Central City Opera in the 1930s, by the late 1940s the disease had been virtually eliminated throughout the country. Dr. Gardiner's vivid description of smallpox in that fifteen-year-old boy in a cabin in western Colorado had finally become a matter of purely historical interest.

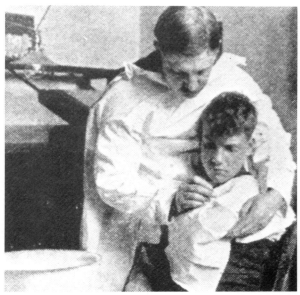

17 PUBLIC HEALTH AND TYPHOID

Notwithstanding its youth, Denver is one of the dirty citys of the country. Filth has been accumulating for nearly twenty years, with but little disturbance.

F. J. Bancroft, M.D. (Denver), 1878[1]

PUBLIC HEALTH WAS NOT a priority issue in early Colorado. Dr. Bancroft's comments referred to Denver, but they might have applied to many of the state's smaller communities as well. The mining camps were, one senses, almost proud of their inattention to sanitation. Such namby-pamby matters were of no concern to miners and prospectors. As for drinking water—what could be purer than a mountain stream? The open sewers, crowded quarters, and general filth simply contributed to frontier town ambience. The agricultural and ranching towns may have been a little more concerned with their appearance, but local taxpayers were not enthusiastic about paying for water treatment plants. The homesteader resisted such measures as quarantine and compulsory vaccination as infringements on his liberty. The farmer had more important things to worry about than the proper location of his privy. The rancher didn't care about the depth of his well—just so long as it didn't run dry. The infectious diseases continued to take their enormous toll, but one by one, medical scientists were demonstrating the etiologic agents, describing the means of spread, and advising on methods to control many of them. Public health measures were being advocated by an increasingly confident medical profession and were being successfully applied to diphtheria, smallpox, tuberculosis, and scarlet fever.

Although sanitation and public health were statewide issues, as Dr. Bancroft suggested, the problems were most apparent in Colorado's largest city. Five years earlier, Bancroft, as city physician, had "respectfully recommended" that

> the city be thoroughly policed as soon as practicable, for there has been much waste matter and filth accumulated in many of the alleys and yards . . . during the winter, which needs only the spring rain to generate miasma.[2]

Denver's major newspaper, the *Rocky Mountain News,* supported the city physician, and urged the city to take appropriate action.[3] That little was done is indicated by Dr. Bancroft's subsequent remark about Denver as "one of the dirty cities of the country." He cited specific examples:

> Waste matter thrown into the Platte . . . lodged along the banks emitting most unwholesome odors.
> Slop-holes, numerous and disagreeable, are everywhere seen . . .
> Whoever will take an early morning drive through the town will not fail to see a dozen or more dead rats . . .
> Privies overflowing and located near wells . . .[4]

Still, little was done. A year after Bancroft's second warning, the *Denver Tribune* commented:

> The lack of sewage and the inefficiency of the means provided for the disposition of waste and offal demand that every precaution be taken. The gutters need cleaning, the alleys need cleaning . . . Garbage and filth are prolific mothers of disease . . . Clean up![5]

177

Years later, a downtown merchant named Strauss, unsuccessful in his efforts to have the city remedy the "cesspool" which periodically collected outside his Larimer Street clothing store, posted a placard accusing the city of ignoring this "breeding place for cholera."[6] Mr. Strauss had been frustrated by two years of fruitless communication with the mayor, board of health, street commissioner, and city engineer. The politicians responded to Mr. Strauss's placard by having him arrested for "obstructing the highway." So much for fighting City Hall.

State Board of Health

Every act of commission or omission which may affect the public health . . . shall be regarded as a nuisance, and the person or persons causing the same shall be held liable accordingly.
Laws of the Union Mining District
(Clear Creek County), 1861[7]

Noble as such early attempts were, Colorado's politicians—whether in Denver, the mining camps, or the countryside—were loathe to enact or enforce public health measures. Finally, in 1876 the legislature created a board of health.[8] Its nine members included the president, Dr. Bancroft, and physicians from around the territory. The first meeting was held in Bancroft's office, and the nine members were apportioned among nine committees devoted to such areas as epidemics, climate, altitude, food, drink and water, and sewers and sewerage.[9] Unfortunately, the board was provided with no facilities and a total budget of only $500. As one of its early members recalled, it was "simply a literary and advisory board . . . absolutely without power."[10] The board was largely ignored, the state auditor refused to sanction its vouchers, and it "received no encouragement or sympathy from the people." The board's president noted that the lack of funds prevented the publication of "the year's proceedings" but "confidently hoped that the Legislature . . . will increase our appropriation so as to facilitate the work of the Board . . . "[11] Unfortunately, "The Legislature failed to appreciate its labors and [the board] died a natural death from inanition in 1880."[12]

In 1892 the threat of a cholera epidemic reminded Colorado that it had no statewide agency available to deal with problems of health and disease. Fortunately, the epidemic did not materialize, but the crisis resulted in the establishment of a new board of health, responsible for the "general supervision of the interests of health and life of the citizens of the State."[13] Again, there was little in the way of money to support this major endeavor. The new board did gather health statistics and published the state's first mortality data.[14] In the early 1900s, it began to participate in national public health activities, and in 1906 the U.S. Bureau of the Census proclaimed that Colorado's vital statistics reports had become sufficiently accurate to warrant their inclusion in the National Registry.[15]

In addition to its national participation, the board began to increase its interactions with local health authorities. In 1898, for example, in addition to assisting local authorities with a number of smallpox outbreaks, the board dealt with:

> Complaints of the disposition of dead cattle at Hillside, requests for permission to exhume dead bodies, the existence of refuse heaps at Westcliffe, and mediation in a dispute as to proper kind of wall paper to be used in school houses in Ouray.[16]

Increasingly, local agencies relied on the state board's expertise in public health matters. Water purification plans submitted by the towns of Hotchkiss, Delta, and Fort Collins were approved by the board, and in 1904 the board was asked to investigate a devastating outbreak of typhoid in Leadville. Sometimes the state board's interactions were unsolicited—as when it investigated unsanitary conditions in Pueblo and reprimanded Glenwood Spings's health officer for alleged carelessness.[17] In 1906 the same year that the board's legitimacy was recognized by the Census Bureau, the dominant role of the state board vis-a-vis local health authorities and boards was settled by a court ruling supporting the board's requirement of compulsory vaccination of schoolchildren in Victor.[18]

Gradually, the board took on additional roles. It was charged with inspecting and licensing hospitals and sanitaria, served as a repository for birth certificates and other data, participated in health education programs, lobbied the legislature for public health reforms, and engaged in a variety of other activities. It was especially proud of its role in "wiping out of existence all irregular lying-in hospitals, whose chief business was to traffic in human flesh," i.e. illegal abortion mills.[19] By 1912 the board had thirteen employees, including a food commissioner, a chemist, a bacteriologist, and several inspectors. These individuals were involved in the board's mission to enforce pure water, food, and drug laws. By 1916 there were 250 local boards for the state board to interact with and, over the next decade, the board established divisions dealing with venereal diseases, child welfare, public health nursing, and other areas.

Denver: Public Health, Politics, and Garbage

In 1880 prompting by Denver's physicians and a typhoid epidemic resulted in legislation defining the city's board of health.[20] The board was to be composed of the mayor, the city physician, members of the city council, and three citizens. In addition to general oversight of the city's health, the board was provided with specific powers. It could require, for example, hotels to report any sick persons on their premises, and once reported, a person with a contagious disease could be removed by the city from his hotel to the County Hospital.

Five years later, the Bureau (later Department) of Health was created and the position of city physician was elevated to that of commissioner of health. The bureau reported to the aforementioned city board of health. In its early years, the inevitable political considerations were somewhat diffused by the statesmanship of the commissioner, Dr. Henry Steele. One of Denver's pioneer physicians, and highly respected, Steele was able to introduce many administrative reforms, scientific methods, and public health measures.[21] Steele worked closely with his two talented assistants, William Munn and Henry Sewall, and with their help and the support of Mayor Platt Rogers, Steele's short tenure as health commissioner marked the "golden age" of public health in Denver. When he died in 1893, it was said that "he was mourned by the public as no other member of our profession in this city has ever been."[22]

The golden age did not last long. In 1892 in a medical society address, Mayor Rogers closed with the wish, "May you [doctors] see to it that . . . the [Denver] health department is not destroyed by partisan hands."[23] In 1893 control of the Bureau of Health was transferred to a politicized city council, and in 1895, when the talented and outspoken Dr. Munn was appointed commissioner, the fireworks began.[24] Munn's 1896 budget requested $59,496 and the city council appropriated ʻ$35,000.[25] Munn charged that the council's parsimony was "for the purpose of crippling the department in its work, handicapping the commissioner in his efforts to control disease and meet emergencies . . ." Munn averred that he had earned the council's displeasure by his refusal to permit them "to dictate the removal of efficient officers because their political activities and beliefs were not suitable to the councilmen." Furthermore, the health commissioner charged, council members had engaged in various dirty tricks, such as "flooding the office with spurious complaints," thereby wasting the time of the bureau's inspectors. Denver's doctors supported Munn and denounced the council and the "hand of the politician—impudent, shameless, and red with the blood of the innocents."[26] The battle with the city council continued until the election of 1899, when both Munn and his patron, Mayor T.S. McMurray, were relieved of their offices.

The battles between Denver's doctors and politicians, and between health and politics, continued into the twentieth century, often focusing on Denver General Hospital (Chapter 7). In 1916 a charter amendment restored the appointment of what was now called the manager of the Department of Health and Charity to the mayor. In 1927 the code was revised, removing the requirement that the position be filled by a physician. Prospective employees of the health department were, once again, being asked such questions as:

> What is your political party? Did you participate in the recent campaign? If yes, state what work you did. In what precinct?[27]

Back in 1878, Dr. Bancroft called for the creation of municipal sanitary districts and the appointment, to each, of a "scavenger":

> The scavenger should gather into heaps all waste matter found in streets and alley . . . There should also be . . . cartmen employed to remove all matter collected by the scavengers, and to take garbage from residences for a small and fixed compensation, say ten cents for each barrel-full.[28]

Two years later, a garbage collection system was initiated, but once again, all sorts of political considerations were interposed. Dr. Munn was especially proud of the system he had introduced—the collection of Denver's garbage by nearby ranchers—to be used as feed for their hogs. This was done at no cost to the city, but was ended when Munn's unorthodox system was later deemed unsanitary.[29]

Contagious Diseases

W. E. Driscoll
County Health Officer
Cripple Creek, Colorado

Dear Doctor:

Please accept our thanks for reports of three cases of scarlet fever. We are pleased to know that you have taken hold of the work vigorously in the management

of contagious diseases and sanitary matters, and feel sure Teller County's health record will be second to none in the state . . .
Taylor HL, M.D., 1905 (Secretary, Colorado State Board of Health)[30]

When an outbreak of a highly contagious disease such as scarlet fever, diphtheria, or smallpox occurred, various measures were taken to contain the disease and prevent its spread. Eventually, some of these measures were enforced by law. Generally, the first step was to report the situation to the local health authorities. Cripple Creek's Dr. Driscoll had the cooperation of the physicians who had reported their cases to him. He, in turn, was required to report to the state board. The grateful tone of the letter from the state board suggests that such reporting was not always accomplished. In such instances, the board was empowered to seek legal action. In 1906, for example, Leadville's Dr. C. M. Erb was fined ten dollars and costs for failing to report a case of diphtheria within twenty-four hours of its diagnosis.[31]

The next step was to isolate the infected persons and their contacts from those who were, as yet, unexposed. School closures were an important part of these efforts. Again, there was resistance. An Arapahoe County teacher was said to have opposed the closing of her schoolhouse during a diphtheria outbreak because making up the lost time would "interfere with her vacation plans."[32] Another method of isolation was to hospitalize the infected person in a contagious disease facility or "pesthouse." Such places were generally unpleasant and, whenever possible, avoided (Chapter 16). Finally, one could place a large sign or "placard" on the home of the infected person. Whether in a country town or the big city, this was a difficult measure to enforce:

> Dr. Eldridge, City Physician of Grand Junction, has resigned his position because the mayor re-

moved a diphtheria quarantine sign from a house . . . [33]

For the past six weeks the Health Department [of Denver] has had a great deal of trouble in West Colfax . . . [with] quarantine. In the average house, no attention whatever is given to the placard, the sick children are allowed to mingle with other children, and visiting is not restricted . . . When an arrest is made, poverty and ignorance is the plea.[34]

The third measure used to stop the spread of contagious disease was disinfection and fumigation. Denver's Dr. Henry McGraw recommended that the patient be washed with a mild disinfectant such as chlorinated soda, his excreta treated with lime, and his bedclothes and clothing rinsed in carbolic acid or corrosive sublimate and then boiled.[35] The walls, floors, and furniture were to be washed with similar disinfectants and all handkerchiefs and rags burnt. Fumigation was accomplished by one of three means—steam, sulphur dioxide, or formaldehyde gas.

Often, when an outbreak occurred, the local authorities turned to the State Board of Health for help. In 1905 when scarlet fever broke out among the "Mexican population" of Las Animas County, the board sent its inspectors:

> A vigorous quarantine was established, a house-to-house canvas was made to discover unreported cases, schools were closed, and public gatherings prohibited.[36]

The county commissioners "cheerfully" supplied guards to enforce the quarantine, and the board was subsequently happy to report the epidemic was limited to about 200 cases.

Sometimes local authorities were not so "cheerful" in their interactions with the state board. When scarlet fever appeared in Leadville, the same year as in Las Animas County, there was opposition to public health measures from the local authorities. Placards were removed and quarantines discontinued. The state board's representatives held a conference with the mayor, city council, and "leading physicians of the town" and informed them that

> if the directions of the Board were not followed, it would be necessary to supercede [the local authorities]. An agreement was then reached, and Leadville was soon free of scarlet fever.[36]

During an outbreak of scarlet fever in Manassa, in the lower San Luis Valley, the state board complained that "this is a Mormon town, the local board of health being composed of faith curists."[37] Interestingly, however, the state board's most serious problems with local authorities appear to have been in Denver.[38]

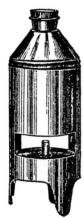

17.1 Disinfection and fumigation were used in the hope of stopping the spread of certain contagious diseases. The Lister fumigator was popular, and formaldehyde was often used as the fumigating agent.

This bedroom has been prepared for fumigation; the fumigator is on the floor to the right.

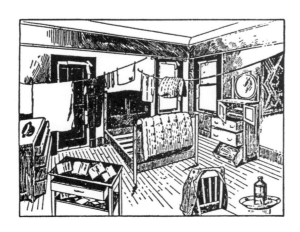

In their efforts to curtail the spread of contagious diseases, boards of health, medical societies, and physicians found themselves in conflict with a variety of institutions and practices. These included the unsanitary conditions of the railroads (Chapter 19), the common practice of spitting (Chapter 15), and the public water fountain. In their zeal, they warned against "the dangers that lurk in our circulating libraries [and] the evils growing out of the handling of infected books"[39] and, "the unprotected [telephone] transmitter and the hot, close and vitiated air of the telephone booth [as] a fertile source of infection."[40] Their greatest efforts, however, were directed against the era's Public Health Enemy Number One—the housefly. The unwary public was warned that:

They are born in filth; they feed on filth; they walk on filth, and then, with filth sticking to their feet, legs, and bodies, they feed and walk on the food [you] eat.[41]

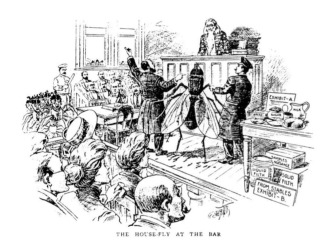

THE HOUSE-FLY AT THE BAR

Air Pollution

On a dry summer's evening an observer will notice in looking down upon the city [Denver] from Capitol Hill . . . that the town appears to be shrouded in an impenetrable mist, above which only the tops of houses and trees are visible. This apparent mist is an enveloping cloud of fine dust, of which the sense of smell becomes principally aware as one descends from the purer atmosphere of the hill.

F. J. Bancroft, M.D. (Denver), 1878[42]

Thus, although its composition and its causes have changed, Denver's infamous "brown cloud" has a long history. The following year, 1879, was even worse. Bancroft's colleague on the State Board of Health, Dr. H. A. Lemen, commented on "foul air" in Denver:

The red rays of the sun, often for days, were the only ones which struggled through the smoke and

dust which hung fog-like over the city . . . It insinuated itself into the recesses of every chamber, and likewise into the eyes, nostrils and lungs . . .[43]

Various factors were invoked to account for the brown cloud. In 1879 forest fires in the mountains were blamed, but that was just a temporary cause. Dr. Lemen mentioned "dust from the filthy, unscraped, unswept, and parsimoniously sprinkled streets." He also referred to "gaseous emanations from masses of filth in numerous cesspools and privy vaults . . . and garbage and offal in the alleys and gutters, all undergoing putrefactive fermentation." Perhaps more important was the fact that Colorado's bituminous coal, virtually the sole source of heat and industrial energy in the early days, produces great quantities of smoke. This was the main reason, said another Denver physician, why "Denver is a very smoky city and, in the winter season, sends a trail of black clouds for miles out over the prairies."[44] The chemical fumes emanating from Denver's smelters contributed to the problem, and Dr. Bancroft wondered about the "gases discharged from the Lixivation Works of West Denver . . . sufficiently powerful to destroy vegetation in the yards of those who reside near them."[45] Some pointed out the irony of advertising Denver as a health resort for pulmonary diseases.

A "smoke ordinance" was passed in 1906, but it was rarely enforced, and by 1913 the problem was of sufficient concern to warrant a meeting of the smoke committee of the Chamber of Commerce, the city's smoke inspector, the commissioner of property, and a member of the art commission. The latter two were present because the major concern over air pollution was not health, but the potential damage to property and the esthetic attractions of the city.[46] The committee recommended that a list of "offending firms" be generated, put much of the blame on the railroads, and urged "strict enforcement of the present ordinance—without imposing an unbearable burden on the owner of the steam or

17.2 The housefly was indicted as the major vector of many contagious diseases and campaigns were initiated to exterminate the pest.

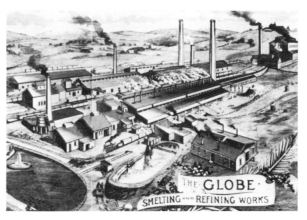

17.3 Air pollution is not a new problem in Denver. In the early days, coal and wood-burning stoves and furnaces and huge smelters used to refine gold and silver ore were the culprits, rather than the automobile. A more true-to-life depiction of this smelter would have shown great clouds of black smoke.

generating plant." Three years later, *Colorado Medicine* described what a visitor that winter would have experienced in the way of Denver's once "invigorating air":

> Wandering through the city, he would breathe a mixture of bituminous smoke and air with considerable carbon monoxide. His sunshine would come filtered through smoke . . . If he should go to City Park or Cheesman Park to view the snowy summits of the Rockies, he would be like to see them, if at all, 'as through a glass darkly.' The city itself would appear enveloped in a murky haze.[47]

The remedy for Denver's brown cloud, said *Colorado Medicine* in 1916, was the combination of a tougher anti-pollution law and "a smoke inspector who will enforce it," and such devices as "automatic stokers, smoke consumers, economizers, etc." The automobile was, as yet, an insignificant contributor to the problem, and ironically, although the dangers of carbon monoxide were stressed, ozone was still considered to be a healthful component of the atmosphere. The editorial concluded with a question of contemporary interest to Denver's citizens:

> How long can the present condition remain or grow worse and Denver maintain her reputation as a health resort or even as a desirable place for well people to live?[47]

It should be mentioned that the problem of air pollution was not limited to Denver. In such cities as Leadville and Durango, where vast quantities of ore were continually being pulverized in giant mills and roasted and refined in huge smelters, great clouds of harmful dust and chemical smoke were perpetually suspended over the streets. In the 1890s a medical visitor to supposedly pristine Colorado Springs wrote that the city was "overhung and enveloped in its own smoke-product, and the view of it from the plains is far from ideal."[48]

Food and Drugs

In nineteenth-century America, those who believed that government should keep its hands off private enterprise were consistently successful. This was certainly true when it came to any regulation of the quality, or even the safety, of food and drugs. Local and state governments had passed a few laws, but these were generally unenforced and ignored.[49] In Denver in 1895, for example, although an ordinance prohibited the sale of "diseased, stale, or unsound fruits, vegetables, meats, fish, or fowl, . . ." Mr. Jacob Baum, the city's lone meat and food inspector complained:

> I am not able to look after the stockyards in addition to the inspection of 275 butcher shops and also the large number of commission [wholesale produce] houses, restaurants, peddling wagons, dairies . . . etc.[50]

The inspector found many problems. Meats and other foods, for example, were left untended, outside of stores, often lying on the sidewalk where

> I have noticed dogs . . . urinating on these provisions. Then there is dust and manure from the streets which blows on [them], and the spitting on the streets from consumptives . . . I have noticed articles so exposed to be literally covered with flies, which is also very unhealthy.[50]

In addition to the filth, the spoilage due to lack of refrigeration, the inclusion of insect parts and other detritus, and the occasional cases of botulism from improperly canned foods, there were the adulterations and "sophistications" practiced by a totally unregulated food industry. In 1905 the *Denver Medical Times* listed some common examples of adulteration—the practice of diluting food products with other materials:

> Spices [with] starches, sawdust, ground shells, dirt, charcoal and hulls, . . . flour with corn meal, confectionary with talc, . . . ground coffee with chickory, and tea leaves with non-tea leaves. 'Lie tea' is made with dust and tea sweepings, starch and gums.[51]

Sophistication referred to the adding of substances, not to increase their bulk, but to improve their appearance or taste. In pre-refrigeration days, attempts were made to preserve or "embalm" meats, fruits, and vegetables through the use of various chemicals—including formaldehyde.[52] Alum was added to whiten and preserve bread; aniline dyes were used to color butter, jellies, and candy; lead salts or Prussian blue was added to tea; and ultramarine to sugar to give it a bluish-white color.

17.4 Prior to the enactment of regulatory legislation, Colorado's hundreds of dairies were uncontrolled. They were generally filthy and the cattle were often diseased.

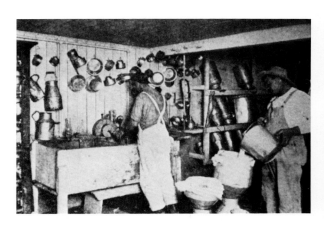

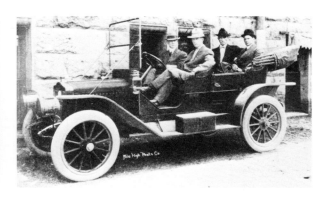

The turn of the century was marked by intensive efforts at reforming many "wrongs" in the American system. Not the least of these was what *Colorado Medicine* called "the pure food agitation."[53] Nationally, horror stories filled the pages of muckraking newspapers (such as the infamous one about the disappearance of the Chicago sausage maker's wife) and novels such as Upton Sinclair's *The Jungle*. Colorado had its own horror stories. In one incident, a batch of corned beef had been "preserved" with an excessive amount of formaldehyde, resulting in the severe illness of a number of persons in Arvada, a Denver suburb.[54] In 1906 Congress passed the Pure Food and Drugs Act—a consumer protection milestone which provided for the sanitary processing and marketing of foods, the elimination of many harmful additives and deceptive adulterations, accurate labeling, inspections and scientific analyses, and seizures and criminal actions for violations. The chief inspector of Colorado's Board of Health commented that "no law ever passed in the United States has been so far-reaching or widespread in its provisions."[55]

Three years later, the chief inspector was reporting mixed results.[56] Some 2,640 inspections (groceries, butcher shops, dairies, etc.) had been accomplished in 140 Colorado communities in 1909, resulting in forty-three hearings and nineteen prosecutions. Convictions were virtually impossible to obtain. His inspections showed that lard was still being adulterated, dried fruits were frequently wormy, and "conditions pertaining to the sale of eggs [was in] a very bad state of affairs."

> Some commission houses admitted that they sold three classes of eggs—fresh, seconds, and rots . . . Also, peddlers were visiting the city dumps and gathering the eggs discarded by the commission houses, and selling them to small dealers. The worst conditions were found on [Denver's] West Colfax Avenue, where 95 per cent of the eggs purchased by our inspectors were so vile that we gagged while examining them.[56]

In other areas, the inspector did find improvements. The adulteration of spices had "practi-

cally ceased," jams and jellies were not being artificially colored, and coffee "made from biscuit dough, as well as from various grains labeled 'health coffee' is now as scarce as hen's teeth." He was especially proud of one accomplishment.

> Probably the most notable betterment has been in the condition of oysters. [In the past] 25 to 75 per cent of oysters sold were nothing but water. In addition to the dishonesty of it, the unsanitary methods of adding ice and water was the cause of a great deal of sickness.[56]

According to another Colorado physician, a "most reprehensible practice," the adding of formaldehyde to preserve oysters was "now fortunately disappearing."[57] Gradually, as the Pure Food and Drug Law was enforced, and as other legislation was enacted, other reprehensible practices were eliminated from the food industry. Of interest, in light of recent concerns, in 1918 Colorado's State Board of Health ruled that saccharine could not be used as a sugar substitute in soft drinks "on the ground that it is injurious to health."[58]

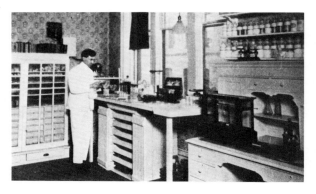

17.5 Some of Denver's health inspectors on the way to an inspection site.

17.7 Tests for water purity, bacterial contamination of milk, and for sophistications and adulterations of foods were conducted in the Department of Health's laboratories at Denver General Hospital.

17.6 Denver's wide-open city market was a favorite target of the inspectors.

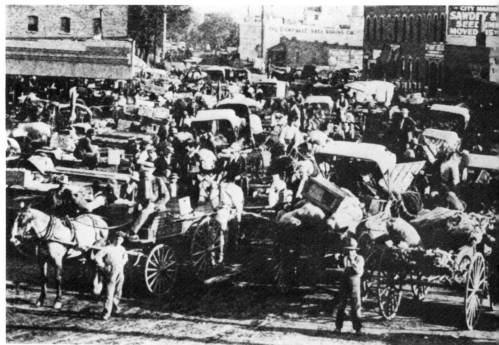

Water and Typhoid

The Denver Water Company now supplies the city with an abundance of water as pure as that leaping forth from the mountain canons.
     Denver Chamber of Commerce, 1886[59]

Typhoid fever has followed the well-remembered advice of Horace Greeley to go West and grow up with the country.
     D. W. McLauthlin, M.D. (Denver) 1887[60]

Typhoid is the ultimate "filth" disease. The bacterial agent, Salmonella typhosa, is maintained in the gall bladder and intestines of resistant human carriers and excreted in their feces.[61] When food or water contaminated with such bacteria-laden excrement is ingested by susceptible persons, typhoid may result. The gradual onset of flu-like symptoms leads to high fever, prostration, and the result of intestinal lesions, diarrhea, abdominal pain, and distension. By two weeks, the patient is severely ill and often delirious. In the majority of cases, recovery occurs during the third week, but in the absence of treatment, at least ten percent of patients die.[62] The disease is now treated with antibiotics. Man is virtually the only species susceptible to typhoid, and human carriers serve as the reservoir for the bacterium. In the early 1900s, Mary Mallon, better known as "Typhoid Mary," spread the disease as she made her peripatetic way working as a cook.

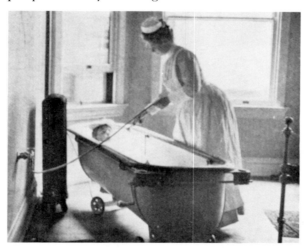

17.8 Typhoid killed thousands of Coloradans. Various measures were used to "break" the fever, including cold baths.

Nationally, prior to the introduction of rigorous public health measures, typhoid was a common disease. In the 1890s there were 300,000 to 400,000 cases each year in the U.S.A. and tens of thousands of deaths.[63] Typhoid was especially common in Colorado early on largely, as elsewhere, as the result of ignorance. Later, when the bacterial etiology and epidemiology of the disease became understood, typhoid's predelic-

tion for Colorado was the result of resistance by public and private authorities to instituting proper sewage disposal and adequate water purification. The disease occurred sporadically on farms and ranches and in devastating outbreaks in rural towns, mining camps, and cities.

Although such foods as shellfish (grown in sewage-contaminated beds) and milk (adulterated with contaminated water) have contributed to the spread of typhoid, the major source has been drinking water. Limited outbreaks occurred when shallow wells were contaminated by an improperly located or constructed privy or cesspool. Most communities obtained their water from streams and rivers, directly or via irrigation ditches, and with minimal or no attempts at purification. Little attention was paid to the fact that such sources contained raw sewage dumped into the water from communities upstream. Thus, periodic outbreaks of typhoid occurred in the 1860s and '70s—sometimes called mountain fever, sometimes dysentery, or other names. As the population increased—and sanitation measures did not—oubreaks became more common. Typhoid continued to be a problem in Colorado until well into the twentieth century. The first major outbreak occurred in Denver in 1879-1880.

Denver's physicians had warned of the dangers for years. With Colorado's silver boom, the city's population swelled to about 35,000. There were thousands of privies and cesspools, many of them draining into the two streams which flowed through town—the South Platte River and its tributary, Cherry Creek. Denver still had no sewers, and refuse was carried in open ditches which ran through residential and business districts to the river and creek. The season had been unusually dry, the streams were low and stagnant, and the doctors warned it was just a question of time before typhoid would strike. As the hot summer months progressed, the disease began to appear—sporadically at first, and then increasingly until, when the epidemic had played itself out by early winter, as many as one in twenty Denver residents had had the disease. There were, by conservative estimate, about forty fatalities—the proportional equivalent, in today's metropolitan Denver, of about 1,600 deaths.

Denver's drinking water was obtained from the South Platte River. The State Board of Health's Dr. H. A. Lemen described the contamination of that source.[64] It was well known, he pointed out, that "liquid waste" from the city's "hotels, restaurants, saloons . . ." and other businesses was emptied into the South

Platte. Cherry Creek, he added, was the "receptacle of thousands upon thousands of cart loads of filth." The "fluid wastes from laundries and mills, from stables and pig sties, from cow yards and privies, and drainage from residences" emptied almost directly into "ditches which wended their way to Cherry Creek and the South Platte." Untreated sewage from the county jail emptied directly into the creek—"mingling its abominations directly with water in the stream."

The Denver Water Company, a private corporation whose board consisted of some of the city's most powerful citizens, was franchised to provide the city's water. Since 1872, it had used the highly publicized (but primitive) Holly filtration process to purify the city's water supply.[65] In July a number of Denver physicians complained that the Water Company was pumping its water from polluted sources. The company denied this and, supported by the mayor, claimed that its sources were well above the inflow of Cherry Creek, the contaminated ditches, and the sewers. As reported by Dr. Lemen:

On December 7, 1879, Dr. Charles Denison . . . discovered that such was not the case, and Dr. J. Culver Davis and [I] confirmed his observation . . . The public were made cognizant of the facts . . . through publication in the daily press . . . A perfect storm of indignation over the discovery was engendered. Some bitter recriminations ensued between members of the Denver Medical Association and the officers of the Water Company.[66]

In meetings of the Denver Medical Association and in articles and letters to the editor with such provocative titles as "Water of Death" and "Scourge of Filth," the doctors attacked the Denver Water Company and placed the blame for the typhoid epidemic squarely upon its shoulders.[67] Dr. James J. McDonald was quoted as saying, "Our water is not only filthy, but it is damned filthy; not only opaque, but it stinks."[68] Dr. Lemen added that Denver's water "stinks in the nostrils of all men having properly constituted olfactory organs" and that if improvements were not made, Denver would either have to bury up to one hundred typhoid victims a month or "do as the president of the water company does—drink less water."[69]

The Water Company attempted to answer the attacks. First, they hired a chemist to analyze the water. He reported it to be chemically "pure." This, the doctors pointed out, was irrelevant—typhoid was not due to a chemical impurity but to an infectious agent. The battle heated up and the president of the Water Company, Colonel James B. Archer, an Englishman unused to the rough and tumble ways of the frontier, began to answer in kind. Noting that the company had "received some pretty rough handling at the hands of the M.D.s," the Colonel gave his opinion of the typical doctor—"A young man who is too lazy to be a mechanic [or] lacks the brains to be a lawyer . . ."[69] What, he asked Denver's citizens, has the medical association done for you? "Met in solemn conclave to determine that the company is responsible for the ill-success of their experiments on your bodies, which experiments have sent so many to fill our cemetaries." The association's Dr. J.C. Davis responded, "It was your experiments, James, with the waters of the west Denver mill ditch and Cherry Creek that has sent so many to fill our cemetaries, not ours."[70]

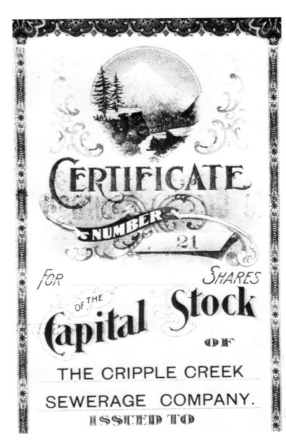

17.9 Some communities attempted to provide adequate sewage and pure water facilities, but these were generally private enterprises and subject to financial rather than public health considerations.

The city approved a new sewer system that fall, and improvements were promised by the Water Company. When a committee, including the mayor, visited the new water works the following spring, they found that the old works were still in use and that the new facility was "as stiff as the grave."[71] When Colonel Archer was asked about this he became furious, blamed the city for any contamination of its water, and refused to activate the new works. That summer and fall there were several hundred additional cases of typhoid in Denver.

17.10 In Denver in 1879-1880, a devastating outbreak of typhoid resulted in a battle between the Denver Water Company and Denver's doctors. Some outstanding detective work by Drs. Denison, Culver, and Lemen demonstrated the direct contamination of Denver's water supply by raw sewage from a hotel (E), the county jail (G), and other sources.

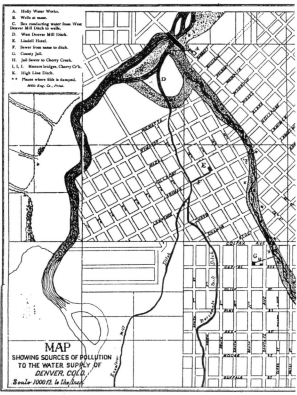

A. Holly Water Works.
B. Wells at same.
C. Box conducting water from West Denver Mill Ditch to wells.
D. West Denver Mill Ditch.
E. Lindell Hotel.
F. Sewer from same to ditch.
G. County Jail.
H. Jail Sewer to Cherry Creek.
I, I, I. Manure bridges, Cherry Cr'k.
K. High Line Ditch.
** Places where filth is dumped.
Mills Eng. Co., Print.

MAP
SHOWING SOURCES OF POLLUTION TO THE WATER SUPPLY OF DENVER, COLO.
Scale 1000 ft. to the inch.

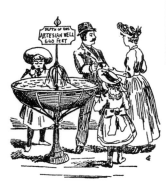

17.11 Fearful of Denver's water, some hotels, businesses, and wealthy families resorted to artesian wells, to tap the water table deep beneath the city. This one was located near Elitch Gardens in northwestern Denver.

17.12 The water pumping station at Denver's main reservoir, Lake Archer in central Denver. Some improvements were made by the water company, but the new station continued to pump sewage-contaminated water into Denver's taps in the 1890s. Typhoid continued to be a problem into the twentieth century.

In 1883 Colonel Archer died, and a competing company, the Citizen's Water Company was founded. The discovery of a deep underground water table led to the digging of artesian wells, some of them 1,000 feet deep, but this source provided water to a small number of consumers. Although water pipes were laid and the sewage system extended, most of Denver continued to rely on a contaminated water supply—and typhoid became even more common. In 1890 there were 287 deaths due to the disease, accounting for more than ten percent of the city's mortality.[72] The following spring, the city engineer reported that "great improvements have been made by the Denver Water Company, which will assure a continuous and lasting supply of pure and wholesome water."[73] Indeed, the typhoid mortality rate was reduced by more than half that year, but in the five-year period between 1891 and 1895, there were 336 deaths due to typhoid in Denver. At the same time, the Chamber of Commerce was proclaiming that: "The water supply of Denver is the best, purest, and cheapest of any city in the world."[74]

By 1894 the newly formed Denver Union Water Company had achieved a monopoly as the sole supplier of the city's water. It soon attempted to relax the relatively stringent sanitary requirements which had been enacted by the city. In 1896 summer floods resulted in more than the usual contamination of Denver's water supply. The *Denver Medical Times* was soon reporting that "Typhoid fever is rampant in Den-

ver at the present time."[75] The County Hospital itself had been subjected to an outbreak of the disease, affecting half of the hospital's staff and resulting in the death of its twenty-six year old chief resident and its chief nurse.[76] Ultimately, there were more than 600 cases that year and eighty-eight deaths.[77] Denver's health commissioner, Dr. Munn, made a detailed inspection of the Water Company's facilities, found evidence of contamination, and made a number of recommendations.[78] There ensued a conflict between the outspoken Munn, his supporter, Mayor McMurray, and the company. As in 1879, the battle soon became bitter. The *Colorado Medical Journal* reported that Dr. Munn's investigations

> reveal a state of water pollution which is something frightful. For years we have been led to believe that we were drinking pure mountain water piped directly from the snow-capped peaks in the mountains. [So] monstrous a lie was never before circulated. Instead of pipes, are open ditches; instead of mountain water, . . . contaminated river water.[79]

A physician visiting from St. Louis published an article in the *Denver Medical Times* lauding the purity of Denver's water.[80] Dr. Munn expressed his "regret" that the author did not bother to mention that he happened to be the guest—and relative—of the Water Company's attorney. There ensued a series of published recriminations between the two physicians. And so it went . . . until Mayor McMurray and Dr. Munn were forced out of office in 1899. In 1903 the Water Company instituted Munn's suggestion of "the slow sand method of filtration." In 1911 calcium hypochlorite was added to Denver's water, and by 1916 chlorination had been introduced. Typhoid continued to occur in Denver in the 1920s, but at a much lower rate than previously.

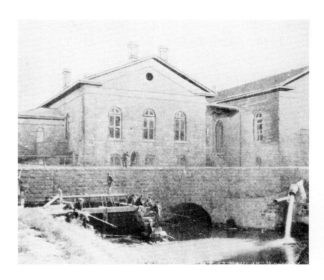

Rural Colorado was, by no means, spared from typhoid, and it was said, "not infrequently in the country, it is more difficult to get good water than poor beer."[81] At the same time that Denver was beginning to show improvement in its typhoid record, increasingly severe outbreaks were occurring in the mining camps and rural towns. In Fort Collins in 1900, "as victim after victim was stricken down . . . the inhabitants became almost panic stricken."[82] Nearly 300 cases occurred in the town during a single week. The outbreak was traced to a transient who came down with the disease while boarding in a farmhouse upstream on the Poudre River. According to an investigating physician from the State Board of Health, the outbreak resulted from:

> An ignorant nurse, contrary to the doctor's orders, emptying the discharges from her patient, laden with its pernicious freight of typhoid germs, into a little ditch . . . which empties directly into the Poudre.[83]

In 1904 an outbreak of typhoid at the Camp Bird Mine in the San Juan mountains was followed by an epidemic at Montrose, downstream on the Uncompahgre River.[84] The board of health noted that untreated sewage from the Camp Bird was dumped into the river, the source of Montrose's untreated drinking water.

The coal camps, with their frequently unsanitary water supplies (Chapter 8) were often the sites of typhoid outbreaks. In 1906 a typical outbreak occurred in the coal camp of Marshall in Boulder County.[85] There were thirty-five cases in the tiny community, including the doctor, and two deaths. The doctor noted that while Marshall's water was obtained from an open ditch, another nearby camp, Mitchell, obtained its water from an eight-hundred-foot deep well and had not had a single case.

What may have been Colorado's worst outbreak of typhoid occurred in Leadville in 1904.[86] The first indication of a problem was received at the State Board of Health in early January, in the form of a phone call from Leadville's Dr. Sol Kahn. The board sent an investigator to the town, who soon confirmed Dr. Kahn's diagnosis and estimated that there were at least 300 cases. Some of Leadville's doctors disagreed with the diagnosis, believing the disease to be the flu or some other "fever." The city's newspapers also denied the possibility of typhoid, fearful, perhaps, of the damage such news might have on commercial activities. The board recommended various public health measures, including the employment of Dr. W. C. Mitchell, the

state bacteriologist, to examine the city's water supply. The mayor refused, and the number of cases, and deaths, continued to increase. Finally, under public pressure, an emergency meeting of the town council was held, and the board was invited to come to town and conduct an investigation. By then, as one newspaper reported, "the people had resigned themselves to the fact that Leadville has an epidemic of typhoid fever."[87] Some remarkable detective work resulted in the following analysis of the outbreak, which eventually resulted in about 600 cases and thirty-five deaths.

The first case had been in a man who had come to town from Breckenridge and was hospitalized at St. Vincent's Hospital. He survived, but Sister Ann Regina, who had nursed this patient, came down with the disease and died. Soon afterward, additional cases began to appear in town and many of them were hospitalized at St. Vincent's. The board's inspectors soon found that sewage from the hospital was deposited, without any attempt at disinfection, in an unlined settling tank, several feet above the water pipes which supplied the city. During the period preceding the outbreak, these water pipes were emptied and flushed several times, allowing the hospital's sewage to seep into the city's drinking water and, within a period of several weeks, an epidemic of typhoid.

By 1922, although Denver's mortality due to typhoid had continued to fall, forty-nine other American cities had a lower rate.[88] Outside of Denver, the typhoid mortality rate was higher, and only seven states had higher rates than Colorado. It was not until years later that typhoid finally disappeared from the state.

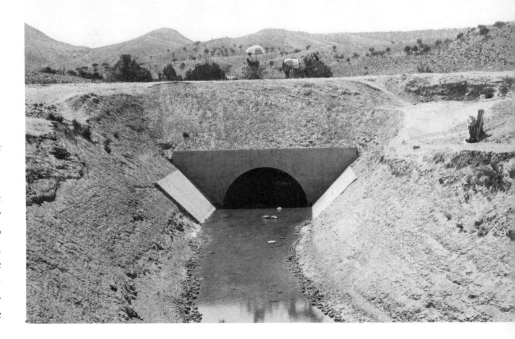

17.13 Impure drinking water and typhoid were by no means limited to Denver. Many of Colorado's rural towns and farms obtained their water from streams and irrigation ditches containing the untreated effluvia of their upstream neighbors.

18 SOCIAL DISEASES

Oh, how they drink!

General William Larimer (Describing his fellow pioneers in Denver City), 1859[1]

ALCOHOL ARRIVED WITH COLORADO'S earliest settlers. In 1858 ex-mountain man and tyro entrepreneur, Dick Wootten, achieved immortality in Colorado when he imported a large quantity of New Mexico whiskey, the legendary Taos Lightning, to help Denverites celebrate Christmas. Saloons, first in tents, later in cabins and more substantial structures, were always among the first, and most important, features of any mining camp, railroad town, or ranching community. They were the focus of the miner's, cowboy's, and working man's social activities. Much has been written on the colorful aspects of drink and drinking, of the saloon and saloonkeepers, of dance hall girls, gamblers, and shoot-'em-ups, and even the social-political aspects have been discussed. Little attention, however, has been paid to the medical aspects of alcohol and alcoholism in early Colorado and the West.

Alcohol has been used medicinally, mainly as a stimulant or tonic, throughout the ages by physicians and lay persons alike. In small doses it makes people feel better—or at least they think they feel better. In the nineteenth century, when there was so little in the way of effective therapy available to physicians, this was no mean accomplishment. When the patient felt better, the family felt better, and so did the doctor. In larger doses, alcohol was used as an anaesthetic—especially before the introduction of ether and chloroform.

Virtually every nineteenth-century home medicine chest included some "medicinal spirits." Goldseekers heading for Colorado were advised to include a little alcohol in their packs—but not too much. Reed's 1859 guidebook, for example, suggested:

> Have but little liquor along, no more than is sufficient for medicinal purposes, as it is generally apt to create disturbance; having . . . the peculiar effect of giving to those who use it the disposition to finger [i.e. gouge out] each other's eyes . . .[2]

Once in Denver, the immigrant found alcohol much more easily than he found gold. Virtually all of Denver's early chroniclers commented on the number of saloons and the amount of drinking in the frontier town. "Everywhere [in Denver] are saloons . . . It is the custom to partake freely, several times a day, of the sacramental glass of whisky . . ."[3] Those who preferred to drink in private could head for any one of a number of establishments. In 1859 Larimer Street's City Drug Store advertised: "A constant supply of pure wines and brandies, *especially* for medicinal purposes."[4]

Alcoholism, common in Denver, was rampant in the mining camps. The suburb of a particularly bibulous camp, Creede, was named Gintown.[5] In Leadville, it was noted:

> There is an uncontrollable desire for mountain dew, or liquid refreshments. A friend coined the word that expresses habitual inebriation—"whisketarians." Other localities have their vegetarians, but Leadville has her "whisketarians."[6]

In more succinct language, a Leadville physician summarized: "Our mining camps have the reputation of consuming large quantities of into-xicating beverages."[7] He attributed this to the fact that, in the mining camps,

> a large proportion of unmarried men, and the lack of innocent amusements, induces many to seek the excitement and recreation of the saloon . . . where a false sense of sociability and generosity rebounds to the benefit of the liquor vendor.[7]

To put it another way, when a man wasn't working, what else was there to do but drink? Reverend J. J. Gibbons saw many cases of de-lirium tremens among the San Juan District miners. His description of one such case is vivid:

> I found him like a maniac laid on a bed, strong straps binding his wrists and ankles . . . foaming at the mouth like a vicious dog. One moment hor-rid despair sat upon him, the next, his eyes set in his head from hideous fright . . . His cries, moans, and howls were unearthly. It was a dreadful pre-sence to watch and the doctor said that there was no hope.[8]

In the farming and ranching communities of the plains, where family and religion played a larger role, liquor was sometimes a little more difficult to obtain. In Peyton, Colorado, for example, a number of "cow gentlemen" had to resort to drinking patent medicines to satify their thirst.[9] Unfortunately, they found enough to get drunk and wound up in a shooting fray.

As for Denver, one physician commented: "What must impress itself on every observer in Denver is the immense number suffering from the chronic effects of alcohol."[10] According to some members of the clergy, the indiscriminate prescribing of alcohol-containing tonics and medications by physicians was contributing to the prevalence of alcoholism. In 1878 the issue became public when the Reverend Dr. Frank M. Ellis, described as "an eloquent but irrespon-sible temperance advocate," charged the medi-cal profession with being "accountable for more drunkenness than any other class of citizens."[11] Similar accusations resulted in a gradually in-creasing anger among Denver's medical com-munity and culminated, several months later, in a special meeting of the Denver Medical So-ciety. At the meeting were a number of lay guests, including Bishop John F. Spalding, the chairman of the Board of County Commission-ers, and members of the press. The proceedings began with three of Denver's most respected physicians, Richard Buckingham, H. A. Lemen, and Henry K. Steele, responding to Reverend Ellis's charges.

Dr. Buckingham began conservatively, em-phasizing the "sacrificial and philanthropic" na-

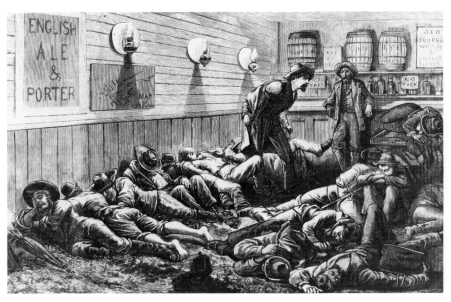

ture of the medical profession and pointing out that, as a "temperance man" himself, "he had never made a drunkard or knew of one made by a brother physician." Next, Dr. Lemen rose and advanced to the front of the room "with a roll of manuscript which frightened the repor-ters." Although he defended the judicious use of alcohol for medicinal purposes, he denied that he had "ever made a drunkard." Those who asserted that alcoholism was the result of physi-cians' care were simply lying or, at best, mista-ken. Lemen felt that doctors who were totally opposed to any medicinal use of alcohol might be better suited to being Sunday school superin-tendents. Finally, he suggested, the abolition of alcohol might lead to the expanded use of to-bacco and opium. Dr. Steele added some com-ments on the frequency of alcoholism among clergymen.

Bishop Spalding "responded with good temper." He wished that physicians would dis-card alcohol from their therapeutic regimens, but he was willing to concede that "physicians alone were the proper judges of medical value and use." If a patient continued to use a physi-cian's prescription for alcohol after leaving the doctor's care, it was the patient's responsibility, not the doctor's. Finally, he had always been convinced that physicians rarely prescribed al-cohol and was delighted to find that this was, indeed, the case. An understanding had been reached between Denver's physicians and cler-gymen, and the evening ended amicably.

Although most physicians continued to pre-scribe alcohol, they generally did so in modera-tion. They admitted that medicinal alcohol could, under unusual circumstances, lead to al-coholism, and Denver's Dr. Galen Hassenplug reported the case of a young girl who had become

18.1 Alcoholism was rampant in the mining camps. This Leadville saloon provided a place to sleep off the effects of its whiskey.

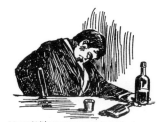

INTEMPERANCE AND OTHER EXCESSES.

18.2 Most of Colorado's physicians either ignored or even agreed with temperance move-ments—until the clergy's attacks were directed against them!

an alcoholic after the prolonged use of brandy to treat her typhoid.[12] Dr. F. G. Byles, in a paper delivered to the Denver Medical Society, conceded that "alcohol is useful, but not necessary."[13] Furthermore, he added, "if doctors do not need alcohol [in the treatment of the sick], they should say so and not be accountable for its sale on every corner under the false impression of its being a necessity to their armamentarium."

While the profession was wavering as to physician-prescribed alcohol, there was no question of its attitude towards the growing and indiscriminate use of non-prescription alcohol- containing tonics, bitters, and nostrums. In 1902 the Colorado Medical Society offered a prize of twenty-five dollars for the best essay on the subject of "Dangers of Self-Drugging With Proprietary Medicines."[14] The winner was Dr. Edward Bumgardner. In his essay entitled "Pro Bono Publico," Dr. Bumgardner pointed out that

> The one poison that is used in nearly all nostrums is alcohol . . . Physicians are recognizing more and more the harm done by alcohol and are coming to use it less.[14]

He went on to list some of the most popular patent medicines, reporting the percentage of alcohol contained in each. These included:

Hood's Sasparilla 18.8%
Schenck's Sea-Weed Tonic 19.5%
Burdock Blood Bitters 25.0%
Hostetter's Stomach Bitters 44.3%

18.3 Both the clergy and the doctors fought the over-the-counter tonics, bitters, and other patented medicines which contained alcohol—sometimes more than 25% by volume.

The last was, therefore, 88.6 proof. Thus, it was little wonder that grandma could abstain from such socially unacceptable sources of alcohol as brandy, bourbon, or gin and didn't even have to resort to the cooking sherry in order to get properly soused. All she had to do was self-medicate her aches and pains with any one of hundreds of tonics, bitters, and other packaged remedies available at the corner drugstore. Some even contained an additional source of comfort in the form of opiates, cocaine, or other narcotics—all of this in the absence of any requirement for the manufacturer to publish the contents of their products, thereby allowing the consumer to remain comfortable in the sanctity of his or her ignorance.

A few years later, the *Denver Medical Times* published the new federal law which required the manufacturers of "intoxicating tonics" to be licensed as distillers. In addition, the contents of their products now had to be printed on their labels. With obvious pleasure, the *Times* concluded:

> This new departure will be a severe blow to the secret medicine interests, not only because of the direct tax on their products, but still more because of the educative effects upon those who are disposed to tipple, sometimes innocently, with such flavored spirits as Peruna, Hostetter's Bitters, and the late Lydia Pinkham's Vegetable Compound.[15]

At the same time, the *Times*, like most physicians, opposed the total abstinence advocated by such organizations as the Anti-Saloon League.[16] With tongue in cheek, the *Times* suggested that prohibitionists of all types should join forces, and that since:

> An automobile kills somebody once in a while. Lets prohibit 'em all.
>
> Theaters often present immoral plays. Prohibit theaters!
>
> Artists paint naughty pictures sometimes. Prohibit art![16]

Humor was not about to stem the tide, however, and in 1920, Colorado and the nation went dry—legally, if not in fact. Alcoholism continued to be a major problem.

Narcotics and Drug Addiction

In every little cooped-up, dingy little cavern of a hut [they] were . . . smoking opium, motionless and with their lustreless eyes turned inward . . . He puts a pellet of opium on the end of a wire, sets it on fire, and plasters it into the pipe, then he applies the bowl to the lamp and proceeds to smoke.

The stewing and frying of the drug and the gurgling of the juices in the stem would well nigh turn the stomach of a statue . . . He takes about two dozen whiffs and then rolls over to dream.

Mark Twain in *Roughing It*, 1872[17]

Mark Twain was describing an opium den in Virginia City, Nevada. The same description could have been applied to any one of a number of similar establishments along the "hop alleys" of Denver and many of Colorado's mining camps. Originally limited to the ruling classes, opium addiction spread to China's masses in the nineteenth century. Governmental attempts to eliminate it were opposed by the British, who profited from the opium trade. Opium was brought into China in quantities so huge that even the most miserable peasant could afford it as a means of escaping the unpleasant realities of serfdom. By the 1850s Chinese workers were being imported to California as railroad workers and laborers, and by the 1870s, they had come to Colorado. They brought the opium habit and the opium den with them.

If the Chinese worker was miserable in his own country, he was even more so in the "land of opportunity." In an alien country away from family and friends, illiterate and unfamiliar with the language, raised in a totally different culture, and generally despised by his hosts, it is not surprising that the Chinese turned to the familiar comforts of the opium den and pipe. Once addicted, the unfortunate was trapped into virtual slavery, forced to pay much of his meager salary to support his habit. Thus, the familiar caricature of "John" the Chinaman, as drawn by Twain and other visitors to the Chinatowns of the American West, nodding in apathetic lethargy, picturesque and pathetic.

White America was willing to tolerate John's vices—as long as he continued to provide a source of cheap labor and kept to himself. Even when white criminals and prostitutes began to frequent the dens, there was little concern. This tolerance quickly faded when middle America's sons and daughters began to dabble with the pipe. Already looked on with disfavor as racially and culturally inferior by the middle and upper classes, as heathen by the religious, and as cheap competition by the working classes, the Chinese were targeted for their "dens of iniquity."

"Incidents" became more frequent. In 1880, in Denver, the death of an eighteen-year-old boy was blamed on opium—and the Chinese. The *Denver Tribune* headlined: "A Young Man Falls Victim to the Prevailing Chinese Vice."[18] A ready populace responded by burning Denver's

18.4 Chinese opium dens were tolerated until they began to attract young middle-class whites.

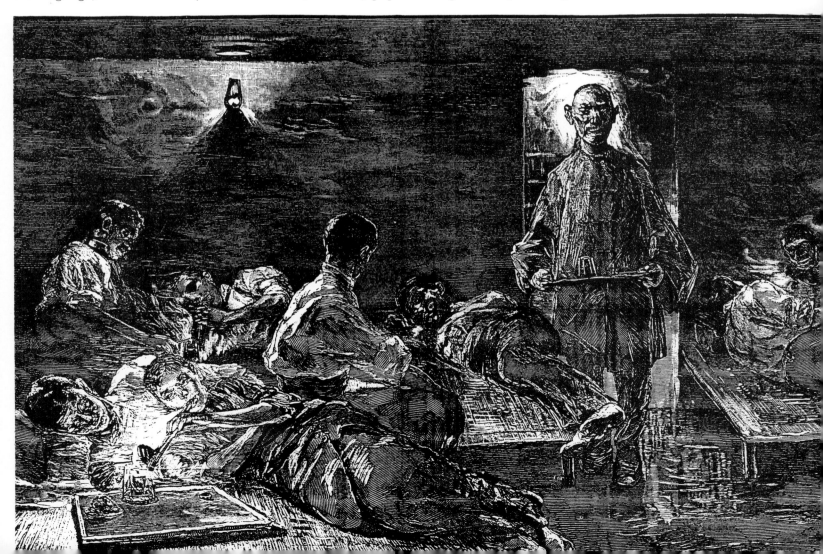

Chinatown and evicting its inhabitants. The Chinese returned, however, and despite periodic raids, municipal restrictions, and the pressures of the press and the pulpit, opium smoking continued. In 1902 Dr. A. L. Bennett, Colorado's medical inspector of Chinese, reported:

> In Denver this fascinating and baneful drug is adding to its victims daily. The drug is sold openly in Chinese stores to white men and women who take it to their homes and smoke. Some strict law [should] be enacted . . . prohibiting the sale of opium to whites. This cursed habit . . . is ruining morally and physically hundreds of whites in Colorado, and in the city of Denver especially.[19]

Colorado's deputy labor commissioner was even more explicit:

> Countless men, women and even children have formed the accursed opium habit, a vice which consigns its victims to a condition of such utter hopelessness that relief is found only through death . . . White men, women, boys, and girls in considerable numbers, many of them from respectable families, are patrons of the opium dens. No slavery is quite so hopeless as that of the . . . opium fiend.[20]

By the turn of the century, drug addiction had indeed become widespread in Colorado and elsewhere in the United States. By then, however, opium smoking and the Chinese connection had become a minor part of the overall problem. A purer and more potent derivative of opium had become readily available in the form of morphine, and another narcotic, cocaine, was becoming increasingly popular.

Opium is obtained from the unripe seed of the poppy by cutting its capsule and collecting the rubbery fluid, drying it, and pressing it into bricks. Raw opium contains a variety of chemicals, the most potent of which is morphine. By the early nineteenth century, morphine had been chemically isolated, thereby making the painkilling and other medicinal benefits of opium more readily available in a concentrated and inexpensive form. Morphine was poorly absorbed when taken orally, but with the invention of the hypodermic needle, the drug could now be administered rapidly and more potently. The Civil War provided ample opportunity to demonstrate morphine's effectiveness as a painkiller. Increasingly, nineteenth-century physicians, whose armamentarium contained little in the way of effective therapy, turned to morphine to relieve their patients' pain and misery. Soon, the number of morphine addicts began to grow, some of them "hooked" as the result of medical care. With the drug readily available from physicians, or over-the-counter from pharmacists and non-professional suppliers, and with little in the way of local or state restrictions, the drug became very popular. In 1896 an article in *Colorado Medicine* referred to "King Morphine" and commented that:

> Everyone . . . is familiar with the devastation produced by the widespread use and abuse of this narcotic and other stimulating poisons. We frequently see the shattered wrecks of once powerful bodies and splendid intellects whose possessors . . . fill untimely and needless graves.[21]

In 1907 Dr. J. E. Courtney described some of the cases of "morphinism" in his Denver practice.[22] One was a fifty-nine- year-old man, a real estate dealer, who had been addicted for eighteen years. He had originally been given morphine to alleviate the pain of "hepatic colic"; now his body was virtually covered by needle scars and "about a hundred small abscesses." A twenty-eight-year-old woman, an addict for eight years, attributed her habit to "grief at deception in a love affair." Particulary upsetting to Dr. Courtney was the case of a thirty-year-old wife of a physician:

> I had to be brought face to face with the difficulties in the subject before I could bring myself to excuse the physician for being to his own wife the instrument of forming and keeping up the morphine habit. She had never had a dose except from his hand![22]

While most addicts injected their dose subcutaneously, another Denver physician reported a pioneer example of "mainlining," i.e. intravenous injection. On examining the arms of his twenty-seven-year-old patient, Dr. William Berlin recalled:

> I found all the veins blackened by constant use of the drug. Each vein showed numerous minute spots, where the needle had left its mark. They were so frequent that it was hard to distinguish one puncture from another.[23]

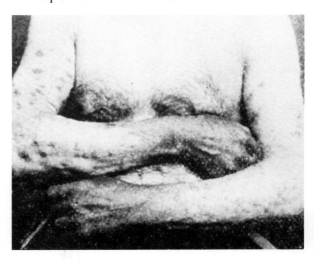

18.5 Narcotics addiction is not a new problem. In 1907 Denver's Dr. Courtney reported this example of a morphine addict whose body was virtually covered by needle scars.

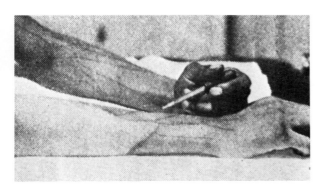

Cocaine was the other addicting drug which was achieving increasing popularity. Among some South American Indians, the chewing of coca leaves produced the same sort of solace that opium smoking had provided for the Chinese. Whether in its raw form, or ingested, injected, or sniffed in its purified form, cocaine is an addicting drug. Although in recent years, it had been minimized as "recreational," its lethal potential, especially in concentrated form, has become all too apparent. Medically, cocaine became widely used as a topical anaesthetic, and because of its abilities to shrink inflamed mucous membranes, many doctors considered it to be the treatment of choice for hay fever. Nevertheless, even in 1911 at least one Colorado physician considered cocaine to be "far worse than morphine . . . It destroys the moral sense, wrecks the mind and body, [and] is a crime producer."[24]

Both cocaine and morphine were readily available to the casual user. In Durango, Colorado, instead of aspirin, people used to buy a dime's worth of cocaine, and morphine was ten cents an ounce and available to anyone.[25] Cocaine was sold in mining camp commissaries for a time.[26] A pinch was often added to a shot of whiskey, it provided the "kick" of many Cola drinks (including the original Coca Cola), and it was often added to tobacco.[27]

Much more common than the classic needle-scarred "dope fiend," was the addict whose habit was covert and who obtained his or her narcotics from the plethora of patent remedies which were available in the late nineteenth century. Hundreds of narcotics-containing "over the counter" remedies—lotions, cough mixtures, tonics, enemas, poultices, and so on—were available for the asking and a few pennies. Morphine, cocaine, and the new, more powerful morphine derivative, heroin, were contained in these prettily packaged, attractively named medications, often in combination with alcohol. Thus, we find, advertised in the standard medical catalogues and journals, as well as in lay publications and newspapers:

Cocaine Compound: Suppositories and Bougies. Unexcelled in the treatment of all uterine, rectal and urethral diseases . . . .

Terp-Heroin . . . Most successfully indicated in the treatment of all diseases of the respiratory tract—pulmonary and laryngeal tuberculosis, pneumonia, emphysema, asthma, etc.[28]

One of the most popular remedies of the day, Wine of Coca, proudly proclaimed that it was made from the freshest coca leaves. It combined the effects of both alcohol and cocaine and was recommended for a variety of ailments. Not surprisingly, such "medicines" made people feel better. They were particularly popular among women. It has been pointed out that, whereas Victorian Age men could participate in a variety of vices which were considered to be more or less socially acceptable, the Victorian Age woman was not allowed such indulgences. Medicinal narcotics, however, like medicinal alcohol, were an acceptable way to deal with the strains and stresses of daily life. Huge quantities of addicting drugs were consumed in this way.

Children were often treated with "soothing syrups" and cough remedies containing narcotics. As early as 1879, Denver's Dr. Arnold Stedman observed that "It is no unusual thing . . . to find children of only a few months old already showing the unmistakable symptoms of the opium habit induced by the administration of

18.6 In 1915 Denver's Dr. Berlin reported what may have been the first example of "mainlining" in Colorado.

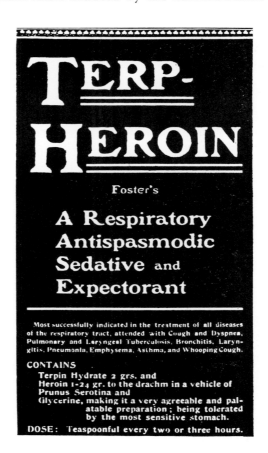

18.7 Innumerable over-the-counter medications contained addicting drugs—even heroin.

. . . soothing syrups and quieting mixtures."[29]

More than twenty years later, another Denver physician deplored the practice:

> Of all the crimes against childhood, few can be greater than that of making helpless infants into opium inebriates. Let no one doubt that this is done in countless cases every year.[30]

Thirty-five years later, these products were still on the market. Denver's Department of Health provided lists of what it termed "baby killers." These included such standbys as:

> Mrs. Winslow's Soothing Syrup (morphine)
> Dr. Fahrney's Teething Syrup (morphine, chloroform)
> Dr. Moffett's Teething Powders (opium)
> Dr. James's Soothing Syrup (heroin)[31]

Overdoses were common in adults as well, both unintentional and in suicides. In the 1890s, over one fourteen-month period, Denver's police surgeon, Dr. Carl Johnson, was called in forty-six suicides.[32] Of these, twenty-eight were ascribed to opiates of one kind or another. Johnson's preference in treating overdoses was "hot, strong coffee [of which] I inject one or two quarts . . . into the stomach . . . I have often used coffee so hot that I could not bear my hand in it . . . The coffee is pumped out as often as it becomes somewhat cooled and replaced with [more]." It must be admitted that this procedure is not without danger.

While Denver's Dr. Johnson preferred coffee for overdoses, Leadville's Dr. Mark Sears used milk—intravenously![33] Having been called to attend to an eighteen-year-old "woman of the

town" in the city jail, the doctor found her moribund, apparently as the result of an overdose. Dr. Sears decided on his milk therapy and, "obtaining a pint of fresh cow's milk and a syringe," began injecting it into a vein. Although she did well initially, Sears reported that his patient suddenly died. Nevertheless, the doctor commented, he preferred his milk therapy to other methods—such as the application of red-hot irons to the feet or "the severe flagellations [which] I practiced myself in the first years of my professional life."

Once "hooked," it was very difficult, then as now, to cure a narcotics addict. Pueblo's Dr. John Inglis had seen hundreds of cases of opiate addiction while a physician in China. He advised that:

> Home treatment of morphinism and cocainism is a failure. Reposing any trust or confidence in the patient himself is [an] error . . . The chronic morphine habitue is a deceptive liar. The patient should be put in charge of a nurse who can live with him 24 hours a day and sixty minutes of each hour.[34]

For the addict who was well-off, any one of a number of private treatment facilities was available. Dr. George E. Pettey maintained one in an elegant home in Denver. He promised "methods [which would] render these addictions the most certainly and readily curable of all the chronic ailments."[35] Interestingly, in light of its more recent history, an Aspen newspaper advertised that town's Keeley Institute as specializing in the "treatment of opium . . . and cocaine habits" in the 1890s.[36] Ladies, it noted, could be treated in their homes.

By 1900 there were at least 250,000 drug addicts in the U.S.A., and Colorado appears to have had more than its share.[37] In 1911 a Colorado physician stated "that the taking of narcotics is on the increase . . . This is especially true among the educated classes."[38] Another noted that in Colorado, "the larger percent of addictions are women."[39] The problem was not limited to any group, however, and physicians and nurses were among the most frequent users. Although one estimate was that fifteen to twenty percent of physicians were either addicts or alcoholics, the *Denver Medical Times* was "willing

18.8 Mrs. Winslow's Soothing Syrup depended on morphine to relieve baby's cough. It was one of many non-prescription "baby killers" which could be purchased at the corner drug store.

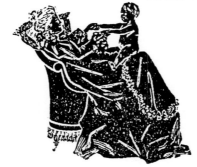

"RIDE A COCK-HORSE TO BANBURY CROSS,
TO SEE A FINE LADY UPON A WHITE HORSE,
RINGS ON HER FINGERS, AND BELLS ON HER TOES,
SHE SHALL HAVE MUSIC WHEREVER SHE GOES."

SO SINGS THE FOND MOTHER IN NURSERY RHYME
TO HER GLAD INFANT, THE WHILE KEEPING TIME;
AND SO CAN ALL MOTHERS WITH TUNEFUL REFRAIN
DELIGHT IN THEIR INFANTS, WHOSE HEALTH THEY MAINTAIN,
THROUGH
MRS. WINSLOW'S SOOTHING SYRUP
OVER FIFTY YEARS SOLD
TO MILLIONS OF MOTHERS IN THE NEW WORLD AND OLD.

18.9 Quack remedies and institutional cures were offered for alcoholism and drug addiction. This one was found in a Pueblo opera house program, circa 1890.

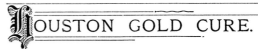

HOUSTON GOLD CURE.

For Drunkenness and the Morphine Habit.

A CURE GUARANTEED   Private treatment given.   Office Room 11, Royal Hotel.
Permanent institute to be established in few days

to believe that from 1 to 2 percent of physicians are morphinists."[40]

In the absence of any national regulations or agencies, Colorado and local governments had enacted laws restricting the sale and use of opiates and other narcotics. As elsewhere in the country, these laws were ineffective and rarely enforced. In 1888, 476 pounds of opium were seized in Denver, but such seizures were exceptional.[41] Finally in 1915, what had come to be known as "the American disease" was addressed by Congress in the form of the Harrison Antinarcotics Law. The new law was strictly enforced in Colorado. One Denver physician, for example, was sentenced to sixty days in the county jail for selling narcotics illegally. The defendent's plea that "he was a Christian man and worked to relieve suffering humanity" was apparently rejected.[42] The Denver Department of Social Welfare reported that an investigation of the "illegal sale of morphine, cocaine, heroin, and their derivatives" had resulted in eighty-two arrests, including twelve physicians and fifteen druggists, with eighty convictions! In some of the cases, the defendants were "given hours to leave town."[43] As enforcement improved, fewer and fewer physicians were willing to risk their professional status in order to supply their patients' habits, and increasingly, addicts began to turn to underworld sources. At the same time, physicians were becoming the victims of the addict's need for a "fix":

> Two Walsenburg physicians recently were victimized by narcotic fiends, and doctors of the . . . district have been warned to keep their offices and automobiles well locked.[44]

Venereal Diseases

When the great educators, teachers, parents and physicians shall be impressed with the importance of imparting a clear knowledge of the . . . ravages caused by venereal diseases, we shall be spared the disgusting spectacle of . . . men in high places pooh-poohing or apologizing for youthful vices.

E. Stuver, M.D. (Fort Collins), 1900[45]

The venereal diseases are those diseases which are spread by sexual contact. Classically, the two major ones have been syphilis and gonorrhea. Although both are venereal and caused by bacterial organisms, they are quite different from each other. Gonorrhea affects the lower urinary tract in men (the penile urethra) and the glandular portions of the lower reproductive tract in women. In men infection is manifest within days of exposure by a discharge or "drip" and may lead, eventually, to urethral stricture. In women the infection is often silent and asymptomatic. However, it may persist, providing a reservoir for future spread of the disease to sexual partners and can lead to infertility. The initial lesion of syphilis is a sore or chancre, usually located on the external genitalia. In the absence of therapy, the disease may silently progress over many years, resulting in severe neurologic or cardiovascular problems. One of the most dreaded sequelae is the dementia known as "general paresis of the insane." In addition, the infection can be transmitted from the infected mother to the fetus. Until the advent of penicillin, the treatment of gonorrhea and syphilis involved a variety of dramatic, often radical and unpleasant and invariably ineffective measures.

Although they are not mentioned in Colorado's early chronicles, it can be assumed that the venereal diseases arrived early, as early as its first visitors. By 1872 Denver's city physician was estimating that "probably every third man who reaches the age of twenty-five has acquired . . . syphilis."[46] Concerned that "this is a disease which he is liable to transmit, not only to his wife . . . but to his progeny," and recognizing that prostitutes served as reservoirs for venereal disease, he urged legislation, including medical inspection, to regulate prostitution. No such legislation was forthcoming, however, and by 1903 the *Denver Medical Times* estimated that half of the city's prostitutes were syphilitic.[47] Denver's Dr. George Stover pointed out, however, that the disease was by no means confined to the demi-monde.

> Enter the palaces of the wealthy and elite, the halls of science and art, even the churches, and the scourge is there, as well as in the miserable hovels of the ignorant, degraded, or criminal.[48]

A strong advocate of public health measures, Stover went a bit far in his warnings:

> No one is exempt from its menace. We are threatened with infection from the baker, butcher, barber, cigarmaker, grocery clerk, launderer, the cook who prepares our food and the waiter who serves it, in hotel, restaurant or home . . .[48]

Similarly, Stover's contemporary, Dr. E. P. Hershey, warned that the disease could be spread by

> wearing a tight fitting hat belonging to another, . . . licking the same envelope that another has licked in order to better seal it, using a neighbor's lead pencil and holding the point between the lips . . . [These] are a few authenticated ways of inoculating the disease.[49]

18.10 The advertising pages of newspapers and popular magazines were filled with claims of cures for syphilis, gonorrhea, and other "private" diseases.

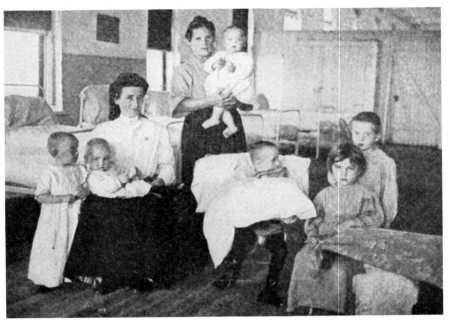

18.11 In 1872 Denver's city physician estimated that one out of every three men had syphilis by the age of twenty-five: "a disease which he is liable to transmit not only to his wife . . . but to his progeny." The "diseased children" in this poorhouse had congenital syphilis.

Finally, there was every grandmother's dreaded sanctum of disease—the public restroom—and its epicenter, the toilet seat. The innocent was warned against:

Using the same soap, same towel, drinking from the same cup that others drink, and sitting upon the same closet seat that every other tenant in the block uses.[49]

Although syphilis was regarded as "one of the most calamitous curses [and] one of the direst maladies in the world," gonorrhea was taken less seriously.[50] The *Denver Medical Times* reported that: "At present most male adolescents regard the 'clap' as a trifling matter to take pride in."[51] The journal warned, however, that while gonorrhea might be asymptomatic in women:

The medical profession has learned to regard gonorrhea as, next to cancer, the most dangerous common disease of womankind. Numberless are the fair victims, the loving young wives, who have gone to their graves, or have lingered through a painful existence of chronic invalidism, because of what seemed to the husband a harmless 'morning drop.'[51]

Pueblo's Dr. R. W. Corwin pleaded for education of the public on the "secret" disease:

When the truth regarding gonorrhea is generally known the disease will be far less prevalent. Boys who now have no dread of it will fear it, girls will be more guarded whom they marry, brothers more willing to protect their sisters.[52]

Fort Collins's Dr. E. Stuver was more explicit, blaming society, and men in particular, for double standards and hypocrisy in their view of the venereal diseases. Such views, in his opinion, served only to maintain the problem.

In the first place a higher moral tone should be inculcated and a single standard of morals for both sexes should be insisted on. Whenever . . . men can be made to feel that the disease leaves the same stigma of shame and disgrace upon them that it inflicts upon their wives and daughters when contracted in the same way, we shall possess a strong inhibitive influence in checking the disease.[53]

In 1860 in Denver, the fee for treating gonorrhea or syphilis was ten to twenty dollars. It was as high as $100 "for curing syphilis."[54] That was a princely sum in 1860, and since the great majority of cases of syphilis either resolved spontaneously or became latent and asymptomatic, the doctor who was fortunate enough to receive payment would have done well indeed. Patients with venereal disease, however, were often deadbeats, and by 1871, the Denver Medical Association was recommending a fee of forty to one hundred dollars to treat syphilis—*paid in advance*, and twenty-five to thirty dollars to treat gonorrhea—*paid in advance*.[55] By 1895, the fee for the first office visit for either disease had been reduced to ten to twenty-five dollars; still high, however, in light of the routine office visit charge of one to five dollars.[56]

Some hospitals refused to admit patients with venereal disease and doctors who specialized in those diseases were often looked upon with disdain by their colleagues. Physicians were cautioned against taking on too many venereal disease patients, lest they be known as "pox doctors" and lose their family practice.

In the absence of any significant public health measures or effective therapy, the venereal diseases continued to wend their way through society, untrammelled by any medical interference. In 1909 *Colorado Medicine* deplored "the foolish sentimentality" towards the venereal diseases which had prevented the introduction of public health measures.[57] With the First World War came documentation of what physicians had already known to be true, the vast numbers of young American men had venereal disease, and soon after, legislation was enacted in Colorado requiring physicians to report infected persons to health authorities.

Prostitution

Women are pure by instinct and by inclination, even as they are trusting and affectionate by nature . . . To mention all the causes that lead to the state of harlotry would be to enumerate all the follies, freaks, eccentricities and naturally mischievous tendencies of the entire human race . . . .

G. W. Cox, M.D. (Denver), 1882[58]

Virtually from their inception, Denver and Colorado's mining camps attracted doctors, lawyers, saloon keepers, preachers, and prostitutes. The frontier, with its paucity of "respectable" women and a population of work-hard, play-hard men whose needs were generally uncomplicated and immediate, made prostitution a growth industry. Single bed cribs expanded into brothels run by entrepreneurial madams, and every community worthy of the name had its red light district.

Much has been written about a few well-known, "class" operations such as Mattie Silks's and Jennie Rogers's parlour houses in Denver. Such enterprises catered to the few who could afford them. The madams who ran fancy houses chose their employees carefully and cared for them accordingly. In considering prostitution it is important to remember that these situations were atypical and that the many idealized and "tongue-in-cheek" accounts of parlour houses are not representative of prostitution as it actually existed. Whether in Denver, the mining camps, or the agricultural-ranching communities of the plains, the majority of consumers were working men, miners, cowboys, and the like. The cribs and bawdy houses which catered to them were often one- or two-room shacks—dirty, drafty, and unsanitary. The great majority of prostitutes were not the "soiled doves" of the parlour houses but, as described by Denver's Dr. George Cox in the 1880s, former "shop girls, milliners, dress-makers, and all those who, by force of circumstances, are compelled to earn their own living. Many of the girls come from the very depths of poverty."[58] Quite a few were European immigrants just off the boat and unable to find legitimate work.

Unlike the mystique and "romance" sometimes said to have attracted the ladies of the parlour houses, for most prostitutes their occupation was simply a matter of day-to-day existence and survival. Once trapped, and "influenced by their associates and surroundings," Dr. Cox found that:

> They soon lose all the native modesty they may have possessed and acquire habits of indolence, filthiness, dishonesty, and intemperance. Smoking, chewing, dipping snuff, drinking, eating opium, and fighting all seem to follow as natural consequences.[58]

Not to mention an isolated and degraded position in the community, venereal disease, unwanted pregnancies and the dangers of illegal abortion, physical abuse, and the realization that for most, the future held the probability of an even more abject poverty than they had left. Even the most naive of the girls was soon educated by her sisters in the details and dangers of venereal disease. Nothing was more damaging to business than word that a woman was "burned." The sensible prostitute, no matter how busy her schedule, found time to douche between contacts. She might use a solution of potassium permanganate, carbolic acid, or bichloride of mercury. She might also insist that her client cleanse himself as well. Such methods, although improving the esthetics of the situation, were generally ineffective in preventing the spread of gonorrhea and syphilis.

Denver's Dr. Frederick Bancroft attributed the prevalence of venereal disease to prostitution. Acknowledging that this "social evil . . . [although] one of the chief causes of the disintegration and downfall of nations," was not likely to be eliminated, he campaigned for "stringent sanitary laws" based on a regulatory system which had recently been introduced in St. Louis.[59] Bancroft proposed that prostitutes be licensed and that periodic medical examinations and treatment of venereal disease be required. Not only would such examinations benefit society, he suggested, they would also help the prostitute who, "When diseased, is sent to a hospital, where she may receive Christian influences and be led to reform."

Bancroft's somewhat revolutionary proposals were opposed by some of Denver's best known physicians and he was denounced in at least one letter to the editor for "supercilious arrogance."[60] Nothing was done and, a quarter of a century later it was noted that "Denver has its full quota [of prostitutes] and about half of them are syphilitic."[61] Years later, the the con-

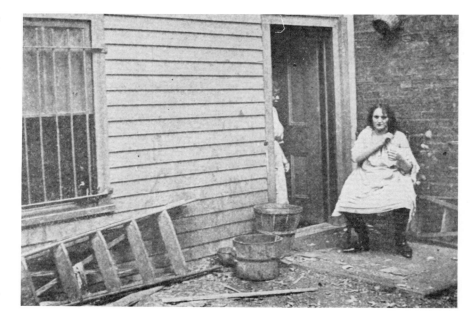

18.12 For most women, prostitution was not the "gilded life."

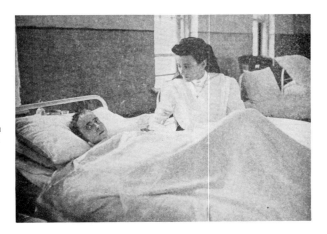

18.13 Illness, and especially venereal disease, was common among prostitutes. This twenty-five year old woman was found by her family three years after she left home, dying of a "loathesome disease" in a poor-house.

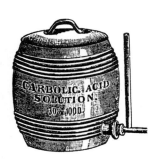

18.14 Carbolic acid, widely used as an antiseptic douche, was a popular means of suicide among prostitutes.

cepts of licensure and medical regulation had been abandoned, and the editor of *Colorado Medicine* was calling for laws to eliminate prostitution as the solution to the problem of venereal disease.[62] Some Colorado communities did insist on medical inspections for prostitutes. In Durango, monthly examinations were required; they cost two dollars, and if she passed the examination, the lady could post a physician's certificate attesting to her (medical) purity.[63] In the mining camp of Victor, Dr. Harry Thomas, as city physician, was responsible for regularly examining the prostitutes of his town. If he found venereal disease, he was authorized to treat the prostitute and her contacts.[64]

Many physicians were concerned about any damage to their professional reputations which might result from their medical care of prostitutes. Having witnessed her deathbed will, and while testifying to that fact in court, one doctor noted that he had been in famed madame Jennie Rogers's house "in a professional capacity, of course."[65] Such concern was certainly justified in the case of a physician who, responsible for examining and certifying the town's prostitutes, made the mistake of allowing them to come to his office. His regular patients soon stopped coming, and according to the story, he "became impoverished and died in the poor house."[66]

The harsh realities of the prostitute's life were relieved by alcohol, morphine, and opium—but only temporarily, and one of prostitution's major occupational hazards was suicide. Carbolic acid, used in diluted form as a douche, was readily available and frequently used as a means of suicide. Lucy Phillips, twenty-four, a prostitute at the Red Light Dance Hall in Victor, for example, swallowed carbolic acid and died. It was said that she had tried to kill herself before.[67]

Carbolic acid was also used by Fay Anderson, "an inmate of Ida Brooks's G Street house in Salida . . . who died, three hours later, in awful agony."[68] On Cripple Creek's infamous Myers Avenue, Annie Rooney was, perhaps, more fortunate:

> [She] endeavored last night to end the ills she knows so well . . . by taking carbolic acid . . . Dr. Wright was summoned and, after an hour's hard work, restored the woman to consciousness. Will she live to reform and thank the doctor, or has he only rescued her for a plunge into greater depths?[69]

Morphine, often in the form of the readily available pain-killer laudanum, was a popular and painless means of suicide. In 1899 a Boulder newspaper reported that:

> One of the demi-monde, evidently tired of life, took a dose of laudanum . . . and came near dying. She is 19 years old and goes by the name of Mamie Myers. She attempted suicide last Wednesday, but Dr. King came to the rescue. Last night her female companions worked over her all night and saved her.[70]

Christmas was a notorious time for suicide attempts in the "red light" districts. It was said that the newspapers wouldn't even print the names of attempted sucides during the holidays, in the belief that the ladies were using this means as a vehicle for advertising.[71]

There are a number of stories which tell of Colorado's prostitutes occasionally assuming the roles of nurses—most often in the mining camps. We have already mentioned the tale of Silverheels and the smallpox epidemic in Buckskin Joe (Chapter 16). When an outbreak of a mysterious illness devastated the miners of Jimtown (near Creede), for example, Mattie Silks turned her parlour house into a hospital, and the ladies donated their two most precious possessions, their nightclothes and their laudanum to the cause.[71] Another story relates that during the influenza epidemic of 1918, Laura Evans shut down her brothels in Salida and sent the girls out to work as nurses.[72] One prostitute, "Jessie," was sent to nurse the minister's wife. In gratitude, the minister offered her a position as housekeeper. Jessie thanked him, but politely refused, adding, "I'll be on my way back to Miss Laura's on Front Street." Jessie's eventual fate is unknown.

19 RAILROAD MEDICINE

THE SURGEON AT THE WRECK

When at last the evil hour feared by
Trainmen comes around,
And that awful earthquake heaving and
That rending, sickening sound,
There's a face that's ever welcome
And he's usually on deck
To save the wounded, soothe the dying
Comes the Surgeon to the wreck.

Anonymous, 1912[1]

I N 1900 IN AMERICA, THE railroads ruled. With nearly 200,000 miles of track, they crossed and recrossed virtually every corner of the country, moving millions of passengers and virtually every commodity on which the nation's economy was based. Their earnings were vast by 1900 standards—nearly one and a half billion dollars that year. The railroads controlled governors, legislators, and judges. They were especially powerful in Colorado, where huge quantities of gold and silver ore, coal, and agricultural products had to be moved across great distances.

Accidents

"Railroad work," said the Colorado Bureau of Labor Statistics, "has always been recognized as a very dangerous form of employment."[2] In 1900, 7,865 people in the U.S.A. were killed and more than 50,000 injured as the result of railroad accidents. Among one million railroad employees in 1900, one in four hundred was killed and four in every hundred were injured. The "high risk" group—engineers, brakemen, firemen and other trainmen who worked with moving stock—had a phenomenally high accident rate. That year, one of every 137 trainmen was killed and one out of eleven was injured. At that rate, during a thirty year career, a trainman had about one chance in five of being killed. If he survived, he would have suffered two or three injuries during his work life.

Collisions and derailments were the most spectacular causes of railroad morbidity and mortality. Mountain routes were especially notorious for brake failures and runaway trains. An example from the 1885 report of Colorado's railroad commissioner:

> On the evening of May 1 . . . the train [Engine 105 and nine cars], immediately on leaving the summit [of Marshall Pass], from some yet unexplained disarrangement of the air brakes, . . . commenced increasing its speed and left the track on a sharp curve . . . knocking down 150 feet of the snow shed.[3]

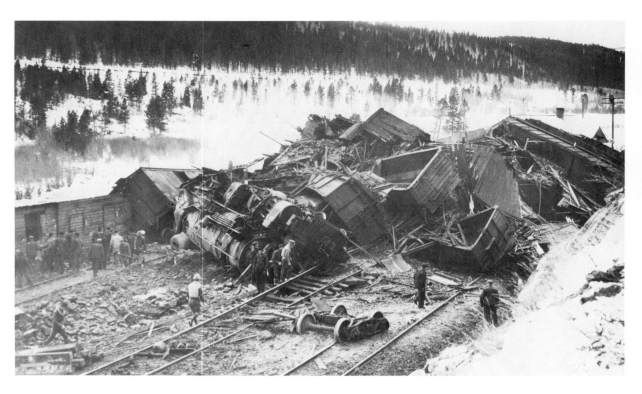

19.1 Mountain routes have always been notorious for brake failures, runaway trains, and spectacular wrecks. This runaway occurred near Rollinsville on the Moffat line.

Two brakemen sustained multiple injuries—fractures, contusions and lacerations. Fortunately, the train remained upright (there were only minor injuries among the rest of the crew and the passengers), and this incident was a minor one in a long list of Colorado train wrecks. That year, 1885, there were thirty-nine deaths and 319 injuries in Colorado railroad accidents.

Less spectacular but far more common than collisions, derailments, and runaways, were everyday encounters between a single worker and the massive, moving equipment. In the locomotive, burns, scaldings, and even boiler explosions were all too common. Away from the engine, the coupling and uncoupling of cars was especially dangerous. In the early days, cars were joined by a ring-like device, the "link," placed into the coupling and fastened by a pin. Many a trainman lost a finger, or worse, or was crushed between the cars while working the couplers. Even after the introduction of automatic coupling, making up a train was dangerous. Couplings sometimes broke apart, sending tons of moving stock rolling down the track. A 1903 Denver coroner's report describes the death of Daniel O'Leary, a brakeman for the Colorado and Southern Railroad.[4] With his train pulling into the South Denver yards, O'Leary, as head brakeman, was standing on the first car behind the engine. When the "knuckle" between the engine and the tender broke, O'Leary fell in front of the cars. Two cars passed over him and his skull was fractured. His death was ruled "accidental" and no blame was assigned.

Just as the miners were usually blamed for mining accidents, the responsibility for railroad accidents was often assigned to the trainmen. In an article on "Railroad accidents: Their cause and prevention," an anonymous "railroad employee" cited some examples:

An engine man failing to test his air brakes in time [or] overcome with drowsiness . . . , A signalman endeavoring to do too many things at one time . . . , Track foremen [careless] in inspecting frogs and switches . . . But, [the cause] that has probably given more concern to railroad officials than all the others combined, is the drink habit.[5]

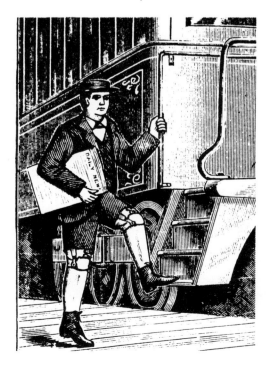

19.2 Trainmen ran a high risk of injury or death sometime during their career. This double-amputee railroad "newsie" may have been a former trainman.

The essayist concluded that the best method of accident prevention was the "encouragement of Christian work among railroad men . . . [for] Christian religion in the hearts of the men will do much to decrease losses of life occasioned by neglect of duty."[5] The journal of railroad medicine, *The Railway Surgeon*, went so far as to state that "nearly all collisions are due to negligence . . . a telegraph operator who failed to deliver an order, . . . a conductor who overlooked a word or figure, . . . an engineman who forgot that a certain order had been delivered to him . . ."[6] The *Journal of the American Medical Association* was not willing to put all the blame on the workers.[7] The railroads, it pointed out, were hiring color-blind men as locomotive engineers—men who were unable to distinguish the red and green of signal lights! This, said JAMA, was criminal negligence.

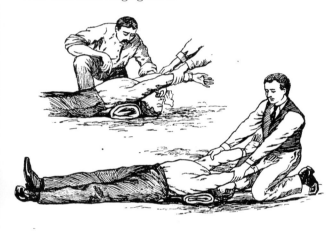

When a medical problem occurred en route, whether a minor ailment in a passenger or a disaster such as a collision, it was the conductor who was expected to administer first aid. In the 1880s, each train on the Denver and Rio Grande Railway was provided with a Conductor's Emergency Chest and a sheet of instructions written by the Railway's Chief Surgeon.[8] The kit contained morphine, ammonia (as a stimulant, e.g. for shock), bicarbonate of sodium (for burns), sutures, sponges, bandages, and dressings. Explicit instructions were given for the first-aid care of wounds, bleeding, fractures, head and chest injuries, burns, scalds, frostbite, and shock. One of the most common problems faced by medic-conductors was "that cinder in your eye," the result of wood and coal burning trains trailing great clouds of dense black smoke in their wake.[9] It was the bane of trainmen and passengers alike. One railroad surgeon described his own experience:

> We hit that cinder with our eye when we are going at thirty miles an hour . . . The collision between the cinder and the eye produces a derailment of

our mental poise . . . Your eye is on fire, and the pain scorches back to the 'angular gyrus' and occipital cortex [of the brain]. It sticks and scratches and hurts and burns.[9]

The best first-aid, the surgeon found, was that suggested by a locomotive engineer: "When you get a cinder in your eye, rub the other eye." In addition, the doctor advised a series of "hands off" manipulations which, he suggested, would result in dislodging the interloper. Matters were not so simple, commented a Denver doctor, when "the cinder is hot and buries itself in the body of the cornea."[10]

Railroad Surgeons

To provide professional medical assistance to trainmen and passengers, the railroads employed a veritable army of railroad surgeons. The railroads felt that their doctors played an important role, and one executive was quoted as saying that he "would just as soon think of parting with his freight department as to dispense with his department of surgery."[11] In 1887, in addition to its chief surgeon, the Denver and Rio Grande had thirty-seven "local surgeons" in towns along its tracks in Colorado.[12] These doctors had their own private practices but were "on call" to the railroad. They were expected to treat their railroad patients "in the same manner as they would a private patient" and "to go to the place of accident, if circumstances demand." In addition, they provided physical examinations for employees, taught first aid, and supervised the sanitation of the trains and stations.[13] Their primary responsibility was to their employer and "to perform all duties in the manner which is most

19.3 The Denver and Rio Grande's conductors were provided with a first-aid kit and some training. They were expected to provide emergency care prior to the arrival of the doctor.

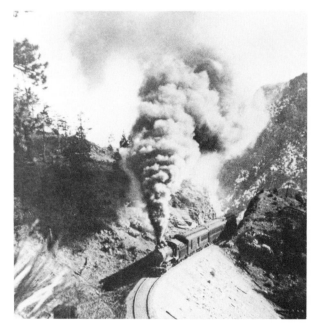

19.4 One common problem was that "cinder in your eye." The traveler on this Cripple Creek Short Line train was as likely to get an eyeful of cinders as scenery.

conducive to the interests of the Company."[14] This was of particular importance in the matter of lawsuits related to railroad accidents. In such situations, the railroad surgeon was expected to help protect the company. He was warned:

> There is probably no passenger train but carries some dangerous freight—men and women who long for a wreck, a jostle, a fall, something on which to base a claim. In the lottery of wreck they hope to win the prize of injury . . . All proper means [should be used] to prevent litigation and claims . . . When a claim is made the subject should be labeled, 'Glass, handle with care.' Only the right word at the right time should be spoken.[15]

Implying that the doctors were expected to keep their mouths shut in such situations, it was pointed out that "the companies employ men for this work. They are experts. They make a study of human nature along these lines."[15] What was called "railway spine" came under this heading. Denver's Dr. W. W. Grant, surgeon to the Chicago, Rock Island and Pacific Railway, described a typical case. Subsequent to a train collision:

> The patient complains of persistent pain at some point of the spinal column, attended with various nervous manifestations due to the 'shock'—[although] there is no evidence of a pathologic or anatomic lesion by any clinical or scientific tests at our command. The element of fear enters largely into these histories [and] there is a distinct appeal to the mental and emotional.[16]

Although some physicians thought that railway spine might have some basis in fact, even if psychological rather than organic, Dr. Grant suggested that in the great majority of cases, recovery was generally associated with a successful financial outcome. In such instances, he suggested, the term "litigation symptoms" might be more appropriate. Grant cited the case of a Denver woman who had been involved in a railway collision. After examining her and finding "only a slight cold," the doctor sensed, "from her manner, [that] she would demand considerable money" from the railroad. Indeed, she soon demanded $2,000, was offered $500, and sued for $15,000. She testified that a year after the accident she was still unable to conduct her business. After examining her again at the time of the trial, Dr. Grant testified that:

> She was as healthy a woman probably as there was in Denver; that if suffering, it was from litigation symptoms and from these she would not recover until the case was fully settled.[16]

The jury rendered a decision in favor of the defendant but awarded her only two hundred

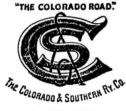

"THE COLORADO ROAD."

F. J. BANCROFT,
CHIEF SURGEON.

19.5 Senior railroad surgeons included some of Colorado's most prominent physicians. Dr. Bancroft was chief surgeon to several railroads.

dollars more than the company had originally offered. By 1914 "railway spine" had been relegated to the category of "traumatic neurosis."[17]

The railroads selected some of Colorado's most outstanding physicians as their chief and senior surgeons. Dr. Frederick Bancroft was chief surgeon to the Denver and Rio Grande. The Rock Island's Dr. Grant and the Union Pacific's Dr. L. E. Lemen served as presidents of the National Association of Railway Surgeons. Such senior surgeons were well paid and treated royally by their employers. The local surgeons were not so well paid. During the fiscal year 1886-1887, the Denver and Rio Grande paid out a total of $10,000, or about $250 per physician, for services to the railroad's employees.[18] The reason why the position of surgeon was coveted by doctors in such railroad towns as La Veta, Basalt, and Westcliff was related more to the prestige and the added business the title brought to their practices. In reality, the railroad surgeon was a "contract doctor," a form of practice which was considered to be unethical by organized medicine and anathema to the "fee for service" doctor. Pueblo's Dr. Will B. Davis asked:

> Why should the surgeon of a railway . . . be permitted to do work for so much per capita and we others not apply the same principles to private practice. Is any man, or set of men, to be privileged above others?[19]

Apparently so, since this form of contract practice was not condemned by the medical societies.

Health Plans and Hospitals

The railroad surgeons provided care to employees as part of company health insurance plans—the "railroad hospital funds." The Denver and Rio Grande's Hospital Fund was typical. For fifty cents a month, the employee was "entitled to medicines and medical attendance . . . or admission to one of the Company Hospitals . . . free of charge, when sick from diseases contracted while in service of the Company or from injuries sustained in the line of duty."[20] Exceptions included "employees sick from venereal diseases, the results of intemperance, vicious habits, or old diseases contracted prior [to employment]." The chief surgeon requested all departments of the railroad to refrain from hiring "persons advanced in years or subject to . . . chronic disease," since such individuals might become a burden to the fund. Those who were already employed and developed a chronic disease might be dropped from the fund at the discretion of the chief surgeon. The interest on

$5,000 was to be applied "to the relief of such employees as have, by long continued service, been worn out, and have become unable to provide for their own comforts and for those who have become needy from the results of severe injuries or long sickness." Thus, an annual amount of about $250 provided the only funds available for disabled or otherwise needy workers among the company's 5,000 employees. In the fiscal year 1886-1887, nearly 4,000 cases were treated at home or in the doctors' offices, at an average cost of less than three dollars per case.

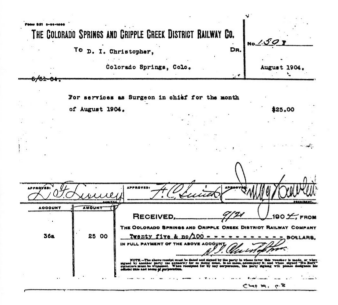

The Denver and Rio Grande's "health plan" also provided for hospitalization. In fiscal year 1886-1887, 270 patients were admitted and treated, at an average cost of thirty-two dollars per case. Although the fund had arrangements with hospitals in Denver, Pueblo, and Durango, most patients were admitted to the Denver and Rio Grande Hospital in Salida, an important railroad junction. Opened in 1885, and one of the country's first railroad hospitals, the three-story brick building was built in the style of a large Victorian house. Valued at more than $20,000, it was so modern that that it had hot running water and, alongside each bed, an electric bell for summoning a nurse.[21]

The hospital maintained strict rules. For example, "Trivial surgical cases, such as the loss of a finger" were rejected as outpatient problems, and the hospital retained the right to discharge patients who "shall become intoxicated . . . or who become insubordinate to the rules of the hospital."[22] By the turn of the century, the railroad's workers and management were engaged in a dispute over the fund and the hos-

pital. According to an anonymous author, the railroad was not abiding by the fund's by-laws and had gained control over its board of trustees.[23] Furthermore, the workers claimed, the chief surgeon

> is a surgeon in name only who we are paying a salary of $3,000 yearly to work against our interests . . . As the company's [employee] . . . all he has to do is please the company—he don't have to please us. His venal attitude was never so completely demonstrated, and the wrath of the employees never reached its climax until [he] discharged, without cause, Dr. [F. N.] Cochems, the idol of all the employees and the ablest and most successful surgeon in the entire West . . . The medical management of the hospital was never in less competent hands than now.[23]

The Brotherhood of Locomotive Firemen passed "strong resolutions" denouncing Dr. Cochems's firing, but to no avail.[24] The "idolized" doctor remained in Salida, however, establishing his Red Cross Hospital and, apparently, remaining a thorn in the side of the railroad. In 1916, for example, Cochems filed suit against the Denver and Rio Grande, alleging improper practices in regard to their distribution of free railroad passes to contract doctors.[25] Despite such setbacks, the Denver and Rio Grande Hospital Fund served as a model for other railroads—with a few individual embellishments. The Colorado and Southern Railway's "Instructions to Surgeons," for example, referred to the medical care, not only of its passengers and workers, but also to another category of person usually ignored by the railroads:

> When tramps are injured while prowling about the yards, or stealing rides—humanity requires that they should be cared for until they can be turned over to the . . . authorities.[26]

By 1927 railroad hospital funds were still a medical bargain. The Atchison, Topeka and Santa Fe Hospital Association, whose hospital was located in La Junta, was still charging only a dollar a month for membership.[27]

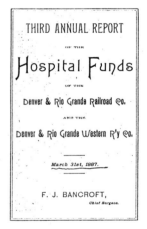

19.6 The railroad surgeon was expected to "perform all duties in the manner which is most conducive to the interests of the company." In return, he received a fee for service—and the prestige attached to being associated with the railroad. (Dr. Michael Arnall)

19.7 The Denver and Rio Grande's hospital fund was a model for the industry.

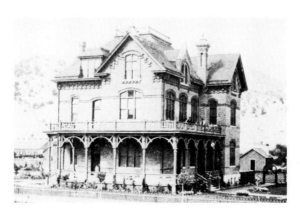

19.8 The Denver and Rio Grande's hospital in Salida was opened in 1885. It was one of the nation's first railroad hospitals.

Sanitation

Sanitation was the one area in which the doctors and the railroads found themselves in conflict. Even the most prominent railway surgeons publicly deplored the unsanitary conditions of passenger cars and coaches. Dr. Grant, in his presidential speech to the American Academy of Railway Surgeons in 1899, commented on the poor ventilation and germ-laden atmosphere to which the railroad traveler was subjected:

> The transom window . . . admits more smoke, cinders, and dirt than pure fresh air, [there are] sudden frequent and extreme changes of temperature, [and], should we examine the air of a Pullman coach with a spectroscope, the myriad living things to the square inch revealed . . . would be enough to cause the shades of Pasteur [and other microbiologists] to weep for the living.[28]

A member of the Colorado Board of Health complained that

> the [drinking] water on the cars is sometimes carried for several trips without any cleaning of the coolers and . . . I have seen a quantity of ice lying on a platform covered with dirt of every nature, then transferred to the water cooler by an employee, with hands not only black from grease, but having been just used to remove tobacco juice from lips and chin, and worse from nostrils.[29]

Unsanitary conditions contrasted sharply with the railroads' marketing campaigns. The Burlington Route, for example, was appealing to the "princesses of Colorado" with advertisements touting their trains' "toilet rooms—dainty as a boudoir."[30] At the same time, Colorado's Board of Health was discussing the unsanitary conditions of "water closets" on railroad cars.[31]

Of special concern was the possible spread of contagious disease by passengers coming to Colorado. In the 1890s, the State Board of Health issued a series of circulars dealing with this and other railroad sanitary issues. Circular No. 6, for example, ordered that:

> If the conductor discovers on the train, any person suffering from cholera, smallpox, diphtheria, scarlet fever or any other contagious disease . . . he will at once communicate by telegraph or telephone with . . . the State Board of Health . . . He must see that the case is detained and kept under surveillance at the nearest station . . .[32]

A published exchange of communications between the general manager of the Colorado Midland Railway and the State Board of Health in 1894, suggests that the railroads simply ignored these edicts.[33] Nevertheless, the pressure for im-

proved sanitation continued, and in 1903, the Colorado Railways Association adopted a rule that:

> No invalid could enter a train in Colorado without a physician's certificate that the bearer was not suffering from any contagious disease. The intention is to protect passengers from infection, and not to depend upon undeveloped diagnostic abilities of conductors, as has been the custom heretofore.[34]

Unfortunately, this simply shifted the onus from the railroad company to the passenger and was, therefore, completely ineffective. The biggest public health problem was with the nation's major provider of railway coaches, the Pullman Company. Dr. Grant described how Pullman cars were cleaned—by simply running compressed air over cushions, blankets, drapery, etc.[35] This procedure removed dust and dirt, but not bacteria. There were no company regulations or instructions regarding hygiene or the protection of passengers from contagious diseases. Grant told how he had recently observed a patient with scarlet fever lying on a berth all day, exposing every person in the car. He also knew of an instance in which a young lady with advanced tuberculosis had been put on a Pullman car, where she "coughed and expectorated continuously." Grant pointed out the ironic fact that, although there were strict rules regarding the transportation of dead bodies, there were few regarding the "transportation of the living subject" with contagious disease, and those few

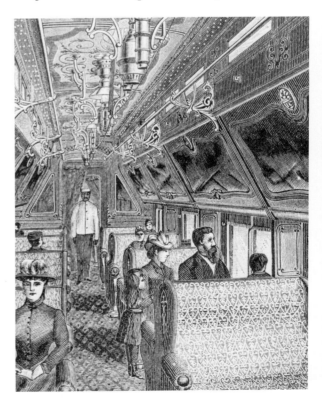

19.9 Dr. W. W. Grant suggested that the plush furnishings of the railroad cars served as a "nidus for the protection and preservation of germs."

rules were generally ignored by railroad personnel. If persons with contagious diseases were going to be allowed passage, it was necessary to "fumigate [the cars] with some antiseptic, such as formaldehyde gas . . ." At the very least, since the materials used in furnishing railway coaches served as a "nidus for the protection and preservation of germs," Grant urged the Pullman Company to use "less carving and embossing, less plush and velvet and drapery . . ." in their cars.

As Colorado's tuberculophobia grew, newspapers began to agitate for reforms and politicians began to react. In 1900 the Denver City Council passed an ordinance requiring the fumigation of all sleeping cars upon their arrival and departure from Denver.[36] The Pullman Company responded by threatening to cancel a facility which they had promised to build in Denver, thereby eliminating four hundred new jobs.[37] The issue was resolved amicably, however, with the company agreeing to adhere to a list of sanitary and fumigation measures proposed by the State Board of Health.[38] Denver's public health officer, Dr. C. E. Cooper, illustrated the problem presented by tuberculous travelers and the new measures being taken by the Pullman Company:

Their linen and blankets cannot help being contaminated and they sometimes expectorate and miss the cuspidor, owing to the motion of the train . . . At the Pullman shops in Denver, when a car comes in, if there is a history [of a passenger with] a contagious disease, the car is fumigated . . . Then they take out all the carpets and hangings . . .[38]

Dr. Cooper went on to describe a complex series of cleansing and disinfecting procedures. With the Pullman Company having adopted such public health measures, Colorado's railroads soon fell into line.

Indeed, railroad medicine was changing. Dr. John W. O'Connor, Salida's pioneer railroad surgeon, recalled, years later, his early days trudging over drifts on snowshoes to see patients.[39] Now he was unable to recruit a resident physician for the Denver and Rio Grande Hospital in Salida, and he complained, the young doctors "won't come out here unless I can assure them of every luxury . . ."

New rules, procedures, and equipment which emphasized safety were reducing railroad morbidity and mortality due to accidents. In 1915 *Colorado Medicine* was able to state that deaths due to railroad accidents, which had been declining for a decade, had reached a new low.[40]

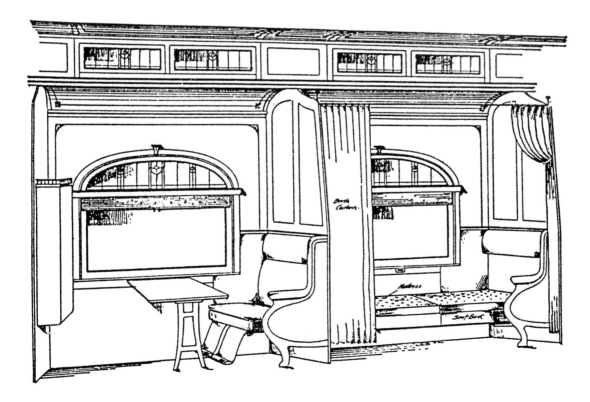

19.10 The influx by train of thousands of consumptives to Colorado led to concerns about the spread of the disease among other passengers. Denver's Dr. Sherman Bonney designed a special passenger car for the transport of consumptives. It is unknown whether his design was ever implemented.

20 LAW AND ORDER

Vice and crime are nothing else than the sickness of the social body, and the physician is the true one to suggest a remedy and apply the treatment. Castration, with our antiseptic surgery and anaesthesia, is painless and safe, and would have a greater deterrent effect on the vicious than our penitentiaries or the gallows . . .

Dr. B.A. Arbogast (Breckenridge), 1895[1]

THE FRONTIER WAS A dangerous place, not only because of a harsh environment and disease and the other vicissitudes of pioneer life, but because of the human violence which accounted for a significant part of the West's designation as "wild." This was especially true of the mining camps and of Colorado's big, bad city—Denver. On the day of his arrival in Denver, Dr. S. D. Hopkins encountered a body hanging from a pole downtown, a murderer who had been lynched.[2] Indeed, in the 1860s, crime had become so rampant in Denver that a secret group of vigilantes had been organized. The vigilantes had their own rules and regulations. Within twenty-four hours of his arrival in Denver, complete with umbrella and silk hat, Dr. John Elsner received an anonymous note tacked to his door. He recalled that:

> With skull and crossbones at the top, underneath was printed, 'Dispose of your hat and umbrella, as it is a violation of the vigilantes.' It was not necessary for me to do this, as the following day I missed my umbrella and discovered my hat cut into two parts. From that time on I wore a felt hat.[3]

Within a short time of his arrival in Creede, "one of the wildest of the frontier settlements . . . where many bad characters flocked," Dr. Henry Van Norman had heard of twenty-five fatal shootouts.[4] In Crested Butte, Dr. Charles Gardiner heard gunfire in the street outside his cabin. On retiring that evening, he found bullet holes in his bed.[5] In Leadville, coroner's cases were so numerous that Dr. G. Law found "his income from this source about as profitable as a gold mine."[6]

There was always the potential for personal violence in medical practice. In his book of advice for a new physician, Dr. D. W. Cathell warned:

> Midnight desperadoes may lead you into their traps by feigning sickness and then rob or murder you; or your brute, crazy with drink; or your homicidal maniac; or your fever-tossed patient who knows not what he does; or your lunatic with a delusion; or the infuriated fellow in whom you have made a wrong diagnosis . . . The unreasoning tiger in whose family you have had sad deaths, or unfortunate surgery . . . The thug, the fanatic, the madman—any blood-thirsty demon may suddenly assault and try to maim or kill you.[7]

Many such incidents can be cited in early Colorado medical history. One day, Dr. Hopkins was accosted in downtown Denver by an irate cattleman. The doctor, who happened to be an expert boxer, floored his assailant.[8] Silver Plume's Dr. F. R. Porter was shot at by the brother of one of his patients, a man who felt that his sister was not recovering quickly enough.[9] Dr. Frederick Bancroft had his own six-shooter ready when a cowboy threatened to shoot him if his brother died as the result of Bancroft's surgery.[10] When Dr. Gardiner, testifying in a murder trial, was threatened by the defendant, the judge, doctor, and eleven of the twelve jurors all drew their guns. The judge granted Gardiner the right to shoot the defendant on sight if their paths ever crossed in the future.[11] Georgetown's Dr. William Burr had his revenge on an outlaw who had led him on a bogus housecall and stole his horse; the doctor later recognized the man and served as a witness at his trial.[12]

Outlaws

There were a number of encounters between Colorado physicians and some of the area's more infamous badmen. Outlaw Ike Stockton, his leg shattered by a sheriff's bullet, had his leg amputated in the Las Animas City jail by Dr. H. A. Clay. Stockton died the next day.[13] Dr. W. F. McClelland managed to salavage Joe Slade's leg when that notorious outlaw was shot by Jules Beni, another outlaw and the namesake of Julesburg, a town in northeastern Colorado. Years later, Slade performed a bit of surgery of his own on Beni, cutting off his ears before shooting him.[14] In Trinidad, Clay Allison was said to have playfully filled Dr. Menger's stovepipe beaver hat full of holes with a sawed-off shotgun. Just to show he was only kidding, the famed outlaw treated the doc to a new Stetson and a drink.[15] According to Sister Blandina Segale, the Menger brothers, along with Dr. Michael Beshoar and another Trinidad physician, were near victims of an angry Billy the Kid.[16] Billy's ire had been aroused by the doctors' refusal to remove a bullet from one of his buddies, and to show his displeasure, he planned to relieve them of their scalps. Many years later, Sister Blandina recalled confronting Billy: "I understand you have come to scalp our Trinidad physicians," she said, "which act I ask you to cancel."[16] Assured by his wounded comrade that the nun was "game," Billy relented, and the doctors remained tonsorially intact.

Some of Colorado's medical encounters with outlaws occurred post-mortem. When Jesse James's killer, Bob Ford, was shot to death in Creede, Dr. Van Norman performed the autopsy. The doctor extracted the bullets from Ford's neck and gave them to a friend as a souvenir.[17] When a posse tracking the infamous Reynolds gang killed one of its members, a Dr. Cooper, one of the posse, used his medical skills to remove the outlaw's head. It was subsequently put on display in Alma, Colorado.[18] It wasn't a physician who removed the head of one of the Espinosa brothers, another notorious outlaw gang, but famed scout, Tom Tobin. The head was taken to Fort Garland, where it remained preserved in alcohol, until it was swiped by the fort's departing surgeon, Dr. Waggoner.[19] While crossing the Sangre de Cristo mountains, the absconding doctor's wagon overturned, breaking the jar. Hoping to replenish the spilled preservative in Pueblo, Waggoner was shocked to find "the town, for the first time in its history . . . without either alcohol or whiskey." Lacking any preservative, Waggoner had to remove the flesh from the skull. He eventually donated his prize to a collection of skulls from other famous murderers.

Medical Witnesses

Physicians were frequently asked to serve as expert witnesses in civil and criminal cases. The *Denver Medical Times* provided some advice to the testifying physician:

> When he goes on the stand he should go there unbiased and unprejudiced, confining his statements to facts, keeping out of deep water. His answers should always be based upon his exact and positive knowledge of the subject, and every answer that might be misconstrued by a designing lawyer should be qualified. He should say as little as possible, be sure he is right, and stick tenaciously to what he says . . . He should be dignified, precise, brief, and to the point and allow no one to confuse or bulldoze him, always remembering that the medical profession . . . is gifted with a higher order of education and intelligence than are the men of the legal profession . . .[20]

Monument's Dr. William McConnell testified, in a murder trial, that the victim had been dead for two minutes by the time he arrived on the scene.[21] The defendant's attorney was unimpressed and challenged the doctor's ability to

20.1 There was ample opportunity for the use of bullet probes and forceps on the frontier.

20.2 In bigger cities more sophisticated devices were available to locate bullets. Denver's Dr. C. B. Lyman reported on the use of an electromagnetic bullet probe to the Colorado Medical Society in 1896.

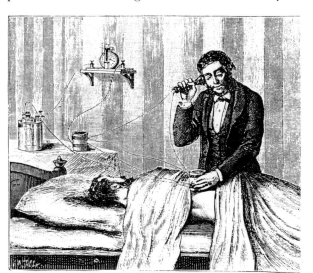

provide so precise a time. He pulled out his timepiece and instructed the doctor to tell him when two minutes had elapsed. The doctor sat quietly in the witness box, his hands in his lap, until precisely two minutes after the lawyer's challenge. The jury was impressed. Some physicians, however, were

> unable to keep an unruffled temper under the sharp proddings of the cross-examiner . . . With such loss of temper comes defeat, as the attorney well knows, for the witness is not then so careful in avoiding the pitfalls prepared for him. He presents a lamentable appearance before the court, and loses greatly in reputation and self-respect.[22]

The *Denver Medical Times* denounced judges who allowed "ignorant, malicious, lying, or drunken lawyers" to mistreat medical witnesses: "Shame on such judges! Shame on such lawyers! Shame on the practice of the court that will permit such abominable proceedings! . . ."[23] In order to minimize such attacks, it was advised that physicians who were willing to provide expert testimony should, indeed, be experts in the area:

> Physicians who are damaged most severely in a medico-legal scrimmage, whom the attorneys dissect, or . . . vivisect, are those who go on the stand claiming to be an expert in some particular department, when in fact, they have no just claims to be so considered.[24]

In rural Sterling, Dr. J. N. Hall acquired a great deal of experience with gunshot wounds. Many were accidental, but some were not. In 1890 he had an opportunity to apply his knowledge in a murder case.[25] The victim was a young man who had been angered by a merchant's

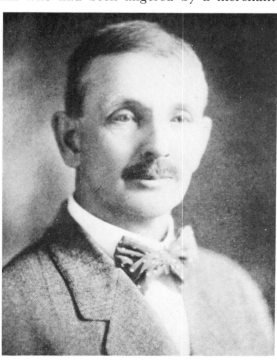

20.3 Remembered today both as a pioneer country practitioner on Colorado's eastern plains and, later, as a professor of medicine and one of Denver's first internists, the multi-talented Dr. J. N. Hall also made a number of important contributions in the field of forensic medicine.

refusal of credit. Some sort of confrontation had occurred, and several witnesses testified, the merchant had put a revolver to the man's head and fired. It seemed like a clear-cut case of murder, and there were murmurings of an impending lynching. One finding bothered Dr. Hall, however: the burn, or "brand," which he found below the bullet wound. Characteristically, Dr. Hall had read, when such burns occurred, they were located above the wound, not below—the result of the "kick" of a fired weapon. After trying some experiments, Hall testified that the gun must have been held upside down. This conclusion was consistent with the accused's claim that he was trying to protect himself by bringing the weapon down on the young man's head, not trying to fire it, and that the gun went off accidentally. The district attorney tried to belittle Hall's "theory," at which point the doctor opened a satchel and spoke to the judge:

> Your honor . . . , I have brought with me thirteen revolvers with suitable ammunition so that the gentleman and every juror can try out . . . the question at issue. I challenge him to do this under your direction.[25]

The defendant was acquitted.

In 1895 a Denver pathologist, Dr. E.R. Axtell, provided expert medical testimony in another spectacular murder case.[26] This time the testimony was to the detriment of the accused. Using microscopy and a battery of laboratory studies, Axtell was able to invalidate the defendant's claim that the blood on his clothes was derived from various animals that he had supposedly killed on a hunting trip. This kind of evidence was sufficiently innovative at the time to warrant the publication of Axtell's paper in the *Journal of the American Medical Association*.

Toxicologic studies were also coming into vogue. In 1904 the astute and apparently ubiquitous Dr. Hall admitted a saloon keeper to Denver's St. Joseph's hospital.[27] The working diagnoses were gastritis and a peripheral neuritis. Hall assumed that the saloon keeper's problems were due to alcoholism, but when the patient's denials were confirmed by his family physician, Hall began to wonder about other possibilities. When Hall learned that his patient drank as many as eight bottles of a particular brand of soda pop every day, he had two bottles sent for chemical analysis. They contained significant amounts of arsenic. These were sufficient, in the quantities imbibed by his patient, to produce gastritis and peripheral neuritis, features which are not only associated with alcoholism but with chronic arsenic poisoning as well.

Coroners

The county coroner system dates back to medieval England and English common law. When Colorado became a state in 1876, its new constitution provided for the election of a county coroner, entitling any citizen who had the right to vote to be eligible to serve in that capacity. No other qualification was required of the official whose job it was to "hold an inquest upon the dead bodies of such persons . . . as are supposed to have died . . . by unlawful means, or the cause of whose death is unknown."[28] The coroner might seek the advice of a "physician or a surgeon" in each case, as he saw fit. Not surprisingly, the position became "purely a political one." Sometimes it was filled by a physician, and in some areas, there was competition among physicians for the job. At one time, for example, Fremont County had two physician-coroners, each claiming that he alone was the legitimately elected official.[29] Most coroners, however, were not physicians, and many were morticians, an occupation with obvious potential for conflicts of interest. Dr. Hall, although he made "no personal allusions regarding coroners in general [and had] no doubt that they perform their duties as well as any person can . . . out of his line of work," was concerned about the system:

> We ask, is it to be supposed that a citizen taken from the ordinary walks of life is to be prepared to pass upon medical questions which tax the best minds in our profession? Is the merchant, the farmer, the politician to decide, without an autopsy, that 'death occurred from apoplexy?'[30]

Hall cited a case, a death near Greeley, which the coroner had ruled a suicide. Two physicians investigated the case and determined that it was probably murder. In another example, a coroner, allegedly concerned about the expense, refused to call for an autopsy in a case of maternal death due to a suspected criminal abortion.[31] Such instances, said Hall, warranted the abolition of the office of coroner and its replacement by that of medical examiner. As in other states, the medical examiner, a physician, would be responsible for investigating each case, and at the request of the district attorney, perform an autopsy when indicated.

Years later, with the coroner system still very much intact, Dr. H. G. Wetherill expressed his opinion:

> The coroner's office is, without exception . . . the most useless, meddlesome, and spectacular bit of political machinery ever invented . . . The place is too commonly filled by some political grafter,

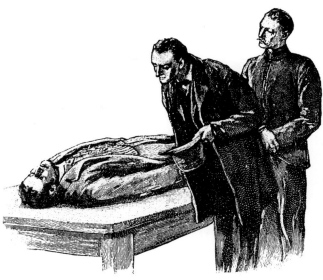

20.4 Coroners were kept busy on the frontier. Colorado's coroner system has remained essentially unchanged for more than a century.

who, for purposes of his own, or in the interests of his friends, finds it profitable to accept the job.[32]

Wetherill, too, called for a medical examiner system, as have others over the years. Nevertheless, and, although many states have adopted such a system, Colorado continues to retain its system of county coroners, essentially unchanged from that of 1876.

Many physicians who took on the job of coroner found it unrewarding and soon left the office. In the 1870s, Dr. Charles Denison, recently arrived and soon to become one of Denver's best-known physicians, found himself "sitting" for three days on several murder victims.[33]

> He got $8 for [the inquest] and it cost him $5 to have his clothes cleaned. This left him a net profit of a dollar a day . . . Dr. Denison likes the office, and especially the emoluments, so well that he handed in his resignation yesterday.

Rural Custer County's coroner, Dr. E. H. Cutts, complained about the "parsimonious tendencies, penny-pinching proclivities, and general jackass propensities of the Democratic members of the Board of County Commissioners" who

> discountenance investigation and practically place [themselves] in an attitude of accessory after the fact. [This] means that there will be more murders in the County. In fact, as soon as the state of affairs become known, all with homicidal desires and a small amount of capital can bring their victims from all parts of the state of Colorado for slaughter.[34]

Unnatural Causes

Early death certificates provide us with some interesting insights into the investigation of "unnatural death" in old Colorado. From a "dusty, dreary prairie village, a cowboy coroner roughly scrawled" that the cause of Pete Hendrick's death was "a big rattlesnake."[35] The cause of death on a certificate from a mining camp was "four tons of dirt," presumably a cave-in. On a certificate from Leadville, it was listed as "a relapse;" from Aspen, "an accident;" from Greeley, "railroads;" and from Rifle, "shotgun." Under "cause of death," a "bright and well-educated man from Huerfano county" wrote, "Ast the doktor."

Death due to unnatural causes was not uncommon in early Colorado. In 1906, for example, Colorado's death rate due to suicide, homicide, and accidents was 40% higher than that of Connecticut, the next state listed in the national registry.[36] In Denver, among 244 cases investigated by the coroner during a six month period in 1913, there were 110 due to unnatural causes.[37] Fifty-eight were accidents, including 17 railroad, 8 street car, 3 automobile, and one "horse falling." There were 9 homicides and 43 suicides. Carbolic acid ingestion was the most frequent means of suicide. The Denver coroner's registry briefly described each of these sad events.[38] On February 10, 1903, for example, Daisy M-----, a twenty-one-year-old divorced white nurse, rented a room in a cheap boarding house on Lawrence Street. The next morning, her landlady smelled gas coming from her room but "thought nothing of it." In the afternoon, Daisy sent a messenger boy for some mineral water and a two ounce bottle of carbolic acid. That evening, her landlady found her barely breathing. A police ambulance took her to County Hospital, but it was too late. No inquest was held and she was given a pauper's burial.

Crooked Doctors and Some Imposters

Although most were presumably honest and a few even served as lawmen, a few doctors were crooks.[39] Some were merely unethical: they split their fees, did uneccessary surgery, promised impossible cures, accepted money for testimonials, and so on. Some took unfair advantage of their professional status. One young schoolmarm, slightly injured in a Denver tramway accident, was promised a favorable medical report from the doctor—if she would be receptive to his advances.[40]

Others broke the law:

> Dr. Frank R----, the smooth young physician . . . who disappeared with a neat sum of his landlady's money . . . is in jail in Chicago charged with bigamy. Besides this, and the charge of embezzlement which the Denver police have against him, he is said to be wanted in other places for forgery.[41]

The wife of Dr. Rudolph B---- of Boulder died recently very suddenly. The coroner's jury brought in a verdict that the doctor had administered poison to her.[42]

In 1891 a visitor to Denver, a Mrs. Barnaby, received a bottle of medicine in the mail from her "friend" and physician back home in Providence, Rhode Island, Dr. Graves. Three days later she was dead of arsenic poisoning. Sent to Denver to stand trial for murder, the doctor committed suicide.[43]

Some medical "outlaws" were actually imposters. Perhaps the most notorious was A. Edward Ryetzel, alias George Elliott, M.D.[44] Ryetzel used a phony diploma to obtain a medical license and opened a "private surgical hospital for women" in Denver, where he performed criminal abortions. He was discovered after causing the death of a young woman and frightening her fiancee into committing suicide. Denver's doctors were warned against a less pernicious medical imposter who was calling on physicians and asking them for handouts. He claimed to be a doctor who was down on his luck, and the editor of the *Denver Medical Times* acknowleged that he had been worked out of a dollar by the pseudo-medical con man.[45] One of Colorado's earliest con men was "Doctor" J. L. Dunn, a "man of pleasing address and smooth exterior," who, when he wasn't selling counterfeit U.S. scrip, was stealing cattle.[46] One of the best known of the breed was "Doc" Baggs.[47] His modus operandi was to work the railroads, dressed in standard physician attire, a Prince Albert coat and a stovepipe hat, and carrying a little black bag. He would diagnose an ailment in a fellow-traveler, provide medication, refuse to accept any fee, and, once having gained his confidence, proceed to sell the sucker some worthless mining stock.

Crime and Punishment

In the early days, most doctors had little to do with criminals, avoiding them when possible and treating them when asked. In his inspection of the state penitentiary at Canon City in 1880, the board of health's Dr. D. H. Dougan commented on the "excellent health" and the low mortality rate of the inmates.[48] Much of this success, said Dr. Dougan, was due to the prison physician, "whose interest in the physical welfare of his unfortunate charge is genuine and sincere." He did find some problems—notably overcrowding ("the corridors are occupied by a large number of sleeping bunks"), the lack of any sewage system or central heating, and the absence of a hospital ("the cells are not suitable places for the sick"). Dougan found that punishment was humane ("the prisoner is tied to a post and the stream from a hose . . . directed against his breast and face . . . until he promises future obedience") and was "only inflicted in the presence of the attending physician." There was, unfortunately, little effort made to distinguish the criminal from the "insane" at the prison and Dr. Dougan commented on "an old colored man of imbecile mind" who was restrained by a ball and chain.

As time went on and as modern concepts of mental illness evolved, many physicians became concerned about the law's attitude towards crimes committed by mentally incompetent persons. In the trial of Orville Turley, "the furnace pipe murderer," seven "expert alienists" testified that the defendant "was afflicted by general paralysis of the insane," the dementia of tertiary syphilis:

> Yet, when the next step was obviously to send the slayer to the insane asylum at Pueblo, [Denver's] mayor took it upon himself to intervene in order to appeal the medical question to a jury of laymen . . . Mayor Bailey is apparently not a believer in medical experts, but has complete faith in the ability of two salesmen, a dry goods clerk, a coal office clerk, and the driver of a laundry wagon.[49]

When the perpetrator was responsible for his crime, there was no question that punishment was in order. Trained to think in terms of cause and effect, some doctors felt that the suitable punishment for rape was castration. That was certainly the opinion of Dr. Arbogast, the physican from Breckenridge who was quoted at the beginning of this chapter. It was also the opinion of a mob in Montrose, Colorado, who ordered two physicians to "mutilate one F. H. Allen, who had been arrested on a charge of criminal assault," presumably rape.[50] The editor of the *Colorado Medical Journal* felt even more strongly about the punishment for rape: "We would suggest for this crime . . . complete castration, with the addition of a brand upon the forehead or cheeks."[51] To the editor of the *Denver Medical Times*, rape was not the only crime which warranted castration. As for anyone who committed an even potentially lethal crime, said the doctor,

> let all such be castrated secundum artem, and the world will soon be better. In this class would come in general burglars and housebreakers, hold-ups, rape-fiends, and last but not least, anarchists.[52]

The concepts of racial improvement and eugenics were very much in vogue in the early twentieth century, and the editor of the *Times* noted that "emasculation is the only certain method of preventing the propagation of criminal breeds." Dr. Arbogast suggested that criminal and other inferior types should not be allowed to breed and that "all professional and confirmed criminals should, before they are liberated [from prison], undergo an operation that would effectively prevent their procreation."[53]

Sometimes people did not wait for the law to mete out justice, and lynchings were an almost routine event on the frontier. The businesslike attitude of one lynching party was described in 1879 by Golden's coroner, Dr. Joseph Anderson.[54] Anderson had been called out to examine the victims of a lynching. One of the mob asked the doctor whether the men were dead. "Yes," said Anderson, "deader than Hell." "All right," said the vigilante, "Hayward is avenged. Good night." Leaving the bodies in the coroner's care, they rode off.

Most of early Colorado's physicians, regardless of how strongly they felt about punishing criminals, were law-and-order men and opposed lynchings. When a Confederate sympathizer in Central City made the mistake of rejoicing at Abraham Lincoln's assassination, a crowd threatened to lynch him.[55] Dr. Worral, assisted by [later Senator] Henry Teller, put his own life on the line and managed to dissuade the mob.

At least some of Colorado's physicians felt that there was a legitimate place in American jurisprudence for the lynch mob. Dr. Thomas Hawkins, the editor of the *Denver Medical Times*,

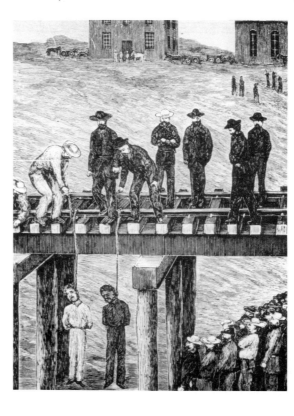

20.5 Coroner Dr. Joseph Anderson confirmed the vigilantes' opinion that the victims of this lynching near Golden were, indeed, dead.

felt that abortionists deserved lynching.[56] In 1900 a young black man was accused of raping and killing a school girl near Limon, Colorado. A week later, "he was seized by the residents of the district and promptly burnt at the stake."[57] In an editorial in the *Times*, Dr. Hawkins supported the lynch mob:

> That the black fiend deserved death no one but a pervert will deny . . . If the chief object of punishment is to deter others . . . then surely this was a shining and fearful warning to evil-doers . . . The summary justice of vigilant committees is to many honest people more satisfactory than the uncertain trickeries of the law's delays.[57]

The following Sunday, a mass meeting was held in a Denver church to protest the lynching. The *Times'* editor reported that "The meeting was conducted by preachers, philanthropists, pettifoggers, and politicians for the benefit of sensationalists."[58] The *Journal of the American Medical Association* took note of this evidence of "mob law in Colorado":

> The proceeding was a disgrace to the age and to the state, and while we can recognize the possibility of a temporary delirium affecting the community, its late condonation [by the Denver Medical Times] has not even this excuse.[59]

Presumably, most of Colorado's doctors agreed.

21 ALTERNATIVE MEDICINE

The majority of the people of these United States are always on the lookout for some one to humbug them. Let some charlatan come along and advertise to tell, for a five dollar note, how to become healthy . . . and the dear humbug-loving public will fall over each other in their mad haste to give the fraud their money.

A. J. Horn, M. D. (Denver), 1898[1]

T HROUGHOUT MOST OF THIS book we have considered medical practice and used the terms "physician" and "doctor" to mean Doctor of Medicine, or M.D. During the nineteenth century, educational standards for the M.D. were raised, licensure requirements were tightened, and medical practice shifted from a theoretical to a scientific basis. Ironically, however, just as "regular" medicine was beginning to make significant progress, a variety of "alternative" forms of medical practice appeared. Some of these, such as homeopathy, were sects within regular medicine, practiced by M.D.s. Most arose outside of the profession, "cults" based on divergent views of health and disease, and practiced by non-M.D.s. Thomsonists depended on botanical remedies, osteopaths and chiropractors relied upon physical manipulation, and Christian Scientists invoked faith and prayer. In addition, all sorts of individuals, ranging from sincere to entrepreneurial to criminal, comprised an army of quacks, charlatans, and "snake oil salesmen." Patent medicines, secret remedies, and nostrums were peddled on streetcorners, advertised in newspapers and magazines, and sold over the counter in drug stores. Itinerant faith healers attracted huge throngs to their healing hands and invocations. Newer "technologies"—electricity, mag-

netism, radiation—were accepted and used by M.D.s and quacks alike.

The M.D.s constantly battled the irregulars and the "alternatives." They pointed with pride to the advances and accomplishments of scientific medicine. It was their sacred duty to protect the public from medical sects and cults, quacks and charlatans. The irregulars and their supporters among the public, the clergy, journalists, and legislators, ascribed different motives to the medical establishment. The doctors simply wanted to suppress competition, they claimed, abrogating the rights of individuals to choose among various forms of health care. The same arguments continue today, periodically focusing on such issues as public health laws, medical licensure requirements, and the eligibility of "alternative" health care providers for payment by governmental agencies and insurance companies.

Homeopathy

Medicine, as practiced by the early nineteenth century M.D. was not only generally ineffective, it was downright unpleasant. Thus, when a New Hampshire farmer named Samuel Thomson introduced a medical system based on botanical remedies, harmless teas, and steam inhalation, it was accepted with gratitude and relief by a populace fed up with being bled, blistered, and purged. Thomsonism gradually faded, but some aspects were incorporated by a few M.D.s into what was called eclectic medicine.

Homeopathy provided a much more challenging and lasting challenge to regular medicine. The creation of a German M.D., Samuel Hahnemann, in the 1790s, homeopathy was based on the concept that "like cures like." Thus fever could be cured by a drug which induced fever if that drug was administered to the patient in diluted, rediluted, and, eventually, infinitesimally small doses. This principle, which sounds so silly today, was, again, a pleasant and harmless alternative to the radical measures of the regulars or, as the homeopaths termed them, "allopaths." Homeopathy became popular among a small but growing number of patients and doctors. Although they were M.D.s, the homeopaths were shunned by the regulars. As the sect prospered, they established their own medical schools, hospitals, journals, and societies. At the height of their success, the homeopaths comprised ten to fifteen percent of the American medical profession.

Sometimes the argument between allopaths and homeopaths grew violent. In 1885, for example, the *Rocky Mountain News* reported on an altercation between two out-of-town physicians in the lobby of Denver's St. James Hotel, one a homeopath, the other a regular.[2] The combatants wound up in Denver's jail. Most of the time, the violence was restricted to the pages of the opposing "schools'" medical journals, which periodically attacked their opposition's most treasured principles and practices. From the *Denver Medical Times*, for example, some comments on Hahnemann's principle of medicinal dilutions:

> The difference between nothing and next-to-nothing is almost nothing; namely, the difference between homeopathic decimal dilutions and no medication at all. [Since] their mode of medication

is of no avail, [they consider that] all medicinal treatment must be useless and might as well be thrown to the dogs; providing, of course, that the society for the prevention of cruelty to animals does not interfere.[3]

The homeopaths, perhaps because they were a small ostracized minority, were more defensive and consistently aggressive. Colorado's homeopathic journal, the *Critique* was filled with attacks on the regulars. Its editor contrasted the "broad, liberal and progressive . . . [homeopaths] reaching out for whatever will aid them in healing the sick . . . ," to

> the allopaths, . . . so bound down by prejudice and sectarianism that they refuse to see good in anything that does not emanate from their own ranks . . . [They] have degenerated into a narrow, bigoted Medical Sect . . .[4]

Another time, the *Critique* pointed out that there had been only one death at the Denver Homeopathic Hospital during the month of August 1903; the same month, there had been twenty-one deaths at the County Hospital, ten at St. Joseph's, five at St. Luke's, and sixteen at St. Anthony's—all allopathic hospitals. The deaths of prominent persons were cited as failures of allopathic medicine:

> Quinine and over-officiousness killed [President] Garfield. Digitalis and over-feeding killed [President] McKinley. Evidently Senator Hanna has followed along the same pathway.[5]

In the late nineteenth century, regular medicine began to make some significant progress, and gradually the foundations of homeopathy began to crumble. Homeopaths ridiculed the germ theory of disease and opposed aseptic technique and public health measures. Appendectomy was regarded, like most surgery, as an unnecessary and dangerous procedure whose sole purpose was the financial gain of allopathic physicians. This opposition to medical progress was summarized by a prominent Denver homeopath in 1899: "It is a matter of supreme satisfaction to be able to say, after the lapse of a century of trial, that homeopathy does not change."[6] Such views, however, were becoming embarrasing to the new generation of homeopathic physicians, many of whom began to envy the scientific and clinical successes of their allopathic colleagues. In Colorado, as in the rest of the country, murmurings were heard in the homeopathic medical school, hospital, and society and a major split developed. Colorado's homeopaths were described as

H. T. F. GATCHELL, M. D.,

{ Homeopathic Physician, }

COLORADO SPRINGS, COL.

Inquiries in Regard to Salubrity of Climate
ANSWERED BY MAIL

21.1 The homeopaths proudly proclaimed their allegiance to their "school" and to Hahnemann's principle of "like cures like."

21.2 Colorado's homeopaths had their own medical society, journals, medical school, and hospital. Denver's Homeopathic Hopital was built in 1898.

engaged in the highly unprofessional pastime of using their professional brethren as targets in a daily gun practice from behind bill boards, from dark alleys, and other unexposed positions of vantage.[7]

Within a few years, and despite a handful of conservative holdouts, Colorado's brand of homeopathy had undergone a revolution. In addition, a rapprochement was developing between the progressive homeopaths and the more liberal regulars. The *Colorado Medical Journal* reported:

> There is rapidly dying out the old spirit of antagonism between these two schools of medicine . . . Both of us have learned that the people want cures, and they don't care through what school they get them . . . Now we find daily consultations between homeopathic and regular physicians . . . It is well the old fight is dying. Good men and fine gentlemen can be found on both sides . . . Let the line fade until there is no longer any.[8]

By 1905 most of Denver's homeopaths had, in de facto fashion at least, accepted most of the principles and practices of regular medicine. A few years later, both the Denver Homeopathic Hospital and the Medical College were closed (1909), and the *Critique* soon followed (1911). In 1925, in his paper on "medical cults," Denver's Dr. Cuthbert Powell reviewed the status of homeopathy:

> Where do they stand today? The so-called homeopathic schools, few of which still survive, teach all branches of medical science. Their graduates practice scientific, rational methods . . . There are today no real homeopaths. The name is still retained by a few stragglers, probably more for sentimental reasons than otherwise.[9]

One reason for the fading of the line between the allopathic and homeopathic M.D.s was the fact that "both schools had so many common enemies that they could not afford to longer quarrel."[10] During the latter part of the nineteenth and well into the twentieth centuries, the M.D.s were faced with a host of challenges from various cults and movements. Dr. Powell divided these into three major categories, "those who cure all diseases by mechanical means . . . osteopaths, chiropracters, etc., . . . those who cure all disease by the exercise of the mind over the body, including mesmerism, spiritualism, Christian Science and the like, and those who manufacture, purvey, and use patent medicines, nostrums, and cures and various electrical, magnetic and radioactive procedures and devices."

Osteopathy

Osteopathy was "discovered" by Andrew T. Still, a country doctor in Baldwin, Missouri. According to a blurb published by the Boulder (Colorado) Osteopathic Infirmary:

> In 1874, Dr. Still, announced to the world his discovery of Osteopathy . . . He first found that he could stop dystentery by manual treatment of the spine . . . One discovery led to another and, by a careful study of anatomy, using the skeleton and the natural body as his text-books, he gradually developed, in spite of calumny and opposition, a system of curing diseases . . . [His] efforts met with such marked success, [that there are now] nearly a dozen new schools, . . . dozens of periodicals, scientific and popular, . . . and over 2,000 graduates practicing in every state and territory . . .[11]

The article provides us with an osteopath's view of "the new science." The premise of osteopathy was that

> all the functions of the body depend . . . on absolute freedom of blood-circulation and nerve-action. The nerves and blood vessels are found to suffer mechanical obstruction along the spine . . . through slight displacements of bony parts, ligaments or tendons, etc., so that blood vessels are compressed and pressure on nerves perverts their action. Disease is the natural result.[11]

The role of the osteopath was to search for these causes of disease and to "remove the obstruction by means of skillful and delicate manipulation of the parts . . . Nature does the rest." The article pointed out that osteopathic treatment was not "rubbing, kneading, tapping or shaking," and that there was no "indelicacy in examination or treatment:"

> Osteopathy treats all diseases . . . It cures any curable disease and many heretofore regarded as incurable, such as exophthalmic goiter, paralysis agitans, locomotor ataxia, etc.. Because the bodily parts are set right, just as any other delicate machine is adjusted and set to running by a skillful machinist. The patient is cured to stay cured.[11]

Colorado's regular physicians did not agree. Dr. George Stover, in considering this "fool system," presented some examples of alleged osteopathic errors which he had encountered in his northern Colorado practice.[12] Miss M.S. of Fort Collins, for example, had received manipulative treatment for what an osteopath had diagnosed as a dislocated hip; she turned out to have "tuberculosis of the hip-joint." Another was a boy who was treated for a dislocated twelfth rib; he, it turned out, had appendicitis.

The Morgan County Medical Society voted to censure any physician who cooperated with osteopaths.[13] The *Colorado Medical Journal* published an article by a professional masseuse which denounced osteopathic manipulation as "the lowest grade of unskilled massage . . . oftentimes of so violent a character that the poor victim is left permanently injured."[14] The *Denver Medical Times* ridiculed the announcement of the opening of Denver's Western Institute of Osteopathy, which, it pointed out, was to be run by a couple named Bolles:[15]

21.3 The *Denver Medical Times* noted that the Western (later the Bolles) Institute of Osteopathy was run by Mr. and Mrs. Bolles.

The Bolles Institute of Osteopathy

Removed to

1457-59 Ogden Street,

Near Colfax Avenue.

May 1st, 1901.

So far as the bulletin shows, there are only two persons in this faculty, Mr. and Mrs. Bolles. It is to be presumed that what Pa Bolles don't know . . . , Ma Bolles does . . . The tuition fee for the course, which is payable strictly in advance, is $500![15]

By 1925 Powell reported that osteopathy no longer limited its therapy to the "physical correction of structural maladjustments" and predicted that "within a few years it will have ceased to exist . . . its followers, like those of Hahnemann having entered the ranks" of regular medicine.[16]

Chiropractic

In his 1925 article, Dr. Powell noted that "with the passing of osteopathy as a distinct therapeutic cult there has arisen another 'adjustment fake' "—chiropractic:

21.4 An M.D.'s view of chiropractic treatment.

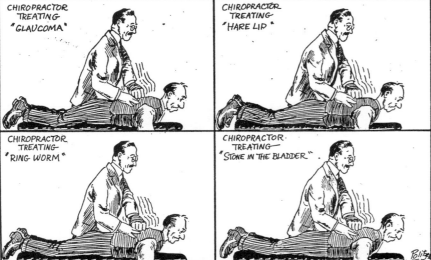

I would really prefer to ignore this new and blatant cult. But by reason of the arrogant position it has assumed and its noxious advertisements, tending to beguile the unsuspecting and gullible public, I may not pass it by unnoticed . . . The chiropractic cult is in no sense of the word a healing cult. It is a business organization.[17]

Chiropractic was the creation of Daniel D. Palmer, a onetime "magnetic healer" in Davenport, Iowa. In 1895, Palmer reported that he had restored the hearing of a deaf man by manipulating his spine and proposed that nearly all of human disease was due to "subluxated vertebrae." This approach evolved into what became known as chiropractic, later defined by the Colorado Chiropractic College as "the science of curing human ailments by locating and relieving impinged nerves."[18] Powell summarized his impressions of chiropractic and its founder:

This ignorant faker, taking advantage of the fact that the human mind, when oppressed by disease or tormented by suffering, is most willing to accept any promise of relief, evolves a pseudo-scientific and fraudulent system of healing, which he foists upon the credible . . .[18]

A more literary view of chiropractic was provided by the *Denver Medical Bulletin* in 1922:

Let's now regard that clever crook,
The wily "Chiroquack."
His Metier is a knowing look,
His Playground's on the back.
He listens with enraptured ear
As every roving spine
Snaps bolt upright in trembling fear,
And then clicks back in line.[19]

Christian Science

Although "cults" such as osteopathy and chiropractic challenged regular medicine, they were, at least, based on the premise of a physical basis for organic disease. The religious cults, on the other hand, regarded disease as a spiritual problem, and their therapeutic approaches were correspondingly spiritual. Although there had always been something of a territorial dispute between the doctors and the clergy, the boundaries were fairly well defined, at least among the established Christian churches and the regular medical profession. From time immemorial, faith healers and even whole movements had come and gone, often after meeting the combined opposition of establishment clergy and physicians.

In the 1870s, regular medicine encountered a new challenge in the form of Christian Science. Founded by Mary Baker Eddy, some of its medically related principles were described by a Colorado spokesman, Mr. E. W. Palmer:

> To a Christian Scientist, it is not logical or conceivable that God . . . created disease, and since he did not create it, it has no real existence but is merely a false conception manifested by the body. Christian Science [looks] to God alone and discards all material aids. Through prayer, the cause and thus the effect [or disease] disappears.[20]

Christian Science proclaimed that it was a "religion and not a system of medicine" and provided healers and "nurses" to pray for those afflicted with the "unrealities" of illness. Like the doctor, the lawyer, and the minister, the "Christian Scientist who gives time and talent . . ." was expected to receive "a small return for his services."[20] Since those services were in the form of prayer (Christian Science taught that such measures as drugs, vaccination, and surgery were useless), it was felt that their efforts should not come under any laws regulating the practice of medicine.

Physicians were angered and frustrated by a group which, on the one hand, denied virtually every fundamental concept and practice of medicine while continuing, not only to survive, but to thrive. The feelings of Colorado's turn-of-the-century physicians were frequently and unequivocally expressed in their medical journals:

> The doctrine of Christian Science is based entirely on an hypothesis which is unreasonable, absurd, and incapable of proof . . . She [Mrs. Eddy] asserts that all so-called diseases are the products of a mind out of joint and that they are all curable by the same means, viz, a little prayer or incantation by a silly woman or a few beatitudes by a sillier patient. The Scientist prays for revenue, while the patient prays for the amusement.

> Christian Science is a good thing for hysteria, but falls down on syphilis. It might help the patient to overcome mild self-limited diseases, but couldn't kill a gonococcus in a thousand years . . . Their cures consist in their ability to make a person believe they are cured.[21]

In a series of alliterative allusions, Dr. H. G. Wetherill referred to the

> material multifariousness of Mother Eddy's misanthropy and her maudlin meandering through meaningless metaphorical monographs on mentality . . . mendacious and monstrous in its monkeying with modern methods of malversation or mental manipulation . . . Money by the millions may methinks be milked from the multitude by Milady's methods.[22]

Colorado's homeopaths and allopaths found themselves united on the issue of Christian Sci-

ence, and their medical journals periodically, and with evident satisfaction, reported instances of the sect's followers turning to medical doctors for help. Even the episode of Mrs. Tweedy and her cow was reported.[23] It seems that Mrs. Tweedy, a resident of Denver, had called on a Christian Science healer to pray for her sick cow. The cow did not improve and Mrs. Tweedy was arrested and fined $100 for "handling the animal in a cruel and inhuman manner." In response, a Christian Science spokeman presented a detailed account of the episode, repeated the tenets of his faith, and asked, "Why should it become a crime to pray for the recovery of a pet cow . . .?"

The issue of greatest concern to physicians, however, was the care, not of free-thinking adults or of animals, but of the children of Christian Scientist parents:

> Their innocent offspring must suffer for the silliness and parsimony of the parents, because, being mute infants, they cannot speak their distress. Many a child has gone to its death because of Christian Science, the modern Moloch of deceitful neglect . . .[24]

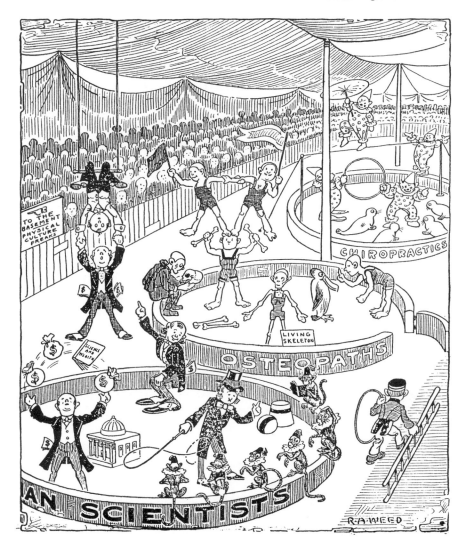

21.5 To the regular physician, chiropractors, osteopaths, and Christian Scientists presented a not-so-entertaining three-ring circus.

Dr. Frank Waxham, whose introduction of endotracheal intubation had saved many
diphtheritic children, vented his anger and frustration. He had been called to see a ten year old
boy with diphtheria who was being "treated"
by Christian Scientists. The Denver doctor described the scene:

> How he fights and struggles for breath. How he
> tosses about the bed and clutches his throat as
> though to tear it open in his great agony and effort
> to breathe . . . The boy is surely and slowly being
> choked to death, and still he is being treated by
> Christian Science. We respond quickly to the hurry
> call, but the boy is now beyond all medical aid
> . . . Christian Science has done its work.[25]

Another disturbance to medical equanimity was
the tendency of Christian Scientists to ignore
public health measures. In the 1920s, the *Denver
Medical Bulletin*, in reporting a severe outbreak
of measles in Denver, commented:

> A certain Park Hill family of Christian Science
> tendencies allowed three children with a rash, sore
> eyes and running noses the freedom of the neigh-
> borhood with the inevitable result. Why is it
> against the law for me to kindle a bonfire in my
> own lot next to my neighbor's house, while such
> cases as these go unpunished and almost un-
> noticed?[26]

Patent Medicines and Secret Nostrums

In addition to "mechano-therapeutic," religious, and other "alternative" approaches to medical care, physicians had to deal with a vast
number of so-called medicines which were being
pushed, advertised, and hailed by everyone from
circus touts to large chemical companies and
manufacturers. Newspapers and magazines received huge amounts of advertising dollars from
the purveyors of all sorts of "patent" (i.e.
patented, over-the-counter) medicines, nostrums (i.e. secret remedies), and the like. Typical of such advertisements was one for Cloud's
Invigorating Cordial and Blood Renewer. The
full page ad, placed in the 1872 *Handbook of Colorado* by its Denver agent, druggist (and later,
prominent business and civic leader), W. S.
Cheesman, described this patent medicine as "a
combination regulated for invalids and convalescents [which] promptly assists to perfect
health."[27] It was, indeed, quite a combination—including blood root (for the liver), man-
drake (for the bowels), wild cherry (for the
stomach and lungs), wild potato (for the kidneys
and bladder), and a mysterious ingredient called
"GOLDEN SEAL" (for "mucous surfaces").

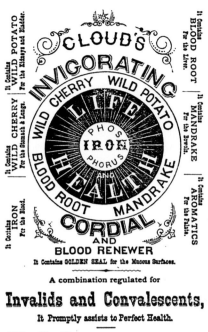

21.6 W. S. Cheesman's pharmacy advertised the benefits of Cloud's Invigorating Cordial and Blood Renewer promi-nently in the 1872 *Handbook of Colorado.*

There were hundreds, and perhaps thousands,
of such concoctions, and their claims filled the
advertising pages of Colorado's newspapers.
From the *Golden City Transcript* of 1875:

> Winter has commenced. Cough, cough, cough is
> the order of the day. All that is needed to cure the
> husky throats and restore sore lungs to health and
> soundness is Hale's Honey of Hore-hound and
> Tar.[28]

From the *Aspen Daily Times* of 1893, an advertisement which included the following testimonial:

> My children insist on having Dr. Gunn's Onion
> Syrup . . . It is without the taste or smell of onions.
> Sold for 50 cents by A.S. Lamb, The Druggist.[29]

From the *Rocky Mountain News* of 1895:

> Animal Extracts: Cerebrine, from the brain;
> Medulline, from the spinal cord; Cardine, from
> the heart; Testine, . . . Ovarine, . . . Thyroidine,
> . . . etc., all sold by the Scholtz Drug Company of
> Denver.[30]

It should be noted that advertising for such
"wonder drugs" was not limited to non-medical
publications. The *Colorado Medical Journal*, for
example, carried ads for Arsenauro:

> "Well, Well, Well!!! No Wonder My Diabetic Pa-
> tient Is No Better—This is *Not* Arsenauro, It is a
> *Fraud* . . . 109 Cases of Diabetes Mellitus Cured.[31]

Some patent medicines and secret nostrums
were Colorado products. Radio-Sulpho, for
example, was manufactured in Denver and was
widely advertised:

Dissolves and absorbs all poisons from the Human system. It is a powerful germicide, antiseptic and pore cleaner. Principally used for uric acid, urinemia, poisons, rheumatism, swellings, blood poisons, cancers, etc. Is successful in the hands of anybody, when directions are followed.[32]

A bottle of Radio-Sulpho cost one dollar. The *Denver Medical Times* reported that the "remedy," which was to be used both internally and externally, consisted mainly "of an aqueous solution of sodium sulphide . . . a substance having no recognition in medicine, but employed in tanneries for removing the hair from hides."[33]

Iodium, another local product, was said to have been the result of "the life study" of Dr. J. B. Blanchard of Denver. Dr. Blanchard's advertisement asked:

Do you cough? Are you weak and spiritless? Do you have catarrh? Do you have night sweats? . . . Take no risks. Consumption may have marked you for its own. Send your name to Dr. Blanchard and learn how Iodium will cure you . . . Consumption is not a disease to dally with . . .[34]

Perhaps the most famous of Colorado's remedies was Marach, better known as Denver Mud. Useful in "all cases of inflammation and congestion," Denver Mud was marketed nationally, and available in containers ranging from "small," at twenty-five cents, to the large five pound package at $2.25. Denver Mud contained powdered silicate of aluminum, glycerin, resorcin, boracic acid, and peppermint, wintergreen, and eucalyptus oils.[35]

Physicians were constantly bombarded by letters, circulars, and pamphlets urging them to try various products. The papers of Dr. W. E. Driscoll, a physician in Goldfield, a mining camp in the Cripple Creek District, include many such mailings. The manufacturers of tonics, "tissue builders," digestive aids, and nutritional concentrates were especially aggressive. Dr. Driscoll, for example, received a promotional letter, informational booklet, and sample of Pronuclein Special Tablets, a product which, it was claimed, would "build up the cells and thus increase the physiological resistance of the body . . ."[36] The same company offered a long list of similar agents, including Peptenzyme, Zymocide, Lacto Preparata, Pancrobiln, Analeptine, and Kumsysgen. Some products, although they many have had some medicinal value, were promoted with the same unbridled enthusiasm as the most blatant quack remedies. Dr. Driscoll's mail included a sample of Hagee's Cordial of Cod Liver Oil. The accompanying letter claimed that the cordial "is an ideal tonic, stimulant, alterative, reconstructive, nutritive and digestive . . . and is of utmost value in the treatment of phthisis, scrofula, chronic pectoral complaints, coughs, colds, brain exhaustion, nervous debility, palsy, chronic cutaneous eruptions, and impaired digestion."[36]

The highest mark of success was attained when the promoter of a remedy obtained the endorsement of reputable physicians. Something of a scandal occurred when a Dr. Dunn, a "well-known quack of Denver" and the promotor of something called "Dunn's Uterine

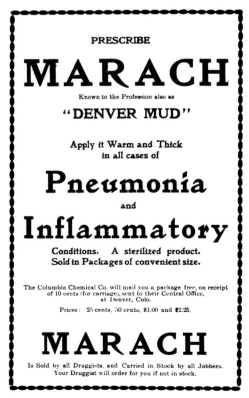

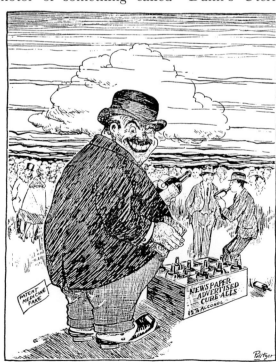

S-A-A-Y, BARNUM WAS RIGHT!

21.7 Famed Denver Mud could be purchased in five-pound containers.

21.8 A typical patent medicine salesman—as viewed by an M.D. He was also referred to as "snake oil salesman."

Evacuant—the ideal uterine cleaner," advertised his product in Denver's newspapers.[37] Among his clients, he listed Drs. F. M. Smith of Holyoke, B. F. Haskins of La Junta, D. S. Hoffman of Lake City, W. O. Patterson of Pueblo, and D. W. Clark of Del Norte, Colorado. The advertisement was reported by the state medical society's journal, and this was followed by letters from each of the physicians cited, emphatically denying that they had provided any such endorsement. The doctor from Holyoke, in fact, emphasized that "I have never given permission for my name to be used in connection with any medicine, nor have I ever given a testimonial, nor do I ever expect to."

Magnetism, Electricity, and Radiation

Magnetic therapy was introduced by an Austrian physician, Franz Mesmer, in 1774. According to Mesmer, illness, and especially nervous diseases, were due to the maldistribution of a magnetic fluid which flowed through the body. Medical therapy required the redistribution of the body's magnetic forces through the use of magnets and other measures. Mesmer's theories were introduced to the United States in the 1830s and were utilized by a number of so-called "magnetic healers."

In the late nineteenth century, magnetism was supplemented and largely replaced by another mysterious physical "force." Electricity's medical potentials were hailed, not only by quacks, but by reputable physicians. In 1893 the *Denver Medical Times* noted:

> Not only in mechanics, but in the healing arts as well are the miracles of the chained thunderbolt made manifest . . . Clinical experience bears out

all the claims which scientific operators make for electricity. In neurology, for paralysis, atrophies, dystrophies, neuralgias, and hysteria; in surgery, for cauterization and chronic joints disease; in gynecology, for dysmenorrhea, ovarian neuralgia and uterine hyperplasia; in dermatology, for psoriasis, herpes, pemphigus, prurigo, alopecia . . . in general medicine, for constipation, indigestion, diabetes and muscular rheumatism . . .[38]

The medical use of Faradism, Galvanism, electromagnetism, and other "-isms" became very popular. Physicians rushed to buy all sorts of sparkling, crackling, and electro-shocking machines for their offices, some costing several hundred dollars. Nor was the use of electricity limited to Denver and its specialists. In Cripple Creek, for example, Dr. V. R. Pennock, presented a detailed paper on the use of "electricity in general practice" to his colleagues.[39] Within a few years, however, the therapeutic promises of electricity had not materialized. In 1905 Dr. Stover reported:

> I still hear occasionally some physician say that he has, or will get, an electric machine . . . [because] he believes that such an apparatus will impress patients . . . This man will later be heard stating that 'there is nothing to electricity; he has tried it and it didn't do any good.'[40]

Indeed, *Colorado Medicine* complained, some physicians were using electricity inappropriately.[41] A Denver doctor, for example, whose "window reads, 'Nose, Throat, and Electricity' " was treating an entire family with the "miraculous, life-giving rays"—the father for apoplexy, the mother for nervous prostration, and the daughter for dysmenorrhea and acne. "Great is electricity," commented the journal, "and great is the specialist who can make grist of every case that comes to his mill."

Non-physician quacks were not far behind. Many of them favored the use of electric and electromagnetic belts which were worn around the waist, neck, head, ankle, wrist, or other parts of the anatomy. A particularly "flaring" newspaper advertisement for electrotherapy was cited by the *Colorado Medical Journal*:

> The claim is made that electricity is nerve and vital force. When that is lost all is lost, and can only be replaced by wearing copious chunks of electricity buckled to some part of the body. The nerve and vital force, in the form of electric fluid, is made to course up and down a man's back-bone like a cloud-burst in a mountain stream. After a certain amount of fluid is absorbed by the spinal canal the patient is promised complete restoration

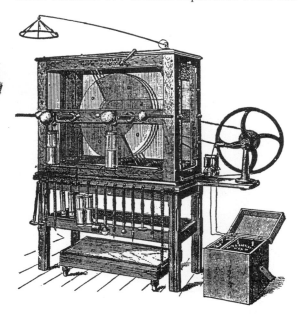

21.9 All sorts of electrical devices were advertised in the standard medical catalogues. They ranged from small and inexpensive to huge apparatuses capable of generating enormous charges. As electricity's therapeutic ineffectiveness became apparent, it was gradually discarded by most physicians—only to be adopted by the medical quacks.

to health. The enumeration of diseases subject to cure by this process is enough to set the cast-iron stomach of a successful Klondike miner.[42]

Electric belts were especially promoted for such disorders as "lost manhood, sexual weakness, spermatorrhea, undeveloped parts, and last of all, et cetera."[42] The patient of one doctor, after reading such advertisements for electric belts, became convinced that he had lost his manhood, and "when seen, was on the border of a driveling idiocy."[42] The "Common Sense" electric belt was advertised as curing paralysis, dyspepsia, fever and ague, seminal weakness, female complaints, malaria, liver complaint and kidney diseases; it cost between three and five dollars.[43]

In the early 1900s, many physicians were entranced by the therapeutic potentials of radiation, and especially the newly discovered element, radium (Chapter 13). One Denver physician, for example, claimed that he had seen "cancers that you would have pronounced hopeless cured in three weeks" of radium therapy.[44] As the limitations, as well as the dangers, of radium therapy became apparent, responsible physicians became concerned about "the exaggerated reputation of radium as a cure for cancer." They also called attention to the fact that "the amazing metal . . . offers strong inducements to quackery and deception."[45] Indeed, as physicians began to limit their use of radium, the quacks began to take their place. One Denver surgeon referred to the latter group as "men, drunk with cupidity, [who are] worse than the locust pest."[46]

Such admonitions did not bother Tom Curran, a radium prospector who had struck it rich on Colorado's western slope and had taken up residence in Denver's elegant Brown Palace Hotel.[47] Not about to retire on his mining income, and presumably believing in the curative powers of radium, Old Tom peddled tiny bottles of powdered radium ore, carnotite, from his hotel room at two bits a bottle. To obtain a maximum dose of radiation, the purchaser was advised to keep the bottle under his pillow at night. Denver's Radium Water Company was a much more ambitious enterprise. Radium "charged" water was prepared by washing the ore and bottling the rinse for use as a medicinal drink, surgical wash, or other salutory purposes. Prepared by Mr. Ben J. Kister, "naturalist and chemist," Kister's Water advertised:

> Surgeons and Physicians should use it in all their Operations. Destroys all Germ Life. Builds up Live, Healthy Tissue. Nothing finer for Burns and Scalds. Can be applied to and injected into the

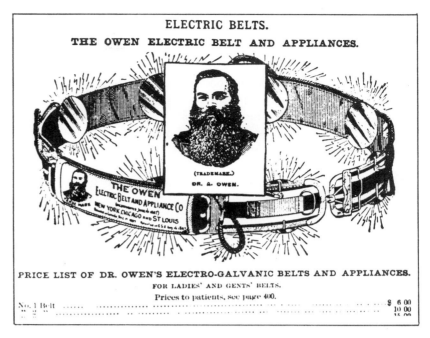

PRICE LIST OF DR. OWEN'S ELECTRO-GALVANIC BELTS AND APPLIANCES.
FOR LADIES' AND GENTS' BELTS.
Prices to patients, see page 400.

No. 1 Belt .... $ 6 00
.... 10 00

most delicate parts of the body . . . Heals all Diseases.[48]

A two gallon jug of Kister's Radium Charged Water cost three dollars. The amount of radiation in this and similar preparations was, fortunately, probably quite small.

21.10 Magnetic, electrical, and electromagnetic belts were popular in the late nineteenth century, especially in the treatment of "manhood" problems.

Quacks, Charlatans, and Mountebanks

The term "quack" was defined by Pueblo's Dr. Will Davis as "a pretender of medical or surgical knowledge and skill not possessed."[49] Although he noted fine distinctions between the quack and the medical charlatan and mountebank, and that the words were frequently used synonymously, Davis pointed out that the term "quack" could be applied to "any and all kinds of medical pretenders, from whatever part of the broad territory of quackdom they may hail . . ."

In an earlier essay on "Charlatanism in Colorado," pioneer physician Jesse Hawes described some of the quacks he had encountered in Colorado's early days.[50] One was "an oily, plausible, soft-handed man who, in his whole life, had never given a month's study to the action of drugs." In his ignorance, said Dr. Hawes, the

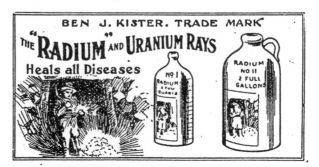

21.11 One of Colorado's promotional pamphlets hailed it as "The Radium State."

quack had prescribed a large dose of morphine for a newborn baby. The baby died; nevertheless, the quack received his two dollar fee. Another was an "unlettered butcher" from the midwest. He had bought a "little book of medical receipts [prescriptions], a silk hat, a fashionable suit, joined the Pike's Peak army . . . " and arrived at a mining camp on Clear Creek. Here he set up his practice. One day, he "plunged a bistoury [a surgical cutting instrument] into an inguinal hernia with deadly effect," the patient presumably dying of peritonitis. In those pre-licensing days, neither "doctor" was subject to legal action. Furthermore, the first doctor had received, not only his fee, but a "kindly, 'Good morning, Doctor'," from the grieving but still grateful parents. "The chronicles of charlatanism are an amusing study for the curious," Dr. Hawes noted in his plea for more restrictive licensing laws. But, he added, the most remarkable aspect is that "toward charlatanism the attitude of the public is an enigma." Colorado's physicians and medical societies continued to fight the quacks over the years, but an indifferent and gullible public, frightened legislators, liberal press, and vested interests continued to make the Centennial State a haven for all sorts of Dr. Hawes's charlatans.

Some were M.D.s. Dr. J. Flatterty advertised in the *Denver Tribune* that he could provide "immediate and scientific medical relief and cure of Diseases of a Special, General, Chronic, Sexual or Difficult character."[51] These included

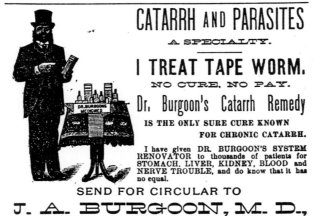

21.13 Quacks and charlatans unabashedly hawked their wares and services wherever they could buy advertising space.

Cases of Secrecy and Impure and Poisoned Blood, Sore Throat, Eyes, Ears and Other Disorders, Self Abuse and Indiscretion, Seminal Weakness, Loss of Vigor, Low Spirits, Pimples and Blotches, Pain in the Head and Back, Dull Expression and Symptoms leading to Insanity, Female Troubles, Irregularities and Sufferings.[51]

The patient was instructed to come to Flattery's office on Lawrence Street or, if he preferred, to "tell your troubles by letter. Medicines will be fowarded free from observation with plain directions to guarantee a cure at home." Dr. Flattery's armamentarium included "certain Harveyan Nerve and and Blood Remedies."

Dr. Flattery was not a member of the State Medical Society. Dr. H. W. Allen was, however, and when he ran a number of advertisements in the Boulder newspapers for such "quack remedies" as Allen's Magic Relief, Allen's Worm Lozenges, Allen's Concentrated Essence of Jamaica Ginger, and Allen's Little Giant Liver Pills, he was expelled from the society.[52]

For every M.D. who engaged in such activities there must have been a hundred non-M.D. providers of "alternative" medicine. Some called themselves "Doctor." The editor of *Colorado Medicine*, deploring the "abuse of the title," commented that " the dignity of anyone who owns a Faradic battery, a bath cabinet, or who massages folks is very much offended if one neglects to address him as 'doctor'."[53]

Schlatter, The Healer

The most famous of Denver's faith healers was Schlatter, "The Healer."[54] Francis Schlatter was born to German parents in Alsace-Lorraine in 1856. Having emigrated to the United States, he was working as a shoemaker in downtown Denver when, at the age of thirty-five, "he received his first spiritual communication." Soon after, he was told to close his business and go out to heal the sick. He went as far as Hot Springs, Arkansas, where, "in bare head and bare feet, begrimed with dust, and presenting the appearance of a demented person," he was arrested, judged insane, and imprisoned for nearly six months. Released, he headed west, and after wandering about, began his healing career. In New Mexico, he healed hundreds and, in August 1895, now known as the "New Mexico Messiah," he returned to Denver. He set up his headquarters in North Denver, and within a short time, huge numbers of Coloradans were coming to receive his therapeutic blessings.

Schlatter presented a striking appearance—tall and ascetic, blue eyes and a delicate mouth, long flowing dark hair parted in the middle, and a full dark beard—all, according to a promotional pamphlet, giving him a "striking resemblance to the likeness of our Savior." Each day, the same scene was repeated in front of his house. Kept in order by specially constructed railings, the line of supplicants extended, several abreast, for many blocks. Some had stood in place since the preceding evening. At the head of the line was a crowd of onlookers. Some came bearing the handkerchiefs of those too ill to come themselves (handkerchiefs blessed by the healer were said to be as effective as direct contact). Promptly at 9 A.M. the Healer appeared:

> Slowly the line files past him, the treatment lasting from one to three minutes [and up to thirty minutes in severe cases] . . . All are treated alike, but the effect is different. With some the contact with his hand is like a shock of electricity, causing the patient to writhe and groan in agony, while with others it is imperceptible.[54]

The atmosphere was compared to a "country fair," with tents, lunch stands, and great masses of humanity. In the afternoon, Schlatter attended those who remained in their carriages, returning to his house to answer some of the 1,500 letters which were arriving daily. Many "cures" were cited: Miss Maud Ward of Longmont had had her vision restored, Mr. D. M. Powers of Georgetown had been cured of rheumatism, and Mr. William Roach of Globeville was no longer paralyzed and threw away his crutches.

The *Denver Times* described Schlatter as "a man with great personal magnetism, clear head,

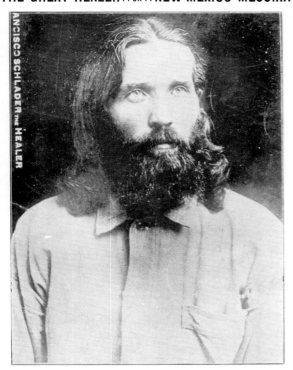

. . . LIFE OF . . .
FRANCIS SCHLATTER
THE GREAT HEALER . . OR . . NEW MEXICO MESSIAH

PUBLISHED BY THE KNOX CO., ROOM 606 COOPER BLDG., DENVER, COLO.
MAILED TO ANY ADDRESS ON RECEIPT OF 25 CENTS

Copyright applied for by The Knox Co.

strong mental individuality, and a great degree of native shrewdness and knowledge of human nature."[55] To a professor at the University of Denver, Schlatter appeared "idiotic," while to others he was "saintly, transcendent, seraphic."[56] Although a promotional pamphlet said that he would accept no money, one Denver resident recalled that as a boy, his father had asked him to take several handkerchiefs to Schlatter for his blessing, and that people left a quarter with the Healer as a "gift."[57] The view of the medical profession was succinct—this "religious fanatic" had undoubtedly "created quite a sensation in Denver" and Schlatter was "either insane or a humbug."[58] The *Denver Medical Times* had no evidence that he had "made any money out of this business," but "there is no question in our mind—and we took some little pains to investigate—that there were others back of Schlatter."[58] At any rate, threatened with arrest, Schlatter suddenly disappeared. Years later he was reported to have died in an insane asylum.

Cancer and Other Cures

Certain diseases were "favorites" of the quacks. In Colorado, in particular, there were innumerable charlatans ready to treat asthma and tuberculosis. Other favorites were the venereal and various skin diseases. Female "problems" were treated by such bizarre procedures as "colpo-hysterectomy, colpo-hysteropexy, and colparrhaphy."[59] Non-surgical "cures" for inguinal hernia were widely advertised. "Professor" O. E. Miller, for example, ran full page advertisements for his "twelve room . . . handsomely appointed offices" in Denver's Tabor Opera House Block where, he claimed, he had "cured 1,000 men, women and children" without the use of "knife or syringe."[60]

The biggest, and perhaps the cruelest, hoaxes were the cancer cures. One Denver man with carcinoma of the tongue was told by a "cancer doctor" that he could be cured and that the treatment would require no surgery and would cost only thirty dollars. Three months and five hundred dollars later, the victim came to a physician in a terminal state.[61] A Denver doctor listed some of the quack methods of curing cancer—arsenic, locally injected acids (called "lymph" or "serum" in the scientific parlance of the age), and various "vesicants and escorotic salves and ointments." The latter, because of their inflammatory and necrotizing effects, deceptively appeared to destroy a cancer. The manufacturer of Denver's Radio-Sulpho Brew (a mixture of epsom salts, alcohol, rhubarb, and

21.14 Schlatter the Healer, pictured on one of his promotional pamphlets.

boneset) advocated its use, combined with poultices of cheese and glycerin, to treat cancer.[62]

Fads, Enterprises, and Institutes

Over the years, innumerable health fads have appeared on the medical scene, some of them recurring in almost predictable and cyclic fashion. One particularly bizarre food fad was reported by the *Rocky Mountain News* in 1875.[63] While visiting a slaughterhouse in Denver, the reporter encountered no less than "six refined and spiritual looking ladies drinking, without any apparent disrelish, the blood that five minutes before, had been palpitating in the veins of a bovine." The reporter inquired as to their unusal lunch habits. The ladies responded that drinking blood "was beneficial in cases of consumption and dyspepsia . . . toned the system up so that all natural functions were performed better, and . . . improved the complexion."

Countless health fads and "movements" continued to appear, disappear, and reappear. Some were based on the public's fascination with non-Western systems of medicine. In many areas of the country, American Indian remedies (in most cases, actually the concoctions of Anglo entrepreneurs) were touted as "natural" ways to maintain or restore health. In Colorado, fascination with the mysteries of the Orient led to the highly successful Gun Wa scam of the late 1880s. Gun Wa was advertised as a "great Chinese physician" who had recently arrived in Denver. Dressed in "full oriental costume, and occupying gorgeously furnished" offices, he was "heralded through the press . . . and [soon] his spacious waiting rooms were filled to overflowing . . ."[64] During the more than two years of Gun Wa's professional life, it was said that his daily office receipts were in the thousands. According to Denver's newspapers, one physician recalled, "you would be led to believe that a demi-god had come to earth, and that all that was necessary to banish disease was to consult this great physician."[65] Gun Wa's treatments were, indeed, unorthodox. In response to one woman's complaints, the Chinese "doctor" recommended daily baths in a mixture of alcohol and turpentine; only later did she discover that she had actually been pregnant.[66] Other Gun Wa remedies, one Denver doctor asserted, were so "loathesome" that "If some of Gun Wa's refined patrons . . . knew their contents . . . , how their delicate stomachs would heave at the very thought of it!"[66] The Gun Wa enterprise was said to be the creation of

21.15 The Keeley Institute was one of many "institutes" which offered cures for drug addiction, alcoholism, and other habits. Its patented, secret gold cure was available at its institutes in Denver, Colorado Springs, Durango, and Aspen.

the owner and manager of a gambling house in Pueblo, Colorado. He had in his employ, in the capacity of general scrubber and spittoon cleaner, a Chinese coolie . . . whom he had dressed up and advertised as the celebrated Chinese doctor, Gun Wa.[67]

The scam was so successful that is was said that, while one "Gun Wa" was kept in Denver, others were installed in Omaha, Dallas, Salt Lake City, and San Francisco. This interstate activity ultimately led to the intervention of federal authorities and the demise of the Gun Wa enterprise.[68]

Less colorful, but equally enterprising, were some of the "medical institutes." In the 1880s, Dr. Leslie E. Keeley came to Tin Cup, Colorado, in search of gold.[69] Finding none, he moved to Colorado Springs and struck pay dirt with his secret "Double Chloride of Gold Remedies" for opium addiction and alcoholism.[70] Through use of the remedy and hospitalization at one of the Keeley Institutes, it was claimed that "hundreds of individuals have been been reclaimed from drunkeness and the opium habit . . ." A number of clergymen supported the Keeley cure, and Colorado's legislature, never known for excessive generosity in the support of medical care, came dangerously close to subsidizing the Keeley Institutes. There were four in Colorado:

A RATIONAL AND SCIENTIFIC TREATMENT

—FOR THE—

Liquor, Opium and Tobacco Habits,

—USING A—

SPECIFIC REMEDY

By which the Poison is eliminated from the body and the Nervous System is restored to its

NORMAL CONDITION

so that there is no longer any necessity for

ALCOHOL OR DRUGS.

We have ample facilities for the treatment and care of male and female patients. Physicians sending cases to us may know that we will give them every possible care and when desired will mail a report of progress every week. Send for circulars.

The Keeley Institute,

at Colorado Springs, Aspen, Durango and Denver. Organized as franchises, these were not small-time operations. The mayor and his wife ran the Colorado Springs Institute, and its board of directors included some of the city's most prominent citizens.[71] Durango's Keeley Institute was described as having been furnished

> . . . comfortably and luxuriously. The floors are carpeted with rich stuffs, the furniture is elegant, [and] the walls are lined with pictures of artistic merit.[72]

"Antis"

We have already discussed early Colorado's doctors' battles with the press, politicians and governors, clergy, and with some of the "antis"—such as those who opposed vaccination and various public health measures. Another group of "antis" fought against the use of animals for medical experimentation. In 1897 the *Rocky Mountain News*, under the banner headline, "Doctors Hard Hit," ran an anti-vivisectionist communication.[73] This was part of a national campaign to prohibit the use of experimental animals. Colorado's doctors fought the "sentimental crankism" and "hysterical influence" of the anti-vivisectionists. The *Denver Medical Times* asked of "these humane and tender-hearted creatures who every now and then raise such a hue and cry about the horrors of vivisection . . .":

> Who . . . is the greater philanthropist, he who seeks to protect some insignificant animals from the so-called cruelty of the vivisectionist, or he who blesses his fellow men by discovering some further means of bringing health and comfort to the sick and suffering?[74]

The most dangerous of the anti-medicine groups appeared in 1910, when many of the enemies of regular medicine combined to form the League for Medical Freedom. That year, the Colorado branch of the league held an organizational meeting at Denver's Albany Hotel. The *Denver Medical Times* described the proceedings, at which there were some fifty people, including Christian Scientists, osteopaths, homeopaths, and a few "all-round fakers":

> The chief orator of the evening was the redoubtable J. Cook, Jr., who, if we are rightly informed, was wont to dispense various kinds of 'dope' on the street corners for a consideration, and with the aid of a ventriloquist. He affirmed that he didn't wish to say anything harsh, but he was satisfied that three-fourths of all the deaths in Denver were due to the doctors.[75]

According to *Colorado Medicine*, the league's purpose was to "discredit the regular medical profession in the eyes of the public."[76] Apparently the league was well financed, receiving "its financial support from the patent and proprietary medicine interests" and "its moral support from the various healing cults . . ." In addition, said *Colorado Medicine*, it received the cooperation of "certain unscrupulous newspapers" who appreciated their extensive advertising.[77] In summary, the doctors viewed the league as an "unholy alliance made up of medico-religious fanatics, quacks and crooks of irregular pathies, and advertising patent medicine fakirs . . ."

Colorado Medicine cited a typical member of the league, Mr. M.D.P., the treasurer of its Pueblo branch.[78] Mr. P. was known for his anti-vivisectionist speeches and had run afoul of the law when some overzealous members of his organization pasted posters proclaiming "Refuse and Resist," the anti-vaccination slogan, on mailboxes. He had boasted, "I am in the fight for medical liberty to the finish, and will force the enemy out of his last trench, and fifty feet beyond." Mr. P. denounced the germ theory and was in the process of bringing suit against Pueblo's public schools to force them to admit his children without vaccination. When diphtheria broke out in his family, he applied "medical massages to the neck," rather than call in a physician. Then, Mr. P., himself, became ill and died. In reporting his death, *Colorado Medicine* could not help but note "the word 'diphtheria'" on his death certificate—an irony which "confutes his work and his League. Poor P . . . !"

The quacks and charlatans, the sects, cults, and faith healers, the fads and fakes, and the "antis" did not disappear with the passing of Colorado's early days.

22 TWENTIETH CENTURY

Dr. A.W. Rew of Fort Collins is at Fort Sam Houston, Texas, in command of an ambulance company . . . He will start for the 'hot place' shortly after the first of the year.

News Notes, Colorado Medicine, 1918[1]

WHEN THE UNITED STATES FINALLY entered World War I, there were only 200,000 men in the army. By the Armistice, eighteen months later, nearly 5 million had served, including 2 million who had been sent to Europe.[2] There were 230,000 Americans wounded and 112,000 deaths. Disease was common, and more American troops died from illness than from war wounds.

The medical requirements of a fighting force are much greater than those of a peacetime population, and many thousands of physicians were needed. As in the rest of the nation, Colorado's physicians were called upon to volunteer to serve in the military. Some, impressed with the medical needs of Europe's civilians, had gone overseas to help early in the war. Boulder's Dr. W. A. Jolley, for example, joined other American Red Cross volunteers at a hospital in Serbia two years before America's entry.[3]

Soon after President Wilson's declaration of war, a call went out for 20,000 physicians. Some of Colorado's physicians volunteered immediately, and each issue of *Colorado Medicine* proudly listed doctors entering the service from around the state. The University of Colorado School of Medicine, under Dr. John Amesse, organized a military hospital which included twenty-two doctors. They set sail on July 4, 1918, and established Base Hospital No. 29 at Tottenham, England.[4] Pueblo surgeon J. Crum Epler wrote home, "I am a very busy man . . . Two of us have done 364 major operations this

22.1 Many Colorado physicians served in World War I, including those at Base Hospital No. 29 in England.

month."[5] The unit eventually returned to Denver in March 1919 to be demobilized.

Six months after the declaration of war, the state society's president, Dr. (now Major) A. C. Magruder, stressed the need for additional medical volunteers. He urged his colleagues: "Don't think whether you are going to be a lieutenant, captain, or major. Enter the work for the work's sake . . ."[6] and reassured them:

> Don't think that because you are not at the top you will have to 'kow-tow' to the many above you. Officers of the regular army as well as medical officers greet you cheerfully and welcome you as one of them.[6]

Major Magruder pointed out that Colorado's military quota was 243 out of a physician-population of 1,733. Thus far, 126 had been recom-

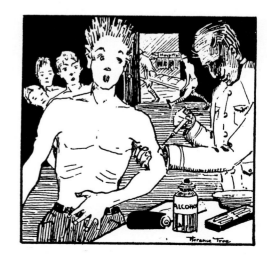

mended for commissions, and although most had accepted, a few had not. Magruder did not have a high opinion of the latter group:

> The doctor who [has his military commission] framed and hung on his office wall, but who fails to accept it and take the oath, is the poorest type that can be imagined. I have heard that some members of this Society have done that very thing.[6]

Finally, he pointed out:

> I do not want to shame you into doing your duty. I don't want even to seem to be persuading you to do what deep down in your hearts you know is your duty; but Colorado stands [with regard to medical volunteers], I am sorry to tell you, forty-sixth [out of forty-eight states].[6]

By November of 1918, the month of the Armistice, about one-sixth of the state's physicians were serving in the military, and although Colorado still ranked low nationally, this may have reflected the fact that many of her doctors had come to the state because of tuberculosis and were medically unfit for military service.[7]

As for Colorado's women physicians, Dr. Margaret Fraser noted that "when our government finally awakes to the value of its trained women, it will find a well organized body of physicians . . ."[8] Dr. Fraser and her colleagues organized the Colorado Medical Women's War Service League, "gathered and shipped nearly one thousand pounds of clothing for children in France and Belgium," and worked for the admission of women physicians to the medical reserves. Frustrated in her efforts to enlist, she went to France and, with other American women physicians, helped to establish a military hospital under the auspices of the French army.[9]

Many doctors who remained at home supported the war effort in other ways. The Volunteer Medical Service Corps was organized to relieve the strains created by the depletion of civilian physicians. At the Medical School, senior students were awarded "certificates of graduation" in lieu of diplomas and left early to join the military.[10] Later, the curriculum was adjusted in order to allow for early graduation.

When the draft was instituted, virtually all of the country's young men underwent a medical examination. The nation was shocked by the large number of medical rejections.[11] Another surprise was the high frequency of venereal disease, a finding which led to legislation requiring the reporting of venereal diseases and to a statewide program of public health measures designed to deal with the problem.[12]

Influenza

[Denver's] manager of Health . . . characterizes the epidemic as the worst in the history of the nation, and compares it to the Black Plague [of] medieval Europe.
                    Municipal Facts (Denver), 1918[13]

We have become used to the influenza epidemics which periodically ricochet around the nation, and to the exotic names of new viral strains, calls for flu shots, depleted classrooms and working places, and warnings of increased risks in the elderly and other susceptible persons. In recent years (1957-1984), seventeen flu epidemics have resulted in a total of about 10,000 deaths in the U.S.A.[14]

Influenza is not a new disease and outbreaks of what was called "la grippe," appeared around the world in earlier times. A particularly bad one struck Colorado in the 1890s. In the fall of 1918, shortly before the end of the war, there began a world wide outbreak, or pandemic, of enormous proportions. Before it was over, it had killed an estimated 20 million people, more than the war itself. In the United States, it was estimated that as many as 500,000 people died of influenza, usually as the result of complicating pneumonia.[15] In addition to its astounding and still unexplainably high mortality was the fact that the disease was most devastating not among infants or the elderly, but among young, previously healthy, adults—especially young men.

Colorado had one of the the highest influenza death rates in the nation.[16] Within weeks, the disease spread throughout the state, devastating cities, towns, mining camps, and even isolated farms and ranches. During the ten months between September 1918, when the first cases appeared, and June 1919, more than 6,000 Coloradans died of influenza.

As the first cases began to appear in Denver, the mayor "took extreme steps—the nature of which were not surpassed by any city in the United States."[17] Public meetings were banned, schools, theaters, and clubs closed, and Sunday church services suspended. Even private gatherings such as dinner parties were officially discouraged. In one week, that ending October 26, there were 217 influenza deaths in the city, and in the first two months of the epidemic, there were nearly 1,200.[18] Among influenza patients admitted to Denver General Hospital, nearly one in three died.[19]

No part of the state was spared. The most remote towns took all sorts of protective measures: people wore masks; schools, churches, pool halls and saloons were closed; houses were placarded and fumigated. The town of Durango even quarantined incoming railroad workers and passengers. All to no avail. The hospitals overflowed, and hotels, boarding houses, and even city halls were commandeered as emergency care centers. Doctors and nurses worked round the clock, assisted by medical students and other volunteers. The University of Colorado's Board of Regents reported:

> Many [of the students] have been at work . . . almost continuously, many of them have contracted the disease . . . and a few have nearly lost their lives. This record of public service . . . constitutes one in which the university may take pride.[20]

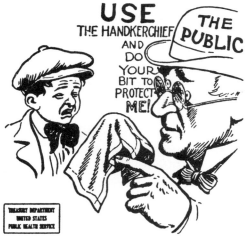

22.2 Posters like this one appeared all over the state during the influenza epidemic of 1918-1919.

Many businesses shut down around the state. The tungsten mines around Nederland were forced to close; in one mine, fifteen of the crew of seventy-five died.[21] From the tiny gold mining camp of Tiger, as many as four bodies a day were brought down to Breckenridge by ore wagon.[22] In Leadville, one funeral home reported more than thirty bodies awaiting burial, and a nearby competitor had nearly that number.[23] Funerals were limited to no more than four mourners. In Cripple Creek, the bodies were stacked outside the mortuary.[24] The town's priests accompanied the doctors on their rounds to save time.

Silverton, a mining camp high in the San Juan mountains, was said to have been the hardest hit community in the state.[25] Despite a variety of preventive measures, including the fumigation of incoming mail, the first two cases appeared on October 18. Within one week, there were forty-two deaths, and in the following week, nearly twice as many. The Town Hall became a hospital—and then "a place to die." When the bodies exceeded the town's ability to produce even rough-hewn coffins, the victims were buried in blankets.[26] Finally, the epidemic subsided, but not before taking 146 lives in the town of about 2,000.

The 1920s

Something is wrong with medical economics . . . The cost of sickness to the public has greatly increased.
            S. B. Childs, M.D. (Denver), 1928[27]

If Colorado's birth was marked by the discovery of gold in Cherry Creek in 1858, then, by 1928, it had reached its biblical lifespan of three score and ten. That year is as good as any to mark the transition from Colorado's early medical years to modern times.

Symbolic of the transition was the change in Colorado's once dominant mining industry. By 1928 gold and silver represented a tiny fraction of the state's annual income, and the few mining camps which remained were nearly moribund, not yet resurrected by later-day tourism and skiing. Coal was still important, but much of Colorado's 5,000 miles of railroad track had become superfluous. On the other hand, the state produced a quarter of a billion dollars in manufactured goods in 1928, and that year it boasted a quarter of a million automobiles.[28]

Nationally, the 1920s were characterized by economic growth, conservatism and isolationism, and some bizarre social, religious, and political activities. Colorado was no exception. Much of the state, for example, was dominated by the KKK for a couple of years, largely under the direction of a prominent Denver physician, Dr. John Galen Locke. Prohibition was still in effect, tariffs were in place, and millionaires and schoolteachers were borrowing money to play the stock market. In Colorado, a high school teacher's salary varied from $30 to $50 a week and, it was estimated, a family of five could live, at a "comfort level," on an income of about $1,200 a year.[28] In Denver in 1928 a quart of milk cost 12¢, sirloin steak was 43¢ a pound, and 15¢ paid for a ten pound sack of potatoes. Colorado's marriage rate was ten percent higher and its divorce rate forty percent higher than the rest of the nation. In that year's presidential election, Herbert Hoover received nearly twice as many Colorado votes as Alfred E. Smith, but Governor Adams, a Democrat, had received an equally impressive margin over his Republican rival.

Colorado's death rate was slightly higher than the national rate.[29] Infectious disease continued to be the leading cause of death (twenty-five percent), and one of every ten Coloradans died of tuberculosis—many of them immigrants to the state. In the 1920s, it was noted that Colorado was one of only five states which did not provide for the sanitarium care of tuberculosis and that the state's T.B. mortality rate was twice that of any other state.[30] In Denver, there were eight deaths from tuberculosis every day.

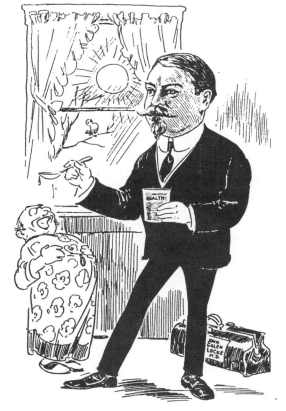

Many "nineteenth century" causes of death were still very much present. In 1928 in Colorado there were 150 deaths ascribed to syphilis, 120 to whooping cough, 82 to puerperal fever, and nearly 50 to scarlet fever. Although there had been severe outbreaks of smallpox and diphtheria in the early 1920s, the widespread use of vaccination and anti-diphtheria immunization had reduced the mortality due to those two diseases drastically. Improvements in sanitation and water purification had been made, but there were forty deaths due to typhoid in 1928. That year, it was said that "Denver water does not meet the [accepted] standard of bacteriological purity . . ." and that "the incidence of intestinal disease in Denver is still higher than that of many other cities in the United States."[31] Furthermore, Denver and other cities were still dumping their raw sewage into rivers which served as the sources of drinking water for communities downstream. Despite the advances of surgery, nearly 250 deaths were attributed to appendicitis. Cancer and heart disease were becoming more prevalent, but still accounted for a total of less than twenty percent of Colorado's mortality. Infant mortality and the risks of prematurity continued to remain high, and Denver's infant mortality was the highest of any city in the country.[32] Denver's maternal mortality

rate was also more than twice that of the rest of the nation.[33] There were 111 deaths due to mining and railroad accidents in Colorado in 1928—still a significant number, but already surpassed by nearly twice as many deaths due to automobile accidents.

In the mid-1920s, there were about 1,800 practicing physicians in Colorado, a physician-to-population ratio of about 1 to 500.[34] The average Colorado physician was white, male, forty-seven years old, and had a farming, business, or professional family background. There were very few minority or women physicians. The general attitude toward women in medicine was expressed in the legend accompanying a *Denver Post* photo of women medical students at the University of Colorado: "Good-looking doctors, like good-looking nurses, are a great help, any psychologist can tell you."[35] Nearly three out of four Colorado physicians had immigrated from outside the state, especially from the Northeast or Midwest. Most had attended college and medical school and had completed their internship outside of Colorado. Although the trend toward specialization was continuing, the majority remained general practitioners. About half of the state's physicians were medical society members.

The housecall was still in vogue, but the automobile had definitely replaced the horse and buggy, and by 1920, at least one physician was using an airplane to circuit ride his farflung eastern Colorado practice.[36] Denver, Colorado Springs, and the larger towns continued to attract large numbers of physicians, but many small rural and mountain communities were without a doctor.

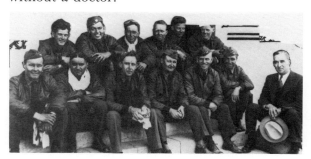

In 1925 the University of Colorado opened its new medical center in Denver. Previously split between the Boulder campus for the basic sciences and Denver General Hospital for clinical training, the school was finally united within a combined medical school–university (Colorado General) hospital building. In addition, the school's new Psychopathic Hospital provided a statewide referral center for psychiatric problems. Denver, with the state's only medical

22.3 Some of the more bizarre aspects of the 1920s are personified in the career of Dr. John Galen Locke, head of Colorado's Ku Klux Klan. The clan virtually ran the state for a couple of years.

22.4 The 1920s continued to see the influx of many talented physicians to Colorado. Dr. Nolie Mumey (front row, second from the left) was not only a distinguished surgeon and a pioneer flight surgeon, but the author and editor of more than one hundred volumes of poetry and Western and medical history.

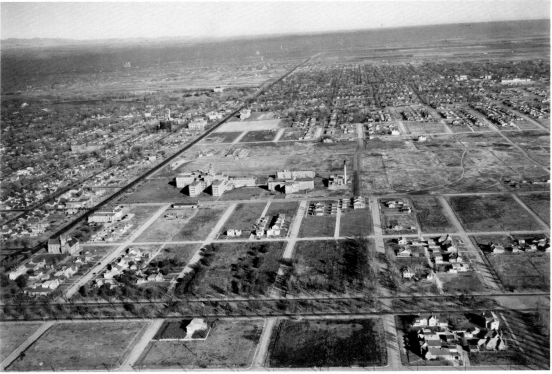

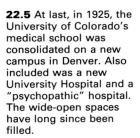

22.5 At last, in 1925, the University of Colorado's medical school was consolidated on a new campus in Denver. Also included was a new University Hospital and a "psychopathic" hospital. The wide-open spaces have long since been filled.

school, its prominent specialists, and its medical library and large hospitals, was very much the center of medicine in Colorado. The Metropolitan Building was the focal point for the state's medical community, its eight stories containing the offices of many of the city's best known physicians as well as the medical society's library and offices. Here, the profession's leaders gathered for formal and informal discussions of the latest in medical advances, legislative maneuvers, and social movements.

About two-thirds of the state's general hospital beds were located in Denver, recently expanded by several new hospitals.[37] This overabundance of hospital beds in Denver led to competition for patients and aggressive marketing by some of the city's hospitals. One hospital offered, for example, cut-rate laboratory fees as an inducement to prospective patients. Next,

said the *Denver Medical Bulletin*, one might expect to see counter offers by other hospitals, such as "On Mondays, Wednesdays, and Fridays, maternity cases delivered at fifty cents on the dollar for boy babies and twenty-five cents for the more dangerous sex."[38]

Major changes were occurring in the practice of medicine. Specialization was definitely on the increase. In addition to the established specialties, Denver's Dr. Charles Spivak was urging physicians to consider concentrating on the care of the newborn (neonatology) and the increasing population of elderly persons (gerontology).[39]

Physicians' conservative attitudes towards certain social and ethical issues were beginning to be tempered somewhat. A 1928 editorial in *Colorado Medicine* denounced abortion, citing the "pretty Leadville girl [who] came down to Denver . . . hoping to avoid ostracism and shame," and who died as the result of an abortion.[40] But, in addition to denouncing abortion, the editor pointed out that a more liberal societal attitude towards illegitimate birth was warranted. In addition, he even commented that the legalization of abortion in the Soviet Union had resulted in a markedly reduced mortality rate! Birth control, once an unmentionable topic in the medical journals, was being discussed publicly. The *Denver Medical Bulletin* reported that the County Medical Society had been addressed by the director of the American Birth Control League and that the speaker had "had no difficulty in holding the attention of his audience for over two hours . . ."[41] It was noted that plans were

22.6 The University (Colorado General) Hospital boasted the very latest in modern medical transportation.

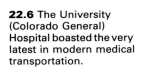

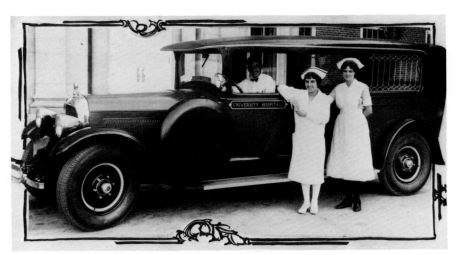

under way to open a birth control clinic in Denver.

In 1928 the average gross income of a physician in private practice was less than $6,500—and less than $5,000 after expenses were deducted.[42] Nevertheless, the cost of medical care was said to be rising precipitously. There was growing concern over how people of "moderate means," let alone the indigent were going to be able to afford these costs. Denver's Dr. Henry Sewell complained that "countless thousands today are paying automobile installments while their long due doctor's bills must wait."[43] Dr. Childs expressed concern over "mounting costs for hospital and nursing care [and] prohibitive charges for surgery . . ."[44]

Another Denver doctor pointed out the inefficiency of individual medical practice and decried the fact that the physician "refuses to recognize the great value of cooperation with his fellow medical men . . . He was born an individual, he prefers to die an individual . . ."[45] Indeed, there was a great deal of concern by physicians over the possibilities of medical control by the government ("socialized" or "state" medicine) and by corporations and insurers ("contract" medicine). The president of Denver's medical society, Dr. Phil Hillkowitz, spoke of some of the concerns of the 1920s physician—"altered conditions under which the doctor and patients are brought together," the disappearance of the family physician, the formation of "medical groups" and contract medicine, and the "rising tide of state medicine."[46]

In addition, and despite the remarkable advances of medicine, the doctors continued to have an image problem. As Dr. Childs commented in 1928,

> The public's attitude toward the profession seems little less than one of distrust. Never before . . . have the leading magazines and newspapers contained so many critical articles, while innumerable attacks upon the integrity of the profession have been made in our state legislatures.[47]

At least some of this was due, said Dr. Hillkowitz, to the "aloofness" of the profession:

> We have not taken the public into our confidence. We have considered it undignified to discuss scientific matters in the lay press . . . Our failure to educate the public is responsible for its unfavorable opinion of the medical profession.[48]

The 1920s also saw a remarkable proliferation of quacks, cultists, food faddists, faith healers, and the like, and Hillkowitz described a medical profession "menaced by the growing power of various cults and vagaries . . ."[48] In 1921, for example, evangelist Aimee Semple McPherson came to Denver and filled its City Auditorium three times a day for several weeks. At about the same time, the anti-medical forces were focusing their efforts on an anti-vivisection bill

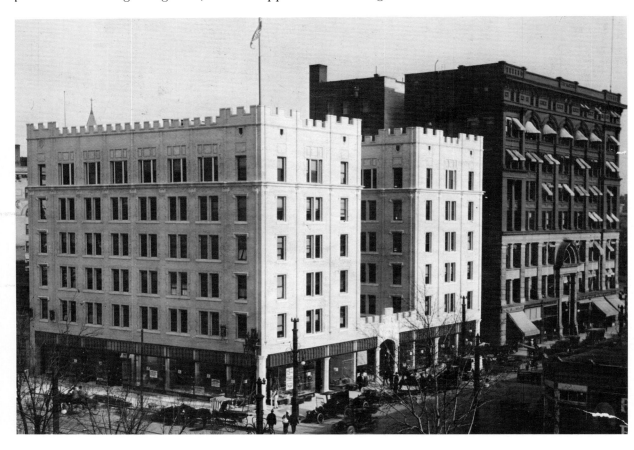

22.7 Denver's Metropolitan Building was the focal point for the state's practicing physicians. Two more stories were added at a later date.

which had been introduced into the state legis- lature. The bill was placed on the ballot and, much to the satisfaction of the doctors, was de- feated by a five-to-one margin, "the largest majority ever recorded in Colorado against an initiated or referred measure."[49]

Dr. Hillkowitz summarized his impressions of medicine in the 1920s.

The old and established forms [of medical prac- tice] are being dislocated and new alignments are being made. The practice of medicine is clearly in a state of flux.[50]

Would anyone question the relevance of the doc- tor's comments, made as Colorado's early med- ical days were coming to a close, to medicine today?

22.8 Medicine was undergoing many changes in the 1920s and there was concern over future developments in the professional, economic, and social aspects of health care. This cartoon suggested a solution to the problem of health care delivery for the middle class. The poor had the "free dispensary" and the rich had the doctor's private office. A compromise, in the form of "cooperative clinics," was offered for the middle class. Some of the problems have changed, but the concerns remain.

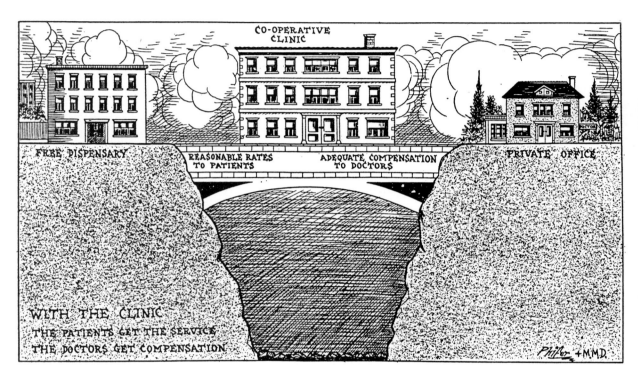

A CO-OPERATIVE, SELF-SUPPORTING CLINIC WOULD BRIDGE THE GAP.

Appendix

FEES

	1860[a]	1871[b]	1895[c]	1909[d]
Office Visit	$2[e]	$2-5	$1-5	$1-5[f]
Housecall[g]	3	4	2-5	2-5[f]
Consultation	10-25	10-12	5-10	5-25
Minor Surgery	10-25	10-50	5-50	10-50
Major Surgery	50-500	100-500	100-500	100-500[h]
Anaesthesia	—	10	5-25	10-25
Delivery	25-200	30	20-50	25-100
Complicated Delivery	50-200	50	30-150	50-200

a. Fee Bill of the Jefferson Medical Society, June 4, 1860.
   (This was the short-lived original medical society in what later became Colorado)

b. Fee Bill of the Denver Medical Association, June 15, 1871.
   (Adopted by the Territorial Medical Society, September 19, 1871)

c. Fee Bill of the Denver and Arapahoe Medical Society, 1895.

d. Fee Bill, Medical Society of the City and County of Denver, 1909.

e. Cited as the minimum fee for a "prescription," presumably equivalent to the minimum charge for an office visit.

f. The charge for the first office visit was $2-10; for the first housecall it was $3-10. The figures cited above were for subsequent office visits and housecalls.

g. Visits beyond the city limits were charged an additional mileage fee. In 1860, this was $2 per mile; by 1909, it was $1-2. Charges were generally higher for night calls.

h. The highest charge cited in any of the fee bills was $1,000—the maximum fee for "removing malignant tumors."

Bibliography and Notes

These frequently cited sources are designated by the following abbreviations:

CM—Colorado Medicine
CMJ—Colorado Medical Journal
DMB—Denver Medical Bulletin
DMT—Denver Medical Times
RMN—Rocky Mountain News
JAMA—Journal of the American Medical Association
Colo Mag—Colorado Magazine
RMMJ—Rocky Mountain Medical Journal
TCTMS—Transactions of the Colorado Territorial Medical Society
TSCMS—Transactions of the Colorado State Medical Society

References to medical journals use standard abbreviations. The volume numbers for Denver Medical Times appear to be inconsistent in different library copies. If there is difficulty in finding a particular article, one should try looking for it in one volume earlier and/or later than indicated in this bibliography.

Chapter 1

1. Holmes OW. In Rothstein WG. *American Physicians in the Nineteenth Century*, 415. Baltimore, 1972.
2. Sappington J. *The Theory and Practice of Fevers*, 188. Arrow Rock, Missouri, 1844.
3. Ibid., 191.
4. Davies NE, Davies GH, Sanders ED. "William Cobbett, Benjamin Rush, and the death of General Washington." JAMA 249:912, 1983.
5. Watson T. *Lectures on the Principles and Practice of Physic*, Third American from the last London edition, revised, with additions by DF Condie. Philadelphia, 1848.

Chapter 2

1. Letter from General James Wilkinson to Lieutenant Z.M. Pike, July 12, 1806. In Jackson D: *The Journals of Zebulon Montgomery Pike*, Vol. 1, 288. Norman: 1966.
2. Hollon WE. *The Lost Pathfinder: Zebulon M. Pike*. Norman, 1949; Carter HL. *Zebulon Montgomery Pike*. Colorado Springs, 1956; Hart SH and Hulbert AB. *Zebulon Pike's Arkansaw Journal*. Colorado Springs, 1932.
3. Saugrain was said to have assisted Lewis and Clark in the medical preparations for their expedition.
4. Letter from Lieutenant Zebulon Pike to General James Wilkinson, July 5, 1807. Jackson, *Journals*, Vol. 2, 243.
5. Wyer MG. "Adventurous physicians." Quart Bull Northwestern University Medical School 20:1, 1946.
6. Cutter IS. "Dr. Edwin James, Great Westerner and Great American." *The Westerners Brand Book*, 1944. Chicago, 1946.
7. James E. *Account of an Expedition from Pittsburgh to the Rocky Mountains . . . .* Philadelphia, 1823.
8. Fuller HM and Hafen LR. *The Journal of Captain John R. Bell*, 152. Glendale, 1973.
9. James, *Account*, Vol. 2, 10.
10. Fuller, *Journal*, 154.
11. Cutter, "Dr. Edwin James," 35.
12. Brandon W. *The Men and the Mountain: Fremont's Fourth Expedition*. New York, 1956.
13. "Diary of Benjamin Kern." In *Fremont's Fourth Expedition. A Documentary Account of the Disaster of 1848-1849*, 102-06. Edited by LR Hafen and AW Hafen. Glendale, 1960.
14. McNitt F. *Navaho Expedition: Journal of a Military Reconnaissance from Santa Fe . . . by Lt. James H. Simpson*, xxxvi-xl. Norman, 1964. The Army surgeon was Dr. Horace R. Wirtz.
15. Mumey N. *John Williams Gunnison*, 23-4. Denver: 1957.
16. Schiel J. "Reise durch die Felsengebirge." In Bachmann FW and Wallace WS. *The Land Between. Dr. James Schiel's Account of the Gunnison-Beckwith Expedition into the West, 1853 - 1854*, 43-44. Los Angeles, 1957.
17. Ashley WH. "The Ashley Narrative." In Dale HC. *The Ashley-Smith Explorations and the Discovery of a Central Route to the Pacific, 1822-1829*, 137. Cleveland, 1918.
18. Ruxton GF. *Adventures in Mexico and the Rocky Mountains*, 274. New York, 1848.
19. Tierney L. *History of the Gold Discoveries on the South Platte River*, 17. 1859. Reprint. Denver, 1949.
20. Ashley, "Narrative," 137.
21. Sage RB. *Rocky Mountain Life*, 307, 316. Boston, 1857.
22. Ruxton, *Adventures*, 208, 225.
23. Sage, *Rocky Mountain Life*, 142.
24. Grant B. *Kit Carson's Own Story of His Life*. Taos, 1926.
25. Sage, *Rocky Mountain Life*, 339.
26. Ferris WA. *Life in the Rocky Mountains*, 40. Denver, 1940.
27. Robb JS. "The mad wolf: A tale of the Rocky Mountains." Graham's Magazine, December, 1846.
28. Russell CP. *Firearms, Traps and Tools of the Mountain Man*, 223-26. New York, 1967; Levine BR. "Lancets on the frontier." The Museum of the Fur Trade Quarterly 12:2, 1976.
29. Museum of the Fur Trade Quarterly 3:9, 1967, 17:10-11, 1981.
30. Sage, *Rocky Mountain Life*, 147, 178-179.
31. Peters DC. *Kit Carson's Life and Adventures*, 76. Hartford, 1874.

32. Conard HL. *"Uncle Dick" Wootten*, 74. Chicago, 1890.

33. Templeton SW. *The Lame Captain - The Life and Adventures of Pegleg Smith*, 72-80. Los Angeles, 1965. Camp CL. *George C. Yount and His Chronicles of the West*, 232-35, 273-4. Denver, 1966; Humphreys AG. "Thomas L. (Pegleg) Smith." In Hafen LR (editor). *The Mountain Men*, Vol. IV, 311. Glendale, 1966; Nunis, DB. "Milton G. Sublette," Ibid., Vol IV, 331.

34. Camp, *George C. Yount*, 232-35.

35. Nunis, "Sublette," 331.

36. Beshoar B. *Hippocrates in a Red Vest*, 123-24. Palo Alto, 1973.

37. Hall JN. *Tales of Pioneer Practice*, 121. Denver, 1937.

38. Hannemann J. "Doctor, compadre, adios!" RMMJ April, 1968; Thompson AW. "The death and last will of Kit Carson." Colo Mag 5:183, 1928; Carter HL. *Dear Old Kit: The Historical Kit Carson*, 177 -79. Norman, 1968. Estergreen MM. *Kit Carson: A Portrait in Courage*, 272 - 80. Norman, 1962.

39. Grant, *Kit Carson*, 10. There is some controversy as to whether Carson was the actual operator, an assistant, or just an observer.

40. Carson's career was chronicled by the army surgeon he had met years before at Fort Massachusetts, Colorado—Colonel De Witt Clinton Peters. Eventually, that friendship resulted in a series of interviews and Carson's only "authorized" biography. Peters DC. *The Story of Kit Carson's Life and Adventures*. Hartford, 1874. The biography was said to have been based on notes dictated to Mrs. Peters by Carson. Dr. Peters died in 1876.

41. Carson's aneurysm was ascribed to an injury he suffered in 1860. It should be noted that aneurysms of the thoracic aorta, especially in the nineteenth century, were usually due to the long term effects of syphilis. Prior to the introduction of penicillin, thoracic aneurysms were not rare, sometimes expanding to enormous size, eroding the sternum, and presenting as a visibly pulsating mass.

42. Henry R. Tilton was a career army surgeon, who after seven previous tours of duty, had been stationed at Fort Lyon. In 1877, while campaigning with the Seventh Cavalry against the Nez Perce, Tilton showed outstanding bravery in rescuing the wounded and was later awarded the Congressional Medal of Honor. He subsequently became Deputy Surgeon General of the Army and retired in 1900. Colonel Tilton died in 1906. Hannemann, "Doctor, compadre," 37.

43. Tilton HR. "Letter to J.S.C. Abbott, Jan. 7, 1874." In Abbott JSC. *Christopher Carson, Known as Kit Carson*, Second edition, 343 - 48. New York, 1901.

44. Ibid., 345. Carson was buried in Taos. The building where he died, Dr. Tilton's tiny four-room home facing the parade grounds, was restored in 1959 and is now the Kit Carson Memorial Chapel.

45. Wislizenus FA. *A Journey to the Rocky Mountains in the Year 1839*, 141. St Louis, 1912. A German physician who came to St. Louis in 1835, Wislizenus joined a trapper's caravan to the Northwest in 1839. On his return, he headed south along the plains fronting Colorado's front range, stopped at Bent's Fort, and then went east along the Arkansas River. In 1846, having caught the wanderlust again, the doctor joined a wagon train to Santa Fe, bypassing Colorado by taking the Cimarron cut-off. He soon found himself in the middle of the Mexican War, joined Doniphan's regiment as surgeon, and wrote up his experiences in another book. Unfortunately, he included virtually nothing of medical interest in either of his books. After returning to St. Louis, Wislizenus married, raised a family and practiced medicine. He died in 1889.

46. Grinnell GB. "Bent's Old Fort and its builders." Collections of the Kans. State Hist. Soc. 15:28, 1923.

47. Hafen, LR. "The W.M. Boggs manuscript about Bent's Fort, Kit Carson, the Far West and Life among the Indians." Colo Mag 7:45, 1930.

48. Thompson E. "Life in an adobe castle, 1833-1849." In *Bent's Old Fort*. Denver, 1978.

49. Garrard LH. *Wah-to-yah and the Taos Trail*, 130. New York, 1850. Reprint. Glendale, 1938.

50. Abert JW. *Report . . . of the Examination of New Mexico*. Sen. Exec. Doc. 23. Washington, D.C., 1848. Aug. 29, 1846.

51. Drum SM. *Down the Santa Fe Trail and into Mexico: The Diary of Susan Shelby Magoffin 1846 - 1847*, 52, 61, 68. New Haven, 1926.

52. Hall, *Tales*, 72.

53. Abert, *Report*, 1.

54. Hughes JT. *Doniphan's Expedition*, 60-61. Cincinnati, 1848.

55. Parkman F. *The Oregon Trail*, 338. Edited by EN Feltskog. Madison, 1969.

Chapter 3

1. Reed VZ. "The Southern Ute Indians of early Colorado." Californian Illustrated Magazine, 1893. Reprint. Golden, Colorado, 1980.

2. Wormington HM. *Prehistoric Indians of the Southwest*, 45. Denver, 1947.

3. Bennett KA. *Skeletal Remains from Mesa Verde National Park, Colorado*. Washington, D. C., 1975. This study, in which 202 skeletons were examined, provides some interesting background data on the Anasazi.

4. Miles JS. *Orthopedic Problems of the Wetherill Mesa Populations. Mesa Verde National Park, Colorado*. Washington, D. C., 1975. Dr. Miles was chairman of the Department of Orthopedic Surgery at the University of Colorado School of Medicine.

5. Freeman L. "Surgery of the ancient inhabitants of the Americas." Art and Archeology 18:21, 1924. Dr. Freeman was a prominent Denver surgeon.

6. Propst NB. *Forgotten People. A History of the South Platte Trail*, 21. Boulder, 1979; Culbertson TA: *Journal of an Expedition to the Mauvaises Terres*, 133. Washington, D. C., 1851.

7. Miller RC. "Annual Report, 1858." *Relations with the Indians of the Plains*, 1857-1861, 168. Edited by LR Hafen and AW Hafen. Glendale, 1959. In the 1820s, when smallpox broke out at Bent's Fort, Colonel Bent warned the Indians to stay away, apparently avoiding an epidemic. Grinnell GB. "Bent's old fort and its builders." Collections of the Kansas State Historical Society 15:43, 1923.

8. Colo Mag 4:151, 1927. The government responded by cutting off their annuity.

9. Taylor MF. *Pioneers of the Picketwire*, 16-17. Pueblo, 1964.

10. RMN Feb 15, 1862.

11. *Report of the Bureau of Indian Affairs, 1863*, 400 - 01. Cited in Coel M. *Chief Left Hand*. Norman, 1981.

12. Miller, "Annual Report."

13. Hafen LR. "The Fort Pueblo massacre." Colo. Mag. 4:56, 1927. Near present-day Pueblo, Colorado.

14. Bowles S. *The Switzerland of America*, 76-77. Springfield, Mass., 1869.

15. The term "Southern Ute" often refers to the Indians of both reservations, in distinction to several "Northern Ute" bands who were exiled to Utah.

16. Stearn EW, Stearn AE. *The Effect of Smallpox on the Destiny of the American Indian*. Boston, 1945.

17. Grinnell GB. *The Cheyenne Indians: Their History and Ways of Life*, Volume 2, 126. New Haven, 1929.

18. Smith AM. *Ethnography of the Northern Utes*, 152. Santa Fe, 1974.

19. Grinnell, *Cheyenne Indians*.

20. Meeker J. *Brave Miss Meeker's Captivity*, 17. Philadelphia, 1879. Reprint. Denver, 1974.

21. Daniels HS. *Ute Medicine-man's Kit*. Durango, 1940. The medicine-man had been jailed in Cortez, Colorado, accused of killing a baby by burying it alive. While in jail, he killed a Mexican boy, for which crime he was sent to the state pententiary at Canon City. The medicine kit had been confiscated by the agency, and lent by it to the library.

22. Jocknick S. *Early Days on the Western Slope of Colorado*, 297. Denver, 1913.

23. Reed, *Southern Ute*, 15.

24. Jocknick, *Early Days*.

25. Pettit J. *Utes: The Mountain People*, 27. Colorado Springs, 1982.

26. Grinnell, *Cheyenne Indians*; Grinnell GB. "Some Cheyenne plant medicines." Amer.Anthropol. 7:37, 1905.

27. Chamberlin RV. "Some plant names of the Ute Indians." Amer Anthropol 11:27, 1909.

28. Jefferson J, et. al. *The Southern Utes, A Tribal History*. Ignacio, Colorado, 1972.

29. Lemley HR. "Among the Arapahoes." Harper's New Monthly Magazine 60:494, 1880.

30. Jefferson, *Southern Utes*.

31. Lemley, *Arapahoes*.

32. Ruxton GF. *Adventures in Mexico and the Rocky Mountains*, 242. New York, 1848.

33. Solly SE. *Manitou, Colorado: Its Mineral Waters and Climate*, 12. St. Louis, 1875.

34. Lynch J. "Pagosa! Pagosa! Healing Water! A Legend from Grateful Utes." *Pioneers of the San Juan*, IV, 452. Denver, 1961.

35. Ibid.; White LC. "Pagosa Springs, Colorado." Colo Mag 9:88, 1932. This reference cites a poem, "Legend of Pagosa Springs" by Ora Garvin, for the legend.

36. "Balneotherapy as practised by the Indians." CMJ 6:453, 1900. The Glenwood doctor was Dr. Richard K. Macalester.

37. Smith, *Ethnography*, 147.

38. Grinnell, *Cheyenne Indians*, I, 130-31.

39. Smith, *Ethnography*, 137.

40. Grinnell, *Cheyenne Indians*, I, 148.

41. Smith, *Ethnography*, 137 - 42.

42. Grinnell, *Cheyenne Indians*, I, 148.

43. Coel, *Chief Left Hand*, 3.

44. James E. *Account of an Expedition from Pittsburgh to the Rocky Mountains*, Vol I, 259 - 71. Philadelphia, 1823.

45. "Testimony in relation to the Ute Indian outbreak," 120. House of Representatives Miscellaneous Document No. 38. Washington, D. C., 1880.

46. Sprague M. *Massacre, The Tragedy at White River*, 123. Boston, 1957. Agent J.B. Thompson would send them to Dr. W.H. Williams for medical care.

47. "Testimony."

48. Sprague, *Massacre*, 259. At least some of the captive women were said to have been raped and at least one was treated for syphilis. Josie Meeker was said to have had subsequent medical and psychiatric problems related to her experiences as a captive and, according to Sprague, was treated by Denver's Dr. Alida Avery.

49. Bancroft MM. "Letter to Caroline Bancroft." Ca. 1930. Mary McLean Bancroft was the doctor's daughter.

50. Blair E. *Leadville. Colorado's Magic City*, 13-14. Boulder, 1980. The prankster was Wolfe Londoner, Colorado pioneer, early mayor of Denver, and himself a colorful character.

51. Hall JN. *Tales of Pioneer Practice*, 95. Denver, 1937. According to Caroline Bancroft, Colorow liked to drink. His problem may actually have been alcoholic cirrhosis.

52. Gunnison Review Sept. 11, 1880. Cited by Wallace B. *Gunnison Country*, 22. Denver, 1960

53. Jocknick, *Early Days*, 215.

54. Bull HR. "Tuberculosis among the Indians." TCSMS 24:314, 1894.

55. Hrdlicka A. *Physiological and Medical Observations Among the Indians of Southwestern United States and Northern Mexico*. Bulletin 34. Bureau of Ethnology. Washington, D. C., 1908.

56. Otis GA "Arrow wounds." *A Report of Surgical Cases Treated in the Army of the United States from 1865 to 1871*, 157. Circular No. 3. Surgeon General's Office, War Department. Washington D. C., 1871.

57. Fraser RW. *Mansfield on the Condition of the Western Forts, 1853-54*, 41. Norman, 1963.

58. Taylor, MF. "Fort Massachusetts." Colo Mag 45:120, 1968.

59. Billings JS. *Report on Barracks and Hospitals*, 320. Circular No. 4. Surgeon General's Office, War Department. Washington, D.C. 1870.

60. "Report to the Surgeon General, 1875." In Nankivell JH. "Fort Garland." Colo Mag 16:17, 1939.

61. Brandes DT. *Military Posts of Colorado*, 20. Fort Collins, Colorado, 1973.

62. Danker DF. *Mollie: The Journal of Mollie Dorsey Sanford in Nebraska and Colorado Territories 1857 - 1866*, 154. Lincoln, 1959. Unfortunately, little information is available on the medical aspects of Colorado's participation in the Civil War, e.g. on the battles in which Coloradans participated in New Mexico. The three regiments of Colorado volunteers each had a surgeon and several assistant surgeons.

63. An excellent review of this topic is provided by Dr. Peter D. Olch's "Medicine in the Indian-fighting Army, 1866 - 1890." Journal of the West 21:32, 1982.

64. Byrne BJ. *A Frontier Army Surgeon*, 155. Cranford, New Jersey, 1935. Byrne had previously served with the Army in the 1870s during the yellow fever outbreaks in Mississippi and Florida. In 1880 he and his unit marched from Santa Fe to southwestern Colorado and built Fort Lewis on the site of the present day Fort Lewis College. In 1888 he and his wife moved back East. Many years later, Mrs. Byrne collected her husband's notes and published the book in a very limited edition. It contains many fascinating tales about the army, Indians, outlaws, and the like, but, unfortunately, little of medical interest.

65. Billings, *Barracks and Hospitals*, 313, 338. Fort Lyon was abandoned in 1889. In 1906, the site was converted into a U.S. Naval Hospital, mainly for servicemen with tuberculosis. In 1922 it became a Veterans Administration Hospital. Boyd LR. *Fort Lyon, Colorado*. No publisher, no date.

66. Cutright PR, Brodhead MJ. *Elliot Coues*. Urbana, 1982; Hume EE. "Ornithologists of the United States Army Medical Corps." Bull Hist Med 8:1301, 1940.

67. Billings, *Barracks and Hospitals*, 340. 315.

68. In the absence of dietary vitamin C, the body's stores are used up and signs of scurvy appear in two to three months. These include cutaneous and gingival bleeding, muscular and joint aches and pains, fatigue, and emotional changes. When vitamin C or antiscorbutic food is introduced into the diet, the disease disappears in several weeks. In severe cases it can be fatal.

69. Bell JR. *The Journal of*, 154. Edited by HM Fuller and LR Hafen. Glendale, 1973.

70. Weir JA. "The Army doctor and the Indian." *Denver Westerners Brand Book*, Volume 31, 356. Edited by Alan J. Stewart. Denver, 1975.

71. Billings JS. *Report on the Hygiene of the United States Army*, xxxvi. Circular No. 8. Surgeon General's Office, War Department. Washington D. C., 1875.

72. Taylor, "Fort Massachusetts."

73. O'Brien EB. "Army life at Fort Sedgwick." Colo Mag 6:174, 1929.

74. Billings, *Hygiene*, xxxvii.

75. Otis, "Arrow wounds," 152. Fort Stevens was a short-lived post built in 1866 at the foot of the Spanish Peaks, west of Trinidad, Colorado.

76. Bill JH. "Arrow wounds." Am. J. Med Sci 44:362, 1862; Coues E. "Some notes on arrow wounds." Med Surg Reporter 14:321, 1866.

77. Brandes, *Military Posts*, 32.

78. Bill, "Arrow wounds."

79. Otis, "Arrow wounds," 162.

80. Coues, "Arrow wounds."

81. Byrne, *Frontier Army Surgeon*, 38.

82. "Report of the Secretary of War, communicating . . . a copy of the evidence taken at Denver and Fort Lyon, Colorado Territory, by a military commission ordered to inquire into the Sand Creek Massacre," 202 - 04. 39th Congress, 2d Session. Sen. Ex. Doc.No. 26. 1867; "Massacre of Cheyenne Indians," 72. Appendix. 38th Congress, Second Session, 1865. Appendix, Ironically, Chivington served as Denver's coroner in his later years.

83. Dunn WR. *War Drum Echoes*, 65 - 82. NP,1979; Forsyth GA. "Thrilling days in Army life." In *The Beecher Island Annual*, Vol 5, 5 - 25. Edited by R. Lynam. Wray, Colo. 1917. This material was originally published in Harper's Magazine in 1900.

84. Ibid., Lynam, 12 - 23. Major Forsyth was thirty years old at the time of the battle. He had enlisted as a private in the Civil War and had received a battlefield promotion to lieutenant. He subsequently served on General Phil Sheridan's staff and was breveted Major General. He retired from the army in 1890.

85. Colo Mag 13:90, 1936.

86. Forsyth, "Thrilling days."

Chapter 4

1. Hill AP. *Tales of Colorado Pioneers*, 31. Denver, 1884.

2. Olch PD. "Treading the elephant's tail: Medical problems on the Overland Trail." Bull Hist Med 59:196, 1985.

3. Clark CM. *A Trip to Pike's Peak*, 2. 1861. Reprint. San Jose, 1958. Clark's reminiscences were originally published in 1861, after his return to Chicago. In the introduction to his book, he stated, "I have endeavored to give a truthful record of the journey over the plains . . . of the troubles and trials that the emigrant encounters. I have nothing exaggerated nor ought set down in malice." Clark served as a surgeon during the Civil War and later at a number

of western forts. He finally returned to Chicago and died sometime after 1903.

4. H.C.P. Missouri Republican Apr. 21, 1859. In *Pike's Peak Gold Rush Guidebooks of 1859*, 298. Edited by LR Hafen. Glendale, 1941.

5. Willing GM. "Diary of a journey to the Pike's Peak gold mines in 1859." Edited by RP Bieber. Miss.Valley Hist. Rev. 14:360, 1927. After unsuccessfully prospecting at Goose Pasture near Central City and briefly practicing medicine and engaging in politics in Denver, Dr. Willing disappeared from view.

6. Redpath J, Hinton RJ. *Hand-book to Kansas Territory and the Rocky Mountain Gold Region*, 16. New York, 1859.

7. Gunn OB. *New Map and Hand-book of Kansas and the Gold Mines*, 12. Pittsburgh, 1859. Reprint. Denver, 1952.

8. Willing, "Diary," 368.

9. Clark, *Trip*, 24.

10. Reed JW. *Map and Guide to the Kansas Gold Region*, 9. 1859. Reprint. Denver, 1959; Marcy RB. *The Prairie Traveler*, 33. New York, 1859.

11. Ibid., Reed, 18.

12. Richardson AD. In Hafen, *Guidebooks*, 303.

13. Richardson AD. "Letters on the Pike's Peak gold region." Edited by L. Barr. Kans Hist Qtly 12:25, 1943.

14. Leavenworth Times, May 7, 1859. In Hafen, *Guidebooks*, 310.

15. Scott NB. "Experiences in Colorado in 1859." Trail 12:11, 1919.

16. Redpath and Hinton, *Handbook*, 14.

17. Marcy, *Prairie Traveler*, 49.

18. Richardson, "Letters," 14.

19. Willing, "Diary," 372.

20. Clark, *Trip*, 25.

21. Willing, "Diary," 366.

22. Marcy, *Prairie Traveler*, 126.

23. Tierney LD. *History of the Gold Discoveries on the South Platte River*, 22. Pacific City, Iowa, 1859. Reprint. Denver, 1949.

24. Marcy, *Prairie Traveler*, 170.

25. Peck RM in Hafen, *Guidebooks*.

26. Wheatley M.L. "Reminiscences of the early sixties." Trail 3:5, 1911.

27. Marcy, *Prairie Traveler*, 170.

28. Parsons WB. *The New Gold Mines of Western Kansas*, 24. Cincinnati, 1859. Reprint. Denver, 1951.

29. Clark, *Trip*, 25.

30. Willing, "Diary," 367.

31. Clark, *Trip*, 24.

32. Harrison EHN. "Diary," 1859. In *Overland Routes to the Goldfields*, 152. Edited by LR Hafen. Glendale, 1942.

33. Gunn, *New Map*.

34. R Cable. Western Weekly Argus, 1859. In Hafen, *Gold Rush*, 353 -54.

35. Harrison, "Diary," 185.

36. Clark, *Trip*, 88.

37. Byers WN, Kellom JH. *Handbook to the Goldfields of Nebraska and Kansas*, 28. Chicago, 1859. Reprint. Denver, 1949.

38. Marcy, *Prairie Traveler*, 62.

39. Clark, *Trip*, 88.

40. The Mountaineer, Sept. 20, 1860.

41. Byers and Kellom, *Handbook*, 72.

42. Central City and Brunswicker, April 6, 1859. Cited by Hafen, *Guidebooks*, 294.

43. Burt SW, Berthoud, EL. *The Rocky Mountain Gold Regions*, 49. Denver, 1861. Reprint. Denver, 1962.

44. "Laws and regulations of Union District, Clear Creek County, Colorado Territory," Article VI, Section 2. October 21, 1861.

45. "Mining laws of Nevada District, Colorado." Article VII, Sections 3 and 5. Colo Mag 36:131, 1959.

46. Smiley J (editor). *History of Denver*, 269-70. Denver, 1901.

47. Clark, *Trip*, 103.

48. Villard H. *The Past and Present of the Pike's Peak Gold Region*, 57. Princeton, 1932.

49. Clark, *Trip*, 49.

50. Villard, *Past and Present*, 57.

51. The Mountaineer, August 9, 1860.

52. Pollak IJ. "Report on diseases peculiar to high altitudes." TCTMS 2:26, 1873.

53. Curtin RG. "Rocky Mountain fever."Trans Amer Climatol Assn 3:190, 1886.

54. Whitmore EA. "Observations on the effects of great altitudes." DMT 18:537, 1898-99.

55. Woodring WW. "Mountain fever, so called." CMJ 7:423, 1901.

56. Brown M. "Digging doctors." Colo Mag 36:242, 1959.

57. Fitzgerald E. "Letter from the mines." In *Colorado Gold Rush, Contemporary Letters and Reports, 1859 - 1865*, 151. Edited by LR Hafen. Glendale, 1942.

58. Wheatley, "Reminiscences."

59. Villard, *Past and Present*, 151.

60. Clark, *Trip*, 25.

61. *Denver City and Auraria, The Commercial Emporium*, St. Louis, 1860.

62. Sagendorf A. In Smiley, *History of Denver*.

63. Spencer, EDR. *Gold Country, 1828-1858*. San Antonio, 1958; Geiser SW. "Dr. L.J. Russell and the Pike's Peak Gold Rush of 1858-1859." Southwest Hist Qtly 48:573, 1945.

64. One of Pollok's patients was the famed Georgetown innkeeper, Louis DuPuy, who had shattered his arm in a mine explosion. After nearly a decade of practice, the Leadville boom rekindled Pollok's mining instincts and he returned to California Gulch "to look after some of his old mining claims". His efforts were apparently unsuccessful, and the Georgetown Miner announced, in 1879, that Dr. Pollok's household goods were to be auctioned off. Pollok's health began to fail and he died in 1882. Baskin OL. *History of Clear Creek and Boulder Valleys*, 526. Chicago, 1880; Carden WD. "Nineteenth century physicians in Clear Creek County, Colorado, 1865 - 1895," 137 - 42. Master's thesis, Yale University, 1968.

65. Brunk IW. "Dr. John Parsons' Colorado Mint." *Denver Westerner's Roundup*, September-October, 1984.

66. RMN, April 23, 1859.

67. Perkin R. "A short sketch of long Dr. Peck." DMB April, 1971.

68. Colo Mag 10:137, 1933.

69. Trail 19:11, 1926.

70. Brown, "Digging doctors."

71. Allen, HW. "Early days in the practice of medicine in Colorado." CM 4:32, 1907.

72. Greenleaf, LN. *King Sham, and Other Atrocities in Verse*. New York, 1868.

73. Majors, A. *Seventy Years on the Frontier*, 264. Chicago, 1893.

74. Hill, *Tales*, 223.

75. Bruyn K. *Aunt Clara Brown: Story of a Black Pioneer*, 69. Boulder, 1970. Colo Mag 26:172, 1949.

76. RMN, November 6, 1868.

77. Gilmore J. *We Came North. A History of the Sisters of Charity of Leavenworth*, 40 - 41. Kansas City, 1961. Denver's St. Joseph's Hospital was opened in 1873.

78. Material regarding St. Luke's Hospital was obtained from the Daily Central City Register, Vol. IX, Dec. 27, 1870 and Jan 13, 28, Feb. 25, June 7, July 20, 1871. I was unable to find the site of the hospital in Central City.

Chapter 5

1. These two chapters and the preceding one discuss the medical aspects of gold and silver mining, i.e. of hard rock mining. Coal mining and the coal camps are discussed in a later chapter.

2. Dougan DH. "Observations at an altitude of 10,025 feet." *Annual Reports of the State Board of Health of Colorado for the Years 1879 and 1880*, 105.

3. RMN, August 15, 1877.

4. Ouray Times, January 11, 1878.

5. Baskin OL. *History of the Arkansas Valley, Colorado*, 53. Chicago, 1881.

6. Gambell FW. "Report to the Mayor and the Board of Health of the City of Leadville." In *Life in Leadville*, 1882, 23. Leadville, 1982.

7. Blair E. *Leadville: Colorado's Magic City*, 160. Boulder, 1980; Willison GF. *Here They Dug the Gold*, 185. New York, 1946.

8. Peterson FC. *Hillside Cemetery, Silverton, San Juan County, Colorado*. Silverton, Colorado, 1981.

9. *Fourth Report of the State Board of Health of Colorado*,

Including the Reports for the Years 1892, 1893, and 1894, 174.

10. Lee H. *Report of the Bureau of Mines, Colorado*, 34. Denver, 1897.

11. Colorado State Board of Health Sanitary Bulletin 4:7, 1904.

12. Leadville Herald Democrat, August 27, 1887, and Buena Vista Democrat, September 8, 1887. Cited in Anderson P. *From Gold to Ghosts, History of St. Elmo*, 58. Gunnison, Colorado, 1983.

13. *Pioneers of the San Juan*, II, 155 - 56. Colorado Springs, 1946.

14. Lee, *Report*, 34.

15. *San Juan*, II, 155.

16. Coleman JW. "Some pathological conditions to which the miner is peculiarly liable." CMJ 3:99, 1902.

17. The Solid Muldoon, September 14, 1888.

18. Exline JW. "The sanitation of mines." TCSMS 26:237, 1896.

19. Darley GM. *Pioneering in the San Juan*, 76. New York, 1899.

20. Gibbons, JJ. *In the San Juan, Colorado: Sketches*, 81 - 82. Chicago, 1898.

21. CMJ 8:570, 1902.

22. Meyer,C. "Pathology of high altitude pneumonia." Gross Med Coll Bull 6:64, 1896.

23. Baskin, *Arkansas Valley*, 308.

24. Blair, *Leadville*, 73.

25. Denver Tribune, March 4, 1880.

26. Manning JF. *Leadville, Lake County, and the Gold Belt*, 12. Denver, 1895.

27. Brown,JW. "Pneumonia in high altitudes and its treatment with jaborandi." JAMA 4:262, 1885.

28. The Solid Muldoon, September 14, 1888.

29. "Proceedings of the Arapahoe County Medical Society, March 20, 1884." DMT 3:355, l884.

30. Ibid.

31. *San Juan*, III, 31. Colorado Springs, 1952.

32. "Proceedings;" Brown, "Pneumonia."

33. Henderson Y. "Physiological observations on Pike's Peak, Colorado, made in the summer of 1911." Trans Amer Climatol Assn 28:11, 1912.

34. Fruyn K. "Dr. M. Klaiber" Colo Mag 33:204, 1956.

35. Wilkinson WW. "Acute articular rheumatism." CM 6:75, 1909.

36. Gibbons, *San Juan*, 186, 124.

37. *Annual Reports of the State Board of Health of Colorado for the Years 1879 and 1889*, 40.

38. Coquoz RL. *The History of Medicine in Leadville and Lake County, Colorado*, 8. NP, 1967.

39. Baskin, *Arkansas Valley*, 52.

40. *Occupation and Health*, II, 108. International Labor Office. Geneva, 1934.

41. *Board of Health, 1892 - 1894*, 172 - 74.

42. Exline, "Sanitation," 235.

43. Colemen, "Pathological conditions."

44. Betts, WW. "Chalicosis pulmonum: Or, chronic interstitial pneumonia induced by stone dust." DMT 19:354, 1899.

45. Ibid., Jones PE, Discussion, 361 - 62.

46. Ibid., Mayo, HM, in Discussion, 363 - 64.

47. Thompson WG. *The Occupational Diseases*, 615. New York, 1914. Citation of a study by S. C. Hotchkiss done for the U. S. Bureau of Mines.

48. Beyer TE. "Silicosis." CM 26:413, 1929.

49. Beyer TE. "The gold rush—its cost in health and life." RMMJ May 1959.

50. Lee, *Report*, 28.

51. Gibbons, *San Juan*, 167.

52. Lee, *Report*, 46 -61.

53. *Biennial Report on Labor Statistics, Colorado, 1901 - 02*, 271. Denver, 1903.

54. The Rico Sun, December 26, 1891.

55. Levine B. *Cities of Gold. History of the Victor-Cripple Creek Mining District*, 49. Denver, 1981.

56. Exline, "Sanitation," 240.

57. Lee, *Report*, 29, 48.

58. Gibbons, *San Juan*, 128, 132.

59. Aspen Daily Times, Dec. 24, 1888.

60. Lee, *Report*, 69.

61. Anderson, *Gold to Ghosts*, 57.

62. Gibbons, *San Juan*, 46.

63. Lee, *Report*, 26.

Chapter 6

1. CMJ 2:96, 1896.

2. Stone WF. *History of Colorado*, I, 769. Chicago, 1918.

3. Kahn SG. "The history of the pioneers in medicine in Lake County." TCSMS 31:488, 1901; Coquoz RL. *The History of Medicine in Leadville and Lake County, Colorado*. NP, 1967; *Corbet, Hoye and Company. Business Directory . . . 1880*, 423 - 25. Denver, 1880.

4. *First Annual Report of the Board of Health of the State of Colorado for the Fiscal Year, Ending September 30, 1876*, 11. Denver, 1877.

5. Baskin OL. *History of the Arkansas Valley, Colorado*, 728. Chicago, 1880.

6. Rico Democrat, November 6, 1891.

7. Carden WD. "Nineteenth century physicians in Clear Creek County, Colorado, 1865 - 1895." Master's thesis, Yale University, 1968.

8. *Pioneers of the San Juan*, II, 169. Colorado Springs, 1946.

9. Hall JN. *Tales of Pioneer Practice*, 24. Denver, 1937.

10. Carden, "Clear Creek County," 40.

11. Griswold DL, Griswold JH. *The Carbonate Camp Called Leadville*, 94. Denver, 1951.

12. Gardiner CF. *Doctor at Timberline*, 25. Caldwell, Idaho, 1938.

13. Crossen F. *Mining Camp Doctor and Other Stories*, 16. Western Yesterdays, IV. Boulder, 1966.

14. Bennett EL. *Boom Town Boy in Old Creede, Colorado*, 83. Chicago, 1966.

15. Collins WR. "Recollections of pioneer life in Colorado—as told to JR Harvey." Colo. Mag. 18:217, 1941. Three quarters of a century later, the future Dr. William, then eight years old, recalled the hardships and adventures of the trip.

16. Digerness DS. *The Mineral Belt*, III, 57 - 58. Silverton, 1982; Horner JM. *Silver Town*, 61-62. Caldwell, Idaho, 1950.

17. Collins, "Recollections"; Carden, "Clear Creek County," 94.

18. Rathmell R. Of Record and Reminiscence - Ouray and Silverton, 67. Ouray, Colorado, 1976; Gibbons JJ. *In the San Juan, Colorado; Sketches*. Chicago, 1898; Herstrom GM. "Holy men in the San Juans." Denver Westerners Brand Book, XX, 239. Edited by FJ Rizzari. Denver, 1965.

19. *Portrait and Biographical Record*, 697. Chicago, 1899.

20. Mumey N. *History of Tin Cup, Colorado*, 147 - 150, 102. Boulder, 1963.

21. Poet SE. "The story of Tincup, Colorado." Colo Mag 9:30, 1932.

22. *Pioneers of the San Juan*, II, 169. Colorado Springs, 1949.

23. Denver Republican, November 6, 1895.

24. Carden, "Clear Creek County."

25. Baskin, *Arkansas Valley*, 728.

26. Thomas L. *Good Evening Everybody*, 23 24. New York, 1976; Levine B. *Cities of Gold. History of the Victor-Cripple Creek Mining District*, 76, 91 - 95. Denver, 1981; Levine B. *Lowell Thomas' Victor*. Colorado Springs, 1982.

27. *Portrait*, 1240; Hambeutel L. *Nuggets from Chalk Creek*. Colorado Springs, 1975. The Mary Murphy was said to have been named for a nurse.

28. Rico Democrat, July 3, 1891.

29. Baskin, *Arkansas Valley*, 749, 405; Carden, "Clear Creek County," 133.

30. CMJ 2:62, 1896.

31. CMJ 2:124, 95, 125 1896.

32. Carden, "Clear Creek County," 46 - 48; *Portrait*, 1245; Baskin, *Arkansas Valley*, 326.

33. Ibid., Carden, 49 - 50.

34. Nicholson E. *Patrick J. Ryan Remembers*. Twin Lakes, Colorado, 1943.

35. *Portrait*, 1245.

36. Carden, "Clear Creek County," 52.

37. Baskin, *Arkansas Valley*, 274.

38. Gambell FW. "Report to the Mayor and the Board of Health of the City of Leadville." In *Life in Leadville, 1882*, 23. Leadville, 1982.

39. Backus H. *Tomboy Bride*, 72. Boulder, 1969.

40. Critique 11:221, 1904.

41. Gimlett PF. *Over Trails of Yesterday*, Book 8, 31. Salida, Colorado, 1949.

42. *Pioneers*, II, 150.

43. Georgetown Courier, April 3, 1879.

44. Fairplay Flume, June 5, 1879. Cited by N. Flynn: *History of the Famous Mosquito Pass*. Denver, 1959.

45. Nicholson, *Patrick J. Ryan*, 9.

46. Gardiner, *Doctor at Timberline*, 45 - 58.

47. Hambeutel, *Chalk Creek*, 57.

48. Anderson P. *From Gold to Ghosts. A History of St. Elmo, Colorado*, 58. Gunnison, 1983.

49. Peterson FC. *Hillside Cemetery, Silverton, San Juan County, Colorado*. Silverton, 1981.

50. Archives of the Society of Leadville Pioneers. Cited in Griswold, *Carbonate Camp*, 92-3.

51. Ingham GT. *Digging Gold Among the Rockies*, 431. Philadelphia, 1882.

52. Shinn JA. "Characteristics of Leadville miners." In Manning JF. *Leadville, Lake County and the Gold Belt*, 50. Denver, 1895.

53. Fish EH: "First aid to injured miners." CMJ 2:41, 1898; CMJ 4:216, 246 1898.

54. Leadville Chronicle December, 1878. In Gilmore J. *We Came North. A History of the Sisters of Charity of Leavenworth*, 53 - 57. Kansas City, 1961.

55. Blair E. *Leadville. Colorado's Magic City*, 124. Boulder, 1980.

56. Baskin, *Arkansas Valley*, 306.

7. Coquoz, RL. *The History of Medicine in Leadville and Lake County, Colorado*, 6. NP, 1967.

58. Manning, *Leadville, Lake City*, 117.

59. Howlett WJ: *Life of the Right Reverend Joseph P. Machebeuf*, 388. Pueblo, 1908.

60. Griswold,DL and JH: *The Carbonate Camp Called Leadville*, 177 - 78. Denver, 1951.

61. Gilmore, *We Came North*, 56.

62. Manning, *Leadville, Lake City*.

63. Baskin OL. *History of Clear Creek and Boulder Valleys, Colorado*, 292. Chicago, 1880.

64. Colorado Miner, May 15, 1880. In Horner, *Silver Town*, 314. The building was part of a complex of structures in Georgetown which included the church, rectory, and parochial school. In 1917 the hospital was torn down and its brick used to build a new church.

65. *Pioneers of the San Juan*, IV, 114.

66. Breckenridge Daily Journal, March 1, 1888. In Fiester M. *Blasted Beloved Breckenridge*, 139-40. Boulder, 1973. No new hospital was forthcoming, however, and the sisters left Breckenridge in 1890. Finally in 1906 a private residence was purchased and converted into a county hospital.

67. Ouray County Historical Museum Archives.

68. Gibbons, *San Juan*, 81.

69. Ouray County Historical Museum Archives. The sisters continued to run the hospital until 1918. The following year they sold it to Dr. C.V. Bates. The Bates Hospital and Sanitarium's claim to fame was its "hot radioactive healing waters [obtained] from natural springs."

70. Typewritten manuscript by Sue Huffman, May 1, 1964. Provided by Dr. James Delaney. The building is now a hotel.

71. *Life in Leadville - 1882*, 15. Leadville, 1981.

72. JAMA 38:1521, 1902.

73. Levine, *Victor*, 74.

74. JAMA 36:821, 1901.

75. Rico Democrat, February 6, 1891.

76. RMN, February 15, 1883.

77. CM 6:460, 1909.

78. Notes in the Aspen Historical Museum, no author cited.

79. Fetter RL, Fetter S. *Telluride*, 188. Caldwell, Idaho, 1979; Denver Times, December 29, 1901; CM 9:87, 1903.

80. Aspen Times, March 26, 1891.

81. Aspen Times, April 12, 1891.

82. Aspen Times, July 22, 1891.

83. Aspen Times, July 18, 1891.

84. Aspen Times, July 21, 1891.

85. Aspen Times, September 12, 1891.

86. *Pioneers of the San Juan*, II, 170.

87. Gilmore, *We Came North*, 212 - 14.

88. Ouray County Historical Museum Archives. Dated 1891.

89. Ouray County Historical Museum Archives.

Chapter 7

1. Simonin LL. *The Rocky Mountain West in 1867*, 32 - 33. Lincoln, 1966.

2. Letter by D.C. Collier, Apr. 9, 1859. In *Pike's Peak Gold Rush Guidebooks of 1859*, 230. Edited by LR Hafen. Glendale, 1941.

3. *Denver City and Auraria, the Commercial Emporium of the Pikes Peak Gold Regions in 1859*, 12. St. Louis, 1860.

4. Letter by William Larimer to The Leavenworth Times. In Hafen, *Colorado Gold Rush*, 249.

5. *Denver City and Auraria*, 26. Apparently there were many more than eight physicians in town. Unlisted in the directory, for example, are a number of physicians whose names appeared in the early newspapers, as in an advertisement for "G.N. Woodward, M.D., Physician and Surgeon, Denver City, K.T." in the April 23, 1859 issue of the Cherry Creek Pioneer. K. T. stood for Kansas Territory, in which early Denver was located in 1859.

6. RMN, May 23, 1860.

7. "Skillful surgical operation." The Mountaineer, Sept. 27, 1860.

8. Zamonski SW, Keller T. *The '59ers: Roaring Denver in the Gold Rush Days*, 2nd Edition, 211. Denver, 1967.

9. Ibid., 56, 194-95, 206. Reference is to to Dr. William M. Bell. However, I was unable to find a physician of that name. Probably, Dr. William Belt.

10. Hill AP. *Colorado Pioneers in Picture and Story*, 125. Denver, 1915. Dr. Cass's interest in gold was not limited to his fee. He subsequently left medicine to become a successful gold broker and banker. Having made a fortune during the Civil War, he invested in Denver real estate and died in 1894, a wealthy man. Stone WF. *History of Colorado*, III, 735. Chicago, 1918.

11. "File No. 4." Colorado Territorial District Court for Arapahoe, Weld and Douglas Counties. August 1, 1861.

12. Lemen LE. "The Medical Profession in Colorado." In Smiley JD, Goudy FC. *Semi-centennial History of Colorado*, I, 666. Chicago, 1913.

13. Boyd LC. "History of the Denver General Hospital, 1860 - 1924." Unpublished typewritten manuscript in the Denver General Hospital library. Boyd states that this building was at the southwest corner of Lawrence and either 7th or 8th streets and that Dr. A.R. Sternberger and his brother had come to the Denver area in 1860.

14. RMN, August 8, 1860. There is also mention of a mysterious "London Hospital" next door to the Jefferson House. RMN, August 27, 1859.

15. RMN, October 17, 1860.

16. Wharton JE. *History of the city of Denver*, 65. Denver, 1866.

17. Boyd, "History." This may have been the smallpox hospital opened by Dr. Cass in 1860 at Larimer and 19th Streets.

18. RMN, October 17, 1860.

19. Smiley JD, editor. *History of Denver*, 770. Denver, 1901.

20. Boyd, "History." The poorhouse was moved in 1867 from 11th Street between Wazee and Market, to 9th and Champa.

21. Hill KL. "A History of Public Health in Denver, 1859 - 1900." Master's thesis, University of Denver,1970. Elsner was County Physician from 1870 to 1873. Bancroft was County Physician from 1866- 69 and City Physician from 1872- 1876 and 1877 - 1878.

22. Hill, *Colorado Pioneers*, 23; Elsner J: "Reminiscences," DMT 28:1, 1908. The first County Hospital was located near 10th and Stout. In 1873 it was relocated to a building across the street from the construction site of the new County Hospital at Sixth and Cherokee.

23. Boyd, "History;" *Denver General Hospital*. A booklet published upon completion of the new Denver General Hospital in 1970. No author cited. In addition to the references cited below, information regarding Denver General Hospital was obtained from these two sources.

24. "County Physician's Report on County Hospital." Weekly RMN, November 11, 1874.

25. Minutes of the Denver Medical Association, Meeting of May 27, 1873. Hill, "Public health," 24.

26. Boyd, "History," 4.

27. Boice J. "Surgical cases treated in the Arapahoe County Hospital." Gross Med Coll Bull 3:117, 1894.

28. Boyd, "History," 6.

29. Colo Climatol 1:48, 1895.

30. Boyd, "History," 6 - 7.

31. Wetherill HG. "An open letter to the Board of County

Commissioners." December 7, 1907.

32. JAMA 41:318, 1903.

33. DMT 30:92, 1910 - 11.

34. For example, Charles A. Johnson's *Denver's Mayor Speer*, Denver, 1969.

35. Boyd, "History."

36. Municipal Facts, November - December, 1925.

37. CM 16:129, 1919.

38. CM 11:471, 1914.

39. DMB, September 30, 1916.

40. Boyd, "History."

41. "Politics in Denver's County Hospital." CM 16:129, 1919.

42. *Second Annual Report of the Social Welfare Department of the City and County of Denver, Colorado for the Year Ending December 31, 1914.*

43. Denver Municipal Facts, November 18, 1911

44. Dean EF. "Serving one-third of the city's population—The Denver General Hospital." Municipal Facts Mar-Apr, 1927.

45. Stauffer DA. "Two bells at the County Hospital." Municipal Facts 3:14, 1920.

46. Dorsett LW. *The Queen City: A History of Denver*, 106. Boulder, 1977. An attempt to establish a tuberculosis sanitarium for blacks near Colorado Springs in 1911 was unsuccessful. JAMA 56:355, 1911. The proposed sanitarium was to be built near Calhan, Colorado, on 480 acres donated by a former slave, James Polk Taylor, and his wife. It was to be called the National Lincoln-Douglas Sanitarium.

47. *Mortality Statistics.* Annual Reports of the Bureau of the Census, 1890 - 1920. U.S. Department of Commerce, Washington, D.C.

48. Dorsett, *Queen City*, 105; De Mund M: *Women Physicians of Colorado*, 34. Denver, 1976; Melrose F. RMN, Feb. 21, 1982. Dr. Ford was born in Illinois and graduated from Chicago's Hering Medical College in 1899.

49. Melrose, RMN. When Dr. Ford applied for her Colorado medical license in 1902, the examiner told her that he regretted charging her a fee, noting that she had two strikes against her—"first you're a lady, and second, you're colored." Dr. Ford's longtime office-home at 2335 Arapahoe Street is being restored. She died in 1952.

50. *Eighth Biennial Report of the Bureau of Labor Statistics of the State of Colorado, 1901 - 1902*, 299. Denver, 1902.

51. Ibid., 299 - 300.

52. Bennett AL. "Report of State Medical Inspector of Chinese." *Sixth Report of the State Board of Health of Colorado, 1901 - 02.*

53. Bennett AL. "Report of the State Medical Inspector of Chinese." *Seventh Report of the State Board of Health of Colorado, 1903 - 04.*

54. *Eighth Biennial Report . . . Bureau of Labor*, 301.

55. Bennett, "Report . . . 1901 - 02."

56. Bennett, "Report . . . 1903 - 04."

57. Bennett, "Report . . . 1901 - 02."

58. Parkhill F. *Wildest of the West*, 113-14. New York, 1951.

59. CMJ 7:564, 1901.

60. Bennett, "Report . . . 1901 - 02."

61. Parkhill, *Wildest of the West*. Bubonic plague was the other exotic disease said to be carried by Chinese and other Orientals. In 1900 reports of this "dread disease" in San Francisco led Colorado to close its borders to all Chinese and Japanese travelers. CMJ 6:366, 1900.

62. Dorsett, *Queen City*, 94, 124.

63. CM 12:438, 915.

64. CMJ 3:432, 1897.

65. *Annual Report of the Superintendent of the County Hospital of the City and County of Denver, 1909.*

66. CM 33:197, 1956.

67. Perilli G. *Colorado and the Italians in Colorado*, 45. Denver, 1922.

68. JAMA 47:598, 1906.

69. Baker J, Hafen LR: *History of Colorado*, V, 682. Denver, 1927.

70. Perilli, *Colorado and the Italians*, 45.

71. *First Annual Report of the Social Welfare Department of the City and County of Denver, Colorado, 1913*, 42.

72. DMT 33:443, 1913-14.

73. In addition to the references cited below, some of the material on these physicians was obtained from the Centennial Editions of the Colorado Medical Society's

Rocky Mountain Medical Journal, Vol. 68, Nos. 4 and 5, 1971.

74. Byers WN. *Encyclopedia of Biography of Colorado*, 446. Chicago, 1901.

75. Elder CS. "Medicine." In *History of Colorado*, III. Edited by JH Baker and LR Hafen. Denver, 1927.

76. In addition to other references cited, much of the material on Elsner was obtained from Hornbein M. "Dr. John Elsner, A Colorado pioneer." Western States Jewish Quarterly; Uchill IL. *Peddlars, Pioneers and Tzadikim*, 25-27, 42 - 48. Denver, 1957; Elsner J: "Reminiscences" DMT 28:1, 1908. Much of the material on Bancroft was obtained from Bancroft C. "Pioneer doctor - F.J. Bancroft" Colo Mag 39:195, 1962; Rogers EJA. "Dr. F.J. Bancroft" DMT 23:24, 1903; and from the Bancroft scrapbooks and from conversations with his grandaughter, Miss Caroline Bancroft.

77. Dr. Elsner kept a record of these circumcisions in a little notebook, indicating name, place, and date, from 1867 until 1905, a valuable record of Colorado Jewish history.

78. Spivak CD. "The Union Catalogue of Medical Books, and some of the private medical libraries in the city of Denver." CMJ 3:214, 1897.

79. Uchill, *Peddlars*, 47. Statement attributed to Amy Salomon Leifton.

80. Historical material on St. Joseph's Hospital was obtained from Gilmore J. *We Came North*; Grant WW. "History of St. Joseph's Hospital" TCSMS 31:519, 1901; "100 years of care." Towerscope, January, 1973; several typewritten manuscripts summarizing the hospital's early admission's books, provided by Dr. James Delaney.

81. Ibid., Towerscope.

82. *St. Joseph's Hospital Report For the Year Ending December 31, 1905.*

83. Some of the historical material relating to St. Luke's was obtained from Peabody O. "The Birth of a Hospital," NP:ND; The Colorado Prospector, Vol. 16, No. 3, 1985.

84. *St. Luke's Hospital, Boulevard, Denver, Colorado.* Undated pamphlet, apparently issued when the hospital was opened in 1881.

85. Ibid., *St. Luke's Hospital; Annual Report of St. Luke's Hospital, 1882.*

86. Ibid., *Annual Report.* It should be noted that not all of St. Luke's patients were socialites. The 1882 report includes, among the hospital's admissions, consumptives from the East ["many dying immediately upon their arrival . . ."] and injured railroad employees and miners from around the state. Worker's expenses for on-the-job injuries were generally paid for by their employers. The *Report* also encouraged contributions so that the hospital could care for "the indigent sick."

87. RMN, July 13, 1882.

88. The original buildings at 19th and Pearl streets have since been replaced.

89. Freeman RB. "History of St. Anthony's Hospital." TCSMS 31:517, 1901.

90. CMJ 8:111, 1902.

91. CMJ 5:339, 1899. It was located at 32nd and Curtis.

92. DMT 20:588, 1901; CMJ 8:226, 1902.

93. Amesse JW. *Children's Hospital*, Denver, 1947.

94. *Fitzsimons General Hospital: The Story of a Great Institution, 1918-1938.* NP, ND; Wier JA. "History of Fitzsimons Army Medical Center. Denver Westerners Roundup, January - February, 1980.

95. Municipal Facts, December, 1918.

96. Municipal Facts 6:12, 1923.

97. Bancroft FJ. "Births and Deaths. Annual Report of the City Physician for 1873." RMN, 1874. (Date unspecified)

98. In 1891, Denver "gained an unenviable notoriety when, from the Marine Hospital Bureau in Washington (the equivalent of today's Public Health Service), a report was circulated putting the death rate of Denver among the highest in the country". The error was due to the inclusion of deaths occuring in the surrounding counties. Steele HK. "The sanitary condition of Denver." *Annual Report of the Denver Real Estate and Stock Exchange, 1891- 1892*, 53. Denver, 1892.

99. *Annual Report and Mortality Statement of the Health Department of the City and County of Denver, 1914.* Denver, 1915.

Chapter 8

1. Chenoweth MS: "Surgery in country practice." DMT 18:495, 1898.

2. These homestead descriptions are derived from Barns CG. *The Sod House*, 57 - 67. Madison, Nebraska, 1930; Long FA. *A Prairie Doctor of the Eighties*, 33 - 43. Norfolk, Nebraska, 1937. Both were written about western Nebraska, but, undoubtedly pertain to neighboring Colorado as well.

3. Bird I. *A Lady's Life in the Rocky Mountains*, 36. New York, 1879.

4. Melvin JT. "Problems in rural sanitation." CMJ 6:77, 1900.

5. CM 20:328, 1923.

6. Davis WB. "Some practical points gathered from sources wise and otherwise" TCSMS 28:288, 1898. A much more serious "country" disease, plague, has become indigenous to parts of Colorado, but only in recent decades.

7. *Pioneers of the San Juan Country*, IV, 226. Denver, 1961.

8. DMT 8B:46, 1889.

9. Hall IC, Gilbert OM. "A survey of botulism in Colorado." CM 26:233, 1929.

10. Axtell ER. "Report of a case of hydrophobia." CMJ 5:456, 1899.

11. Stiles GW. "History of rabies in Colorado." RMMJ 51:102, 1954 #4743)

12. Lemen HA. "Absence of sun-stroke in Colorado." TCSMS 7:76, 1877.

13. Corbett E. *Western Pioneer Days*, 270. Denver, 1974.

14. Hall JN. *Tales of Pioneer Practice*, 109. Denver, 1937.

15. Townshend RB. *Tenderfoot in Colorado*, 161 - 63. London, 1923.

16. Hall JN. "A contribution to the study of accidents from equestrianism." Med News 60:228, 1892.

17. Willis AB. "Queen Ann of Brown's Park." Colo Mag 29:91, 1952.

18. Adams R. *Come an' Get It: The Story of the Old Cowboy Cook*, 40. Norman, Oklahoma, 1952.

19. Townshend, *Tenderfoot*, 57 - 60.

20. Schultz MM. *Tenderfoot Schoolmarm*, 18. Baltimore, 1977.

21. Taylor RF. *Pioneers on the Picketwire*, 53. Pueblo, 1964.

22. Collins M. *Pioneering In The Rockies*, 56. NP, ca. 1910.

23. Propst NB. *Those Strenuous Dames of the Colorado Prairie*, 52, 61. Boulder, 1982.

24. Danielson RW, Danielson, CL. *Basalt: Colorado Midland Town*, 82. Boulder, 1965.

25. *Denver Quaker Cook Book*, Denver, 1905.

26. Hall JN. "A study of the relative frequency of different diseases in private practice." Medicine (Detroit) 2:303, 1896; Hall, *Tales*, 66, 94.

27. Brown RK. "J.N. Hall, Pioneer physician." Denver Westerner's Roundup, July - August, 1981. Hall moved to Denver in 1892, where he became a highly successful internist, professor of medicine, author of many papers and a textbook of medicine, and a leader of Colorado's medical community. He also wrote *Tales of Pioneer Practice*, a collection of medical anecdotes and reminiscences of early Colorado physicians, and a collection of biographies of former presidents of the Colorado Medical Society. After 54 years of practice, Hall died in 1939 at the age of 80, having long since become one of Colorado's best known, respected and beloved physicians.

28. Hall, *Tales*.

29. Law G. "The country doctor in Colorado." DMT 17:433, 1898.

30. CM 12:306, 1915.

31. Hall JN. "Pioneer physicians were a hearty lot." RMN, undated - ca. 1937.

32. Letter from W.A. Hopkins, Nucla, Colorado, to Dr. W.E.Driscoll, Cripple Creek, Colorado. December 18, 1909.

33. Law, "Country doctor"; DMT 30:357, 1910.

34. CMJ 9:87, 1903.

35. DMT 30:358, 1910.

36. CM 13:228, 1916; *The Historical Guide to Routt County*, 48. Steamboat Springs, Colorado, 1979.

37. Law, "Country doctor."

38. Chenoweth, "Surgery."

39. Melvin JT. "The appendicitis question from the standpoint of the country doctor." DMT 16:301, 1896.

40. Gardiner CF. *Doctor at Timberline*, 140. Caldwell,

Idaho, 1938.

41. Hall, *Tales*, 56.

42. *Polk's Medical Registry of the United States and Canada for 1886*. These figures are somewhat deceptive since these physicians also served the surrounding countryside.

43. *Portrait and Biographical Record of the State of Colorado*, 682. Chicago, 1899.

44. Ibid., 1411.

45. Phillips County Historical Society. *Those Were the Days*, 13. Holyoke, Colorado, 1973.

46. Ellis FD. *Come Back to My Valley*, 85. Cortez, Colorado, 1976; Denver Post Aug. 24, 1952; Corbett ER. *West Pioneer Days, . . . Elbert County*, 168. NP, 1974.

47. Harmer WW. "Discussion" CM 5:55, 1908.

48. *Portrait*, 522.

49. Grabow HC. *History of the Fremont County Medical Association*, 1964.

50. Lathrop M. *Don't Fence Me In*, 26. Boulder, 1972.

51. Colo Mag 22:215, 1945.

52. Beshoar B. *Hippocrates in a Red Vest*. Palo Alto, 1973. This full length biography of Dr. Beshoar makes fascinating reading.

53. Byers WN. *Encyclopedia of Biography of Colorado*, 328. Chicago, 1901.

54. Gardiner, *Doctor*, 122.

55. Ellis, *Come Back*.

56. Dunning HM. *Over Hill and Vale*, II, 142. Boulder, 1962.

57. CM 8:115, 1911.

58. CM 5:260, 1908.

59. In later years, Trinidad and its nearby coal camps and towns and Pueblo came to have large Hispanic populations, and still later, Denver and other communities.

60. Law, "Country doctor."

61. *Morgan County Medical Society, 1908 - 1960*, NP, ND.

62. CM 12:351, 1915.

63. Beshoar, *Hippocrates*, 342 - 344.

64. Campa A. "Superstition and witchcraft along the Rio Grande." Denver Westerners Brand Book, V, 172, 181. Edited by Don Bloch. Denver, 1950.

65. Moore M. *Los Remedios de la Gente*. Santa Fe, 1977; Ford KC. *Las Yerbas de la Gente: A Study of Hispano-American Medicinal Plants*. Ann Arbor, 1975; Curtin LSM. *Healing Herbs of the Upper Rio Grande*. Los Angeles, 1965. Some early Hispanic medical attitudes, concepts, and treatments are still in use.

66. Moore, *Los Remedios*.

67. McFadzean J. "The Mexican from the viewpoint of the medical practitioner." CM 4:133, 1907.

68. TCSMS 32:183, 1902.

69. *Twelfth Biennial Report of the Bureau of Labor Statistics of the State of Colorado, 1909 - 1910*, 13. Denver, 1911.

70. *Eighth Biennial Report of the Bureau of Labor Statistics of the State of Colorado, 1901 - 1902, 380*. Denver, 1902.

71. Lemen HA. "A case of so-called phthisis pulmonalis nigra." TCSMS 11:105, 1881.

72. Green FHY, Laqueur WA. "Coal workers' pneumoconiosis." Path Ann 15(2):333, 1980.

73. Editorial. "Carbon monoxide and canaries in mines." New Mex Med J 12:102, 1914.

74. Selekman BM. *Employee's Representation in Coal Mines*, 54. New York, 1924.

75. *Bienn Report, 1909 - 10*, 37.

76. Taylor G. "The conservation of life and property in mines." Indust Survey May 6, 1911.

77. Ibid.

78. *Colorado Year Book, 1932*, 243. Denver, 1933.

79. DMT 32:75, 1912.

80. DMT 32:68, 75; CM 9:246, 1912.

81. Gage WV. "A first-aid packet for miner's use." JAMA 61:768, 1913.

82. *Industrial Relations. Final Report and Testimony Submitted to Congress by the Commission on Industrial Relations*, Vol 9, 8930 - 31. Washington, D. C., 1916.

83. Beshoar M. "Report of Committe on General Hygiene." *Fifth Report of the Colorado State Board of Health, 1894 - 1900*, 84. Denver, 1901.

84. *Industrial Relations*, 8930.

85. *Industrial Relations*, 8500, 8556.

86. Smiley JC, Goudy FC. *Semi-centennial History of Colorado*, II, 182.

87. *Hospital Report of the Colorado Fuel and Iron Company*,

1899 - 1900, 58. In intussusception, a portion of intestine telescopes itself foward into the succeeding portion of intestine. This can result in necrosis of the affected portion of intestine and death.

88. *Industrial Relations*, 8500.

89. *Industrial Relations*, 8498.

90. Beshoar B. *Out of the Depths*, 8. Denver, 1942.

91. Material on the CF & I's medical activities and hospital was derived from several sources, including the early hospital reports of the Colorado Fuel and Iron Company; Scamehorn HL. *Pioneer Steelmaker in the West. The Colorado Fuel and Iron Company, 1872 - 1903*. Boulder, 1976; Taylor RC. *Pueblo*. Pueblo, 1979; Corwin RW. "History of the Colorado Fuel and Iron Company's hospital." TCSMS 31:512, 1901.

92. Corwin's actual employer in the early years was a predecessor of CF & I, the Colorado Coal and Iron Company, and the original hospital was the result of a joint effort by that company and the Denver and Rio Grande Railway.

93. Corwin, "History."

94. Corwin RW. "Thirty years experience with fractures at Minnequa Hospital." JAMA 57:1351, 1911.

95. Smiley, *Colorado*, II, 235; Corwin, "Thirty Years"; Corwin, "History."

96. In 1948, the hospital was given to the Sisters of Charity and their old St. Mary's Hospital was replaced by the new St. Mary-Corwin Hospital. Pueblo's complement of hospitals was also increased by the addition of Parkview Episcopal Hospital, originally founded in 1923.

97. McGovern GS, Guttridge LF. *The Great Coalfield War*, 172 - 74. Boston, 1972.

98. Beshoar, *Hippocrates*, 337.

99. Papanikolas Z. *Buried Unsung: Louis Tikas and the Ludlow Massacre*, 187. Salt Lake City, 1982.

100. Fink WH. *The Ludlow Massacre*, 15. NP, 1915.

101. *Industrial Relations*, 6352.

102. *Industrial Relations*, 6350.

103. *Industrial Relations*, 7367.

104. *Industrial Relations*, 7364.

105. *Industrial Relations*, 7364; West GP. *U. S. Commission on Industrial Relations - Report on the Strike*, 129. Washington, D. C., 1915.

106. CM 11:385, 1914.

107. Wetherill HG. "Letter to the editor of the Philadelphia Public Ledger," November 17, 1914.

108. Selekman, *Employee's Representation*, 10, 131 - 33.

Chapter 9

1. Shollenberger CF. "The physician from a business standpoint." Gross Med Coll Bull 5:13, 1895.

2. Cathell DW. *Book on the Physician Himself*, 4. Philadelphia, 1890. Dr. Cathell's book was a highly popular and widely used compendium of practical advice "on things that concern [the physician's] reputation and success." It was first published in 1882 and, in its multiple editions, was probably used by many of Colorado's early physicians. I have used the "revised and expanded" edition of 1890.

3. Ibid., 5.

4. Ibid., 11 - 13.

5. DMT 4:115, 1885; CMJ 3:385, 1897. Stover became one of Denver's pioneer radiologists, Dean of the Denver and Gross Medical School, and Professor of Radiology at the University of Colorado School of Medicine.

6. Cathell, *Book*, 86.

7. DMT 32:125, 1912 - 1913.

8. Edwards EG. "Working the doctor." JAMA 46:898, 1906.

9. Morgan JW. "Birth registration in Colorado." CM 16:38, 1919.

10. *The Colorado Telephone Company*, 1880. Reprint. NP, ND.

11. CM 5:178, 1908.

12. CM 12:306, 1915.

13. Spivak C. "Medical reprints." JAMA 39:1018, 1902.

14. Spivak CD. "The Union Catalogue of medical books, and some of the private medical libraries in the city of Denver." CMJ 3:214, 1897.

15. Cathell, *Book*, 6 - 24.

16. Fee Bill of the Denver and Arapahoe Medical Society, 1895.

17. Descriptions of saddle bags and other equipment are from various late nineteenth century medical and surgical supply house catalogues.

18. The costs of some of these items in the 1890s is of interest. A stethescope was $2 - 4, a thermometer $1 - 2, and a kit containing various surgical instruments about $20 - 30. A syringe kit was about $2. Steel needles cost 35 cents; they were resharpened and used many times. A gold or platinum needle cost up to $1. A doctor's bag cost from $3 - 5 and saddlebags as much as $10. A pair of obstetrical forceps varied from $3 - 10.

19. DMT 32:185, 1912 - 1913.

20. Corbett ER. *Western Pioneer Days . . . . Elbert County*. NP, 1974. The reference is to Dr. Robert H. Denney of Elbert County.

21. Cathell, *Book*, 22.

22. CM 11:357, 1914.

23. CM 11:176,278,357, 1914.

24. Cathell, *Book*, 287.

25. CMJ 3:357, 1897.

26. Hadsell CA. "Faith." CM 5:455, 1908.

27. Arvada Historical Society. *More Than Gold*, 183 - 84. Boulder, 1976. Based on information supplied by Ruth Foster Hughes.

28. Spivak CD. "A bio-ethnological study of the organized medical profession of the state of Colorado." CM 23:188, 1926. Spivak's study was done in 1925, but since the average age of his respondents was forty-seven, the data provides information on physicians who, on the average, began their practices in the early 1900s. It should be noted that the survey was limited to members of the Colorado Medical Society. It also appears to have been limited to men.

29. Cathell, *Book*, 30, 62.

30. DMT 6:116, 1886.

31. CM 2:95, 1905.

32. TCSMS 15:9, 1885.

33. McMurtrie DC. *Early Printing in Colorado*, 201. Denver, 1935.

34. Spivak, "Bio-ethnological study." Again, Spivak's study was limited to men.

35. Firebaugh EM. *The Physician's Wife*. Philadelphia, 1894. Mrs. Firebaugh, herself, was the wife of a mid-Western physician.

36. Ibid., 17, 59.

37. Ibid., 52, 82.

38. Ibid., 182.

39. Cathell, *Book*, 87-89.

40. CM 9:357, 1912.

41. CMJ 2:297, 1896.

42. Elder CS. "Medicine." In *History of Colorado*, III, 1041. Edited by JH Baker and LR Hafen. Denver, 1927.

43. CM 10:227, 1913.

44. Love MCT. "The lying-in chamber." TCSMS 32:359, 1902.

45. Carden WD. "Nineteenth century physicians in Clear Creek County, Colorado, 1865 - 1895." 153. Master's thesis, Yale University, 1968.

46. Ibid., 82, 145.

47. Williams WH. "Address." TCSMS 7:35, 1877.

48. De Mund M. *Women Physicians of Colorado*, 64. Denver, 1976. Much of the biographical material on women physicians was obtained from this invaluable source and from Dr. Mary Reed Stratton's compilation of biographies of Colorado's women physicians. Manuscript in the Denver Medical Society's library.

49. Ibid., 46. Dr. Lawney, who was 36 years old when she graduated, practiced in Denver for nearly 30 years.

50. *University of Colorado Catalogue and Circular of Information, 1883 - 1884*.

51. JAMA 1:183, 1883.

52. *Directory of Officers and Graduates*. University of Colorado Bulletin, 1921.

53. Melrose F. "Interview with Dr. Agnes Ditson." RMN Jan 31, 1982.

54. Gross Med Coll Bull 5:66, 1895.

55. Critique 10:66, 1903. The comment was in reference to Dr. Frona Abbott, a professor at the Denver Homeopathic Medical College.

56. Steele HK. "Address." TCTMS 5:32, 1875.

57. Love MCT. "Women practitioners of Colorado." TSCMS 32:503, 1901.

58. De Mund, *Women*, 39.

59. Love, "Women practitioners." The office was that of secretary, filled by Drs. Laura Liebhardt, 1895 - 1896, and Minnie C. T. Love, 1897 - 1901.

60. Marrett CB. "On the evolution of women's medical societies." Bull Hist Med 53:434, 1979.

61. CMJ 3:195, 1897. In 1906, the Woman's Medical Society of Denver was incorporated.

62. Love, "Women practitioners."

63. CMJ 6:301, 1900.

64. "M." "The woman physician." CMJ 6:462, 1900.

65. Data collected from *Medical Coloradoana*. Denver, 1922. The first of these appears to have been by Dr. Kate Lobingier - "Mechanical influences in pelvic disorders." TCSMS 21:253, 1891.

66. DMT 11:36, 1892.

67. Love, "Women practitioners."

68. Smith P. "Dr. Mary Solander." The Colorado Daily, May 31, 1982.

69. Love MCT. "Comments." TCSMS 29:454, 1899.

70. Bates ME. "The new movement in dress reform." TCSMS 24:325, 1894.

71. De Mund, *Women*, 14; Bollinger ET. *Rails that Climb. The Story of the Moffat Road*, 130. Santa Fe, 1950.

72. Ibid., De Mund, 52; Brenneman B. "Lady doctor 54 years." RMN Mar. 21, 1957.

73. CMJ 2:56, 1896.

74. De Mund, *Women*, 59, 57, 47. In her later years, Dr. Long wrote several guidebook-histories of the Santa Fe, Oregon, and Smoky Hill trails, based on her extensive automobile explorations.

75. Stratton, "Biographies"; Baker JH, Hafen LR. *History of Colorado*, V, 114. Denver, 1927.

76. De Mund, *Women*, 20; Stratton, "Biographies."

77. Although born in Central City, Dr. Florence Sabin's remarkable accomplishments in research and academic medicine were made at Johns Hopkins and the Rockefeller Institute; it was not until her "retirement" to Colorado in the late 1930s that she began her second career in public health.

78. De Mund, *Women*, 48; Stratton, "Biographies;" Denver Post, May 13, 1942; RMN, May 13, 1942.

79. Ibid., Denver Post.

Chapter 10

1. RMN, June 6, 1860. Cited in Jayne WA. "Historical notes of the Colorado State Medical Society." CM 9:339, 1912. "Jefferson" referred to the proposed name for the territory which later became Colorado.

2. Bancroft FJ."Address as President of the Colorado State Medical Society at its Eleventh Annual Convention." 1881.

3. Gehrung, EC. Personal communication. Cited in *Medical Coloradoana*, 5. Denver, 1922.

4. Bancroft, "Address."

5. "Official minutes of those first meetings [of the Denver Medical Assn]." DMB May 1971.

6. *Report of the Meeting for the Organization of a Territorial Medical Society Held in Denver, Colorado, Tuesday, September 19, 1871*, 4.

7. Kimball JH. "Inaugural address read before the Denver Medical Assn." DMT 2:161, 1883.

8. Cole S. "Address at Third Annual Meeting of the Arapahoe County Medical Society." DMT 5:233, 1885.

9. Hill KL. "A history of public health in Denver," 98. Master's thesis, University of Denver, 1970.

10. Gross Med Coll Bull 6:48, 1896.

11. Fleming CK. "Address." DMT 20:443, 1901.

12. McGraw HR. "The County Society." CM 9:122, 1912.

13. "Report of the Meeting."

14. "Any regular graduate . . ." did not include women during the society's first fourteen years.

15. RMN, September 20, 1871.

16. *Proceedings of the Second Annual Meeting of the Territorial Medical Society, 1872*.

17. *Proceedings of the Third Annual Meeting of the Territorial Medical Society, 1873*.

18. *Proceedings of the Fourth Annual Meeting of the Territorial Medical Society, 1874*.

19. Beshoar B. *Hippocrates in a Red Vest*, 155. Palo Alto, 1973.

20. *By-laws of the Rocky Mountain Medical Association*. Trinidad, Colorado, 1875.

21. Taylor MF. *Trinidad, Colorado Territory*, 140. Trinidad, Colorado, 1966.

22. *Proceedings of the Seventh Annual Meeting of the Territorial Medical Society, 1877*.

23. *Proceedings of the Fifth Annual Meeting of the Territorial Medical Society, 1875*.

24. *Proceedings of the Sixth Annual Meeting of the Colorado State Medical Society, 1876*.

25. *Proceedings of the Tenth Annual Meeting of the Colorado State Medical Society, 1880*.

26. *Proceedings of the Sixteenth Annual Meeting of the Colorado State Medical Society, 1886*.

27. DMT 5:27, 1885.

28. CMJ 2:60, 1896.

29. Councilman WT. "Anatomical consideration of tumors of the brain." CM 12:289, 1915.

30. Johnson, C. "As it looks to a 'Country Doctor'." CM 2:311, 1905.

31. CM 2:287, 1905.

32. Hall JN. *Tales of Pioneer Practice*, 67. Denver, 1937.

33. TCSMS 32:7, 1902.

34. CM 7:389, 1910.

35. Hall, *Tales*, 70.

36. CMJ 4:227, 1898.

37. *Program of the Meeting of the American Medical Association Held in Denver, Colorado, June, 1898*.

38. CMJ 4:227, 1898.

39. CMJ 4:265, 1898.

40. Bancroft, "Address."

41. CM 4:81, 1907.

42. TCSMS 13:5, 1883.

43. CM 5:100, 1908.

44. Epler C. "The medical society." CM 5:45, 1908.

45. CM 5:100, 1908.

46. CM 9:95, 1912.

47. CM 2:143, 1905.

48. Kenney FW. *The History of the Denver Clinical and Pathological Society, 1892 - 1935*. NP, ND.

49. Denver Republican, April 11, 1903.

50. CM 2:112, 1905. The academy was absorbed into the Denver Medical Society in 1909. The Denver Clinical and Pathological Society is alive and well and looking foward to its centenary.

51. Steele HK. "Address." TCTMS 5:32, 1875.

52. Baker SL. "Physician licensure laws in the United States, 1865 - 1915." J Hist Med Allied Sci 39:173, 1984.

53. In the nineteenth century, M.D.s included a majority of "regular," or orthodox physicians and a minority of "irregulars" such as homeopaths, eclectics, and others.

54. Hawes J. "Charlatanism in Colorado." TCSMS 13:37, 1883.

55. Hall JN. "Early registration of physicians in Colorado." CM 65:207, 1935.

56. Hall JN. "The work of the State Board of Medical Examiners for the past year." TCSMS 21:103, 1891.

57. DMT 5:115, 1895 - 96.

58. CM 1:121, 1905.

59. "An Act to Protect the Public Health and Regulate the Practice of Medicine in Colorado, April 20, 1905."

60. CM 2:121, 1905.

61. Church WF. "The Colorado Medical Law in operation." CM 2:303, 1905.

62. CM 2:308, 1905.

63. Ibid.

64. Van Meter SD. "A plea for concerted action of the profession in matters pertaining to medical legislation in Colorado." CM 6:212, 1909.

65. In 1938 the name was changed again, to the *Rocky Mountain Medical Journal* and in 1980, back to *Colorado Medicine*.

66. Actually, for one year, this journal was called the *Rocky Mountain Medical Times*. It subsequently became the *Denver Medical Times* and *Utah Medical Journal* and then, in 1915, reorganized into the more regional *Western Medical Journal*. Some of the most colorful quotes contained in this book were written by Dr. Hawkins and other *Denver Medical Times* editors.

67. The *Colorado Medical Journal* began, in 1894-1895, as

The Colorado Climatologist and Denver Medical News. It ceased publication in 1906. Beggs WN. "The origin and development of the Colorado Medical Journal." TCSMS 31:523, 1901.

68. Beshoar, *Hippocrates,* 291; Rothwell PD. "Sketch of the Health Monitor." TCSMS 31:520, 1901.

69. CM 8:116, 1911.

70. CM 9:65, 1912.

Chapter 11

1. Shollenberger CF. "The physician from a business point of view." Gross Med Coll Bull 5:13, 1895.

2. Rothwell WJ. "Ethics. Address by the Dean to the Graduating Class of Gross Medical College." DMT 22:13, 1902.

3. CM 22:220, 1923.

4. It is also interesting to note that, while today's physician's fees are five to ten times higher than those of 1860 and 1909, they have increased at a much lower rate than hospital costs. Today's hospital costs are hundreds of times higher than they were in the early days.

5. "Schedule of wages paid in Colorado." *Biennial Report, Bureau of Labor Statistics Colorado, 1901 - 02,* 91 - 94.

6. Greenleaf LN. *King Sham, and Other Atrocities in Verse,* 20. New York, 1868.

7. CM 13:228, 1916.

8. Schollenberger, "The physician."

9. Colo Climatol 1:26, 1894-5.

10. Editorial. "The medical profession as an economic factor." Reprinted from Medical World in CMJ 3:151, 1902.

11. Shollenberger, "The physician."

12. CM 9:63, 1912.

13. Fruyn K. "Dr. Matthias Klaiber." Colo Mag. 33:203, 1956.

14. CM 9:127, 1912.

15. Clark CM. *A Trip to Pike's Peak,* 25, 1861. Reprint. San Jose, 1958.

16. "Jefferson Medical Society Fee Bill." Denver, 1860.

17. DMT 28:451, 1908.

18. CM 4:81, 1907; CM 18:277 1921.

19. CMJ 8:396, 1902.

20. JAMA 50:1198, 1908.

21. CMJ 10:88, 1904.

22. DMT 32:185, 1912.

23. CM 8:41, 1911.

24. CMJ 6:494, 1900.

25. CM 14:121, 1917; CM 27:370, 1930.

26. CMJ 2:229, 1896.

27. Goode WH. In Blair DW. "The Early Diaries of Colorado," 79. Master's thesis, University of Denver, 1944.

28. Hawes J. "Presidential address." TCSMS 15:23, 1885.

29. DMT 8:56, 1888.

30. CMJ 2:97, 1896.

31. CMJ 2:58,97 1896.

32. DMT 8:148, 1888; CMJ 4:72, 1898.

33. Stone WG. *The Colorado Handbook.* Denver, 1892.

34. J. B. MacCallum. In GB Webb and D Powell. *Henry Sewall, Physiologist and Physician,* 98. Baltimore, 1946.

35. DMT 21:442, 1902.

36. Blaine JM. "Medical organization - in Colorado." JAMA 41:1289, 1903.

37. DMT 28:282, 1908.

38. CM 3:62, 1906.

39. DMT 3:328, 1884.

40. CMJ 5:341, 1899.

41. CM 4:447, 1907.

42. CM 5:38, 1908.

43. JAMA 39:1398, 1902.

44. DMT 16:19, 1896 - 1897.

45. Rosenberg CE. "Social class and medical care in Nineteenth century America: The rise and fall of the dispensary." J Hist Med Allied Sci 29:32, 1974.

46. Wetherill HG. "A remedy for the dispensary abuse." CMJ 3:433, 1897.

47. DMT 3:279, 1884.

48. CMJ 3:163, 1897.

49. CMJ 9:125, 1903.

50. DMT 15:293, 1895 - 1896.

51. City of Denver 2(11):1, 1914.

52. Edson CE. "The abuse of medical charity." CMJ 3:226, 1897.

53. Critique 8:71, 1901.

54. CM 4:80, 1907.

55. CM 4:304, 1907.

56. Buckingham RG. "President's Address." *Report of the Meeting for the Organization of a Territorial Medical Society, Sept. 19, 1871.* Denver, 1872.

57. Bost Med Surg J 109:473, 1883.

58. JAMA 4:75, 1885. 59. Brown JW. "Pneumonia in high altitudes, and its treatment with jaborandi." JAMA 4:262, 1885; Solly SE. "Temperament." JAMA 12:795, 1889.

59. Brown JW. "Pneumonia in high altitudes, and its treatment with jaborandi." JAMA 4:262, 1885; Solly SE. "Temperament." JAMA 12:795, 1889.

60. Rogers F: Personal communication. These included Drs. E.R. Axtell, A.M. Bucknam, J.T. Eskridge, W.P. Munn, O.J. Pfiefer, E.J.A. Rogers, and H. Sewall.

61. CM 11:245, 1914. These included Dr. Henry Sewall, President of the American Climatological Association and Vice President of the Association of American Physicians; Dr. G. B. Packard, President of the American Orthopedic Association; Dr. Robert Levy, President of the Laryngological, Rhinological and Otological Society; and Dr. Gerald Webb, President of the American Association of Immunologists.

62. *Medical Coloradoana: A Jubilee Volume, 1871-1921.* Denver 1922. Although no author is cited, this listing was largely the work of Denver's Dr. Charles Spivak. Although incomplete, it is an invaluable source of information for anyone interested in Colorado's early medical history. It was published as part of the Colorado Medical Society's fiftieth anniversary celebration.

63. CM 13:228, 1916.

64. DMT 18:121, 1898.

65. DMT 12:576, 1893.

66. DMT 12:488, 1893.

67. DMT 12:576, 1893.

68. CMJ 11:417, 1905.

69. CM 2:259, 1905.

70. Rothwell PD. "What the physicians and people of Colorado need more than a medical bill." CMJ 5:323, 1899.

71. RMN, March 8, 1867.

72. CM 9:66, 1912.

73. Perkin RL. *The First Hundred Years,* 437-45. Garden City, New York, 1959.

74. Wetherill HG. "An open letter to Mr. John C. Shaffer." CM 17:171, 1920.

75. Van Meter SD. "A plea for concerted action of the profession." CM 6:212, 1909.

76. CM 13:97, 1916.

77. DMT 18, 561, 1898 - 1899.

78. Blaine JM. "Letter to the editor." CMJ 5:196, 1899.

79. CMJ 5:200, 1899.

80. DMT 20:413, 1901. The doctors' joy was premature. In 1913, Thomas was appointed to a vacant senate seat, was subsequently elected, and served until 1928. Ironically, his opponent in 1914 was a physician, Dr. Hubert Work.

81. Rothwell PD. In discussion of Andrew CF. "The physician in politics." TCSMS 36:188, 1906.

82. CMJ 3:35, 1897.

83. Law G. "Ethics in malpractice." DMT 11:581, 1892.

84. CMJ 3:122, 1897.

85. CMJ 2:396, 1896.

86. CMJ 3:115, 1897.

87. Wetherill HG. "Letter to the editor." CM 6:52, 1909.

88. Stuver E. "The home and the school." Bull Amer Acad Med 5:53, 1902.

89. CM 19:72, 1922. The author is cited only as "A.C. McC." The only contemporary physician I could find with those initials was Dr. A. C. McClanahan of Victor.

90. Stubbs AL. "Eugenics." DMT 33:454, 1913.

91. CM 13:161, 1916.

92. De Weese JM. "The race question in America and criminal sociology." DMT 30:49, 1910.

93. Solly SE. *The Health Resorts of Colorado Springs and Manitou,* 55. Colorado Springs, 1883.

94. Exline JW. "Religion from a medical standpoint." DMT 11:148, 1892.

95. Stuver, "The home."

Chapter 12

1. The history of medical education in early Colorado is covered much more extensively in Shikes RH, Claman HN. *The University of Colorado School of Medicine. A Centennial History, 1883 - 1983*. Denver, 1983.

2. Elder CS. "Medicine, public health and hospitals." In Hafen LR. *Colorado and Its People*, II, 387. New York, 1948.

3. Sewall H. "Historical sketch of the Medical Department of the University of Colorado School of Medicine." CM 22:364, 1925.

4. Buckingham RG. "President's Address to the First Annual Meeting of the Colorado Territorial Medical Society." 1871

5. *Prospectus and Circular of Information, Medical Department of the University of Colorado, Session of 1883-1884.*

6. JAMA 1:185, 1883

7. DMT 3:254, 1884.

8. Allen FS, et al. *The University of Colorado, 1876 - 1976*, 45. New York, 1976.

9. CMJ 3:284, 1897.

10. DMT 6:52, 1886.

11. DMT 16:61, 146, 1893.

12. TCSMS 24:45, 1894.

13. Munn WP. "Medical education in Denver." Colo Climatol 1:1, 1894.

14. Flexner A. *Medical Education in the United States and Canada. A Report to the Carnegie Foundation for the Advancement of Teaching*. Bulletin No. 4, Carnegie Foundation. New York, 1910.

15. Stover GH. "Mr. Abraham Flexner and the Carnegie Foundation." DMT 30:227, 1910.

16. Flexner, *Medical Education*.

17. Elder CS. "Medicine." In *History of Colorado*, III, 1073. Edited by JH Baker and LR Hafen. Denver, 1927.

18. The Archer mansion was located at 1307 Welton Street in downtown Denver. Ironically, the new medical facility had been the residence of Colonel James Archer, head of Denver's water company and arch-enemy of its physicians during their war against Denver's unsanitary water system (Chapter 17).

19. Memorandum from Dean W.P. Harlow, July 9, 1910.

20. Letters from Dean Meader to President Farrand, April 15, 1915, and February 1, 1916.

21. Elder, "Medicine, public health and hospitals."

22. Silver and Gold, March 15, 1894. This was (and is) the weekly newspaper of the University of Colorado.

23. CM 7:365, 1910; DMT 30:177, 1910.

24. Minutes of the General Faculty, University of Colorado School of Medicine, March 2, 1918.

25. Van Zant CB. "Reminiscences." Typed manuscript, undated.

26. *Catalogue of the Univesity of Colorado, 1889 - 1890.*

27. *Directory, Officers and Graduates, 1877 - 1921*. University of Colorado Bulletin 21:10, 1921. In later years, Dr. Espinosa was listed as a physician in Belen, New Mexico and Dr. Ochiai practiced in Honolulu. I was unable to determine when the first black medical student was admitted or graduated. Mention of a "colored" student in the graduating class of the Homeopathic College was made in 1901; it was noted that, despite the fact that he received many honors at graduation, there did not seem to be any evidence of envy among his classmates. CMJ 7:228, 1901.

28. Ibid., *Directory*.

29. Gross Med Coll Bull 5:66, 1895.

30. Monroe AW. *San Juan Silver*, 82. Grand Junction, Colorado, 1940; *Portrait and Biographical Record of the State of Colorado*, 1331, 1407. Chicago, 1899.

31. Silver and Gold, November 15, 1892.

32. Silver and Gold, May 15, 1894.

33. Silver and Gold, October 31, 1894.

34. Silver and Gold, October 22, 1908.

35. Clapesattle H. *Dr. Webb of Colorado Springs*, 183 - 206. Boulder, 1984. Webb's research activities are described in more detail in Clapesattle's excellent biography.

36. Ibid. Quote attributed to Dr. David Talmage, former dean and distinguished professor of microbiology and medicine at the University of Colorado.

37. Webb had come from England to Colorado because of his wife's tuberculosis. Originally a surgeon, he soon limited his activities to the clinical and research aspects of tuberculosis. His laboratory, located in his home, and the

Colorado Foundation for Research in Tuberculosis, were the antecedents of today's Webb-Waring Institute at the University of Colorado Health Sciences Center.

38. Webb and Desmond Powell subsequently wrote the definitive Sewall biography, *Henry Sewall: Physiologist and Physician*. Baltimore, 1946.

39. Sewall H. "Experiments on the preventive inoculation of rattlesnake venom." J. Physiol. 8:349, 1887; Sabin FR. "The contributions of Charles Denison and Henry Sewall to medicine." Science 86:357, 1937.

40. Connell FG. "Capillarity in intestinal sutures." JAMA 47:405, 1906.

41. Lewis RC. "Medical education in Colorado." RMMJ 70:679, 1956; *Biennial Report of the Board of Regents of the University of Colorado, 1919 - 1920.*

Chapter 13

1. Kickland WA. "Should we all be specialists?" CM 6:82, 1909.

2. Harmer WW. "What's the use?" CM 9:216, 1912.

3. Whitney HB. "Address." CM 5:392, 1908.

4. Haagensen CD, Lloyd WEB. *A Hundred Years of Medicine*. New York, 1943.

5. Grant WW. "The first appendectomy." CM 1:266, 1904.

6. Grant WW. "Appendicitis." TCSMS 22:140, 1892.

7. Grant WW. "The medical and surgical history of the appendix vermiformis." CM 30:280, 1933.

8. Gross Med Coll Bull 2:168, 1894.

9. Perkins IB. "Some thoughts on abdominal surgery." DMT 21:177, 1901.

10. *Laws . . . Second Session of the General Assembly of Colorado, 1879*, 90.

11. McMechan EC. *Life of Governor Evans*, 38. Denver, 1924.

12. Sethman HT. "CMS presidents - The first fifty years. RMMJ 68:74, 1971.

13. *Annual Reports of the State Board of Health of Colorado for the Years 1879 and 1880*, 125 - 26. Denver, 1881; Stone WF. *History of Colorado*, II, 821-22. Chicago, 1918.

14. Eskridge JT. "Needs of the State Insane Asylum." CMJ 2:166, 1896.

15. *Ninth Biennial Report of the Colorado State Insane Asylum*, CMJ 3:75, 1897.

16. Thombs PR. "Insane Asylum." *Second Biennial Report of the Board of Charities and Corrections, Colorado*. Denver, 1894.

17. McDowell WF, Eskridge JT. "Plain facts concerning the financial condition of the Colorado State Insane Asylum." CMJ 4:387, 1898.

18. CMJ 4:431, 1898.

19. Sethman, "CMS presidents." Thombs died two years later.

20. *Second Annual Report of the State Board of Health of Colorado, 1877*, 134 - 40.

21. Thombs PR. "Address." TCSMS 13:18, 1883.

22. Work H. "Home treatment of insanity." DMT 21:209, 1901.

23. Pershing HT. "Nervous disorders in Colorado." DMT 28:158, 1908.

24. Eskridge JT. "The relation of Colorado climate to nervous diseases." Colo Climatol 1:66, 1895.

25. Pershing HT. "The treatment of neurasthenia." CM 1:82, 1904.

26. Oettinger B. "Remarks on treatment of neuresthenia." CM 4:103, 1907; CM 3:23, 1906.

27. Rogers EJA. "The influence of mental attitude in the treatment of diseases." CM 10:232, 1913.

28. "Mr. Dooley on psychotherapeutics." CM 5:507, 1908.

29. Hall JN. *Borderline Diseases: A Study of Medical Diagnosis*, 2 volumes. New York, 1915.

30. Hall JN. "A clinical study of 600 cases of heart disease." Med Rec 76:816, 1909.

31. Hill EC. "Arteriosclerosis." DMT 22:395, 1903.

32. Fisk SA. "Diabetes mellitus." TCSMS 14:71, 1884.

33. Daily Central City Register, June 30, 1871.

34. Bullette WW. "The use of suprarenal capsule extract." DMT 19:234, 1899.

35. Bartlett R. "Oxygen - Nature's remedy." DMT 5:301, 1885.

36. CMJ 2:88, 1896.

37. CMJ 2:152, 1896.

38. Wasson WW. "Radiologic pioneers in Colorado, 1896 - 1918." Unpublished manuscript, 1934.

39. Landa ER. "The first nuclear industry." Sci Amer 247:180, 1982.

40. Bruyn K. *Uranium Country*. Boulder, 1955. This source contains much information on Colorado's radium boom. The laboratory was located at Colfax Avenue and Race Street; the plant was at 1045 Tejon Street near the railroad tracks.

41. Davis AW. *Dr. Kelly of Hopkins*, 126 - 30. Baltimore, 1959.

42. Allen JQ. "The present status of radium therapy." CM 11:18, 1914.

43. Wasson, "Radiologic pioneers."

44. Stover GH. "The therapeutic use of the X-ray." DMT 22:55, 1902.

45. E.C.H. "Dr. George H. Stover." DMT 34:393, 1914.

46. Wasson, "Radiologic Pioneers."

47. Hall JN. *Tales of Pioneer Practice*, 51. Denver, 1937. Although Hall did not recall the doctor's name, it may have been Dr. Arthur E. Bonesteel.

48. *Proceedings of the Second Annual Meeting of the Territorial Medical Society, 1872*.

49. Mumey N. *Dr. Eugene Charles Gehrung*. Denver, 1983.

50. Lemen HA. "A contribution to surgery." TCSMS 14:37, 1884.

51. Hawkins TH. "Abdominal sections in Denver." DMT 3:365, 1884

52. Slick J. "A pessary retained five years." DMT 8:72, 1889.

53. Cole S. "Uterine colic caused by entrance of a leech into the uterus." DMT 1:12, 1882.

54. Love MCT. "Dysmenorrhoea, with report of cases." TCSMS 30:151, 1900.

55. Buckingham R. "Report on obstetrics for the Territorial Medical Society." TCTMS 2:26, 1872.

56. Backus HF. *Tomboy Bride*, 112 - 15. Boulder, 1969.

57. Gardiner CF. *Doctor at Timberline*, 210 - 13. Caldwell, Idaho, 1938.

58. Peden BA. "A case of placenta previa." CMJ 3:381, 1897.

59. Hoffmann KD. "Sewing is for women; horses are for men: The role of German Russian women." In *Germans from Russia in Colorado*, 138. Edited by S. Heitman. Denver, 1978.

60. FitzPatrick VS. *The Last Frontier*, II, 211. Steamboat Springs, Colorado, 1976.

61. Recollection by Hannah Shwayder Berry of her grandmother. In the Denver Post, Empire Magazine, December 10, 1967.

62. Russell AJ. "Puerperal fever." DMT 5:1, 1885.

63. Minden SB. "Puerperal septicemia." DMT 9:266, 1890.

64. CMJ 2:102, 1896. The home was at 635 Pearl Street.

65. Ditson A. "The National Florence Crittenton Mission." DMT 30:88, 1910-11.

66. Hawes J. "Symptoms and sequels of fresh lacerations." TCSMS 29:352, 1899.

67. TCSMS 29:454, 1899.

68. Seaman AB. "Colorado laws relating to criminal abortion." CMJ 9:141, 1903.

69. "Offenses against the person of individuals." 637, Sec. 42. *General Laws of the State of Colorado*, 169. Denver, 1877.

70. CMJ 5:343, 1899.

71. DMT 22:449, 1903.

72. Robe RC. "Abortions." TCSMS 32:287, 1902.

73. Reports of the Coroner of Arapahoe County, 1903.

74. DMT 22:449, 1903.

75. Hawkins TH. "Address." DMT 6:193, 1886.

76. Robe, "Abortions"; Colo Climatol 1:25, 1894; CM 12:72, 1915.

77. Hawkins, "Address."

78. Hawkins HN. "The practical working of the law against criminal abortion." CMJ 9:153, 1903.

79. Work H. "Maternal impressions." TCSMS 24:151, 1894.

80. CMJ 10:22, 1904.

81. Butterfield J. "The incubator doctor in Denver." Denver Westerners Brand Book, 1970, 339. Edited by JC Thode. Denver, 1970. Dr. Couney normally ran a concession at New York's Coney Island amusement park.

82. Taylor AG. "A consideration of the principles of infant feeding." CM 4:306, 1907.

83. Palmer HK. "The incompatibility of higher education with the duties of motherhood." *Annual Reports of the State Board of Health of Colorado for the Years 1879 and 1880*, 93.

84. Whitney HB. In discussion of Taylor, "A consideration."

85. CM 8:55, 1911.

86. Ditson A. "The human stock show." JAMA 61:111, 1913.

87. Melrose F. "Whatever happened to '13 Stock Show baby?" Denver Post, January, 1982.

88. Elsner J: "Diphtheria." DMT 6:65, 1886.

89. Denver Tribune, March 13, 1879; JAMA 35:1286, 1900.

90. Bentley MV. *The Upper Side of the Pie Crust*, 28. Evergreen, Colorado, 1978.

91. Aspen Times, November 1, 1892.

92. Van Zant CB, et al. "In memorium - Frank E. Waxham." CM 8:411, 1911.

93. Waxham FE. "Report of five hundred cases of intubation of the larynx." TCSMS 26:105, 1894.

94. CMJ 2:61, 1896.

95. CMJ 4:58, 1898.

96. Waxham FE. "Plea for the free distribution of diphtheria antitoxin in Colorado." CM 5:474, 1908.

97. "Report of Antitoxin Committee." CM 6:386, 1909.

98. Bates ME. "The Colorado method for the examination and care of public school children." N Y Med J 97:393, 1913; Amesse JW. "The physical examination of school children." DMT 34:421, 1914.

99. Some additional physicians whose names should at least be mentioned include (Pediatrics) Drs. George Cattermole, John Amesse; (Surgery) Clayton Parkhill, Leonard Freeman, Will Swan, J. Crum Epler, Charles Elder, Charles Lyman; (Psychiatry) Edmund Rogers, Edward Delehanty, George Moleen, Franklin Ebaugh; (Internal Medicine) James Arneill, Carroll Edson; (Radiology) Chauncey Tennant, Samuel Childs, W.W. Wasson; (Gynecology) H. Lemen, H.G. Wetherill, Walter Jayne, Francis McNaught; (Obstetrics) Arnold Stedman; (Pathology) Edwin Axtell, Ross Whitman, James Todd, Edward Mugrage, Ward Burdick, Phil Hillkowitz; (Ophthalmology) George Cleary, John Chase, William Bane, G. M. Black, Edward Jackson, Alexander Magruder; (Otolaryngology) Robert Levy, Frank Spencer; (Orthopedics) George Packard; (Dermatology) Arthur Markley; (Neurology) J. T. Eskridge. Others are mentioned elsewhere in the book.

100. *Constitution, By-laws and House Rules of the Citizen's Hospital Association of Pitkin County*. Aspen, Colorado, 1892.

101. As mining declined, so did Aspen and its hospital. By 1921 the Aspen Democrat reported that "The Citizen's Hospital is down to its last dollar" (February 17, 1921). It was taken over by Dr. Warren Twining and run as a private hospital until 1946, when it became Pitkin County Hospital. In the mid-1970s, with Aspen once again thriving, it was replaced by a new facility, Aspen Community Hospital, just outside of town.

Chapter 14

1. Remark made at a "recent lecture in Denver." *Handbook of Colorado*, 1872, 140. Denver, 1872.

2. *First Annual Report of the Denver Chamber of Commerce and Board of Trade - 1883*, 117. Denver, 1884.

3. *Denver City and Auraria, The Commercial Emporium of the Pikes Peak Gold Regions in 1859*, 12. St. Louis, 1860.

4. Colo Mag 16:95, 1939.

5. Bird I. *A Lady's Life in the Rocky Mountains*, 3rd edition, 47 - 8. New York, 1881.

6. St. Louis Med Surg J. 11:129, 1874.

7. *Official Information. Territorial Board of Immigration*, 13. Denver, 1872.

8. Bird, *Lady's Life*.

9. Davis AW. *Dr. Kelly of Hopkins*, 31 - 35. Baltimore, 1959. He was also, in later years, a major participant in Colorado's radium boom (Chapter 13).

10. Byles FG. "Sunlight and health." J. Outdoor Life 3:193, 1906.

11. Munn WP. "Denver's Climate." DMT 18:567, 1898-99.

12. McClelland WF. "Aseptic qualities of the Colorado atmosphere twenty-five years ago." DMT 17:484, 1897-98.

13. McClelland WF. "Miasm, or malaria." TCMS 9:62, 1879.

14. Hawes J. "Malaria. Its existence or non-existence in Colorado." TCSMS 11:76, 1881; Editorial: "The mosquitoes of Colorado." CM 48:161, 1918.

15. Detroit Review of Medicine, September, 1872. Dr. McClelland responded in the Bost Med Surg J 89:44, 1873.

16. Med Surg Report 44:672, 1881.

17. Massey TE. "Report on Climatology." TCTMS 5:48, 1875.

18. Wagner C. "Colorado Springs and Davos-Platz as winter health resorts, compared.". Med Rec 32:567, 1887.

19. Solly SE. The Health Resorts of Colorado Springs and Manitou. Colorado Springs. NP, ND.

20. Denison C. Rocky Mountain Health Resorts. Boston, 1880.

21. Dr. Denison was interested in other areas of medicine as well. He invented an improved stethescope, a rib cutter and other orthopedic instruments, a device to measure breathing capacity, and a ventilator. Denison had a large private practice, specialized in tuberculosis, was the Professor of Diseases of the Chest and of Climatology at the University of Denver, and served as an officer in various societies and professional organizations. His home was said to one of Denver's cultural focal points. Dr. Florence Sabin desribed him as kindly and "interested in people." Sabin FR. "The contributions of Charles Denison and Henry Sewall to medicine." Science 86:357, 1937.

22. Denison C. The Annual and Seasonal Climatic Maps of the United States. Chicago, 1885.

23. JAMA 4:443, 1885.

24. Denison C. "Climatic influences of forests." Colo Climatol 1:79, 1895.

25. "Address of His Excellency, F.W. Pitkin to the . . . Legislature of Colorado." Jan. 14, 1879.

26. Pasquale CJ. One Hundred Years in the Heart of the Rockies, 23. Salida, Colorado, 1980.

27. CM 11:242, 1914.

28. Dougan DH. "Asthma." TCSMS 11:94, 1881.

29. Greenwood G. New Life in New Lands, 95. New York, 1873.

30. RMN, January 6, 1871.

31. Colorado and Asthma. Denver, 1874.

32. Greenwood, New Life.

33. "Resolution of the Denver Medical Association," December 8, 1873. Cited in First Annual Report of the Board of Health of the State of Colorado for the Fiscal Year Ending September 30, 1876. Denver, 1877.

34. Third Annual Report of the Denver Chamber of Commerce, 52. Denver, 1885.

35. Arneill JR. "Asthma." CM 3:45, 1906.

36. Leach S. "Letter. June 21, 1864." Trail 19:19, 1926.

37. Denison C. "The relation of outdoor life to high altitude therapy." TCSMS 31:154, 1901.

38. Swan WH. "Impressions of differences in practice at low and high altitudes." Trans Amer Climatol Assn 18:222, 1902.

39. Hollister OJ. The Mines of Colorado, 41. Springfield, Massachusetts, 1867.

40. Edmondson W. "A few thoughts on acclimation." Annual Reports of the State Board of Health of Colorado for the Years 1879 and 1880. Denver, 1881.

41. Henderson Y. "Physiological observations on Pike's Peak, Colorado, made in the summer of 1911." Trans Amer Climatol Assn 28:11, 1912.

42. Hall JN. "Cardiac dangers in high altitudes." Trans Amer Climatol Assn 24:142, 1908.

43. Jayne WA. "The influence of altitude upon the sexual organs of women." Trans Amer Climatol Assn 11:120, 1895.

44. Henderson, "Physiological observations."

45. Baskin OL. History of the Arkansas Valley, Colorado, 52. Chicago, 1881.

46. James E. Account of an Expedition from Pittsburgh to the Rocky Mountains, II, 23, 46. Philadelphia, 1823.

47. Ibid., 24.

48. Ruxton GF. Adventures in Mexico and the Rocky Mountains, 242. New York, 1848.

49. Baskin OL. History of Clear Creek and Boulder Valleys, Colorado, 294. Chicago, 1880.

50. Taylor B. Colorado: A Summer Trip, 73. New York, 1867.

51. "Mineral Springs of Colorado." First Annual Report of the State Board of Health of Colorado, 56. Denver, 1877.

52. Prentiss JL. "Thermal baths." TCSMS :358, 1894.

53. Urquhart LM. Glenwood Springs: Spa in the Mountains, 77 - 79. Boulder, 1970. The pool remains Glenwood Springs' major tourist attraction.

54. Solly SE. Manitou, Colorado, U.S.A.: Its Mineral Waters and Climate. St.Louis, 1875.

55. Loew was a well known chemist and geologist who had accompanied several of the Wheeler expeditions.

56. An excellent review of Manitou Springs' history as a health resort is provided by Cunningham SA. Manitou: Saratoga of the West. Colorado Springs, 1980.

57. The Clark Magnetic Mineral Spring. NP:ND, ca. 1900. Kindly provided by Ed and Nancy Bathke.

58. Actually, most of Colorado's radium deposits were at some distance from its natural springs—fortunately, otherwise many health-seekers would have been exposed to significant doses of radiation. George RD, et al. Mineral Waters of Colorado. Colorado Geological Survey, Bull. 11. Denver, 1920.

59. Cunningham, Manitou.

60. From an advertisement of the Manitou Mineral Water Company, Manitou Springs, Colorado, ca.1890.

61. DMT and Utah Med J 32:229, 1912 - 13. Other companies were located in Pueblo, Canon City, Golden, Glenwood Springs and Fowler.

62. In recent times, attempts have been made to revive Manitou Springs' bottled water industry.

63. Hill EC. "The mineral water fad." DMT 15:451, 1895 - 96.

Chapter 15

1. Dubos R, Dubos J. The White Plague, Tuberculosis, Man, and Society. Boston, 1952.

2. Fourth Annual Report of the Denver Chamber of Commerce, 52 - 57. Denver, 1887. The next three causes were pneumonia, typhoid, and trauma.

3. Solly S. "Treatment of pulmonary consumption." Trans Amer Climat Assn 7:132, 1890; McConnell JF. "The medical treatment of advanced pulmonary disease." CM 6:310, 1909.

4. CM 6:173, 1909.

5. DMT 16:390, 1886.

6. Critique 10:195, 1903.

7. Solly, "Treatment."

8. Zederbaum A. "Medical treatment of tuberculosis." CMJ 10:171, 1904.

9. The City of Denver, Its Resources and Their Development, 100. Denver, 1891. Meuer's sanitarium was at Broadway and South Jewell.

10. Waring JJ. "History of artifical pneumothorax in America." The procedure was done at Denver's St. Anthony's Hospital. Actually, Dr. Van Zant's approach was a non-surgical version, simply using a twenty-gauge needle and syringe to induce the pneumothorax. Waring reported that the patient was alive and well many years later.

11. Fourth Annual Report.

12. "M." "The medical topography of the Pike's Peak gold region." Kans City Med Surg Rev 1:113, 1860.

13. Colo Mag 8:172, 1931.

14. The Resources and Attractions of Colorado, for the Home Seeker, Capitalist, and Tourist, 57. Omaha, 1888.

15. Fourth Ann Report.

16. Ehrich LR. "Letter to the editor of the New York Tribune," May 22, 1887.

17. Gardiner CF. "Light and air in the treatment of consumption in Colorado." Trans Amer Climat Assn 15:19, 1899.

18. Axtell ER. "Tent life for consumptives." Colo Climatol 1:159, 1895.

19. Wood LH. "The treatment of consumption in Colorado." DMT 6:208, 1886.

20. Galbreath TC. Chasing the Cure in Colorado. Denver, 1908.

21. Gardiner CF. "The sanatory tent and its use in the treatment of pulmonary tuberculosis." Trans Amer Climatol Assn 18:209, 1902; "Early days in Colorado." J Outdoor Life 29:355, 1932.

22. Galbreath, *Chasing the Cure*.

23. Hershey EP. "Out-door sleeping." DMT 33:429, 1914.

24. Denison C. "The sleeping canopy." Trans Amer Climatol Assn 23:183, 1907.

25. Gardiner CF. "Sleeping outdoors in Colorado." J Outdoor Life. 3:49, 1906.

26. Solly SE. "Phthisis." Colo Climatol 1:35, 1895.

27. Gardiner, "Early days."

28. Dodge HO. "Acclimation of the consumptive to the climate of Colorado." Trans Amer Climatol Assn 7:183, 1890.

29. Littlejohn E. "Rocky Mountains, climate, and tuberculosis." Med Rec 63:152, 1892.

30. Anonymous. "Colorado for consumption." Med News 43:278, 1888.

31. Brendamour F. "Report of the Rocky Mountain Tenting Tour Association." Colo Climatol 1:302, 1895.

32. Editorial. "Tubercular physicians not wanted in Oklahoma." CM 8:3, 1911.

33. Galbreath, *Chasing the Cure*.

34. Reports of the Coroner of Arapahoe County, 1901 - 1905.

35. Ralph J. *Our Great West*, 319. New York, 1893.

36. Magruder AC. "Physicians in Colorado for tuberculosis." DMT 28:152, 1908.

37. TCSMS 26:31, 1896. In a later survey of tuberculous physicians in his own huge practice, Dr. J.N. Hall noted a death rate of 39% among tuberculous physicians in Colorado. Hall JN. "Tuberculosis among physicians." Amer J Med Sci 143:75, 1912.

38. Reed J. "Altitude in reference to pneumorrhagia." TCSMS 7:58, 1877; CMJ 3:14, 1897.

39. *History of the Morgan County Medical Society*, NP,ND.

40. Bonney SG. *Pulmonary Tuberculosis and Its Complications*. Philadelphia, 1908.

41. Denison C. Letter in Denison Scrapbook, 1901. Denison Memorial Library, University of Colorado Health Sciences Center.

42. Knight FI. "On the return of cured tubercular patients from high altitudes." Trans Amer Climatol Assn 7:189, 1890.

43. Denison C. *Rocky Mountain Health Resorts*, 114. Boston, 1880.

44. Fisk SA. "President's address." TCSMS 19:14, 1889.

45. Solly SE. "Treatment of pulmonary consumption by residence in Colorado." Trans Amer Climatol Assn 7:132, 1890.

46. Little WT. "Consumptives in Colorado." CM 1:275, 1904.

47. Critique 10:197, 1903.

48. Many such advertisements appeared in Colorado's newspapers as well as local and national journals and other publications. The Maples was located at 2555 West 37th Avenue in Denver; Dr. Beggs' Home was at 133 West Colfax Avenue.

49. FW Oakes. "The Home and Heartsease." CMJ 3:399, 1897.

50. The home was located at West 32nd Avenue and Eliot Street. The buildings were contructed in an elegant Classic Revival style. In 1934 Reverend Oakes retired and the home was closed, having cared for about 20,000 patients. Later it became a Catholic convent and home for the elderly. It was torn down in 1974. Wiberg RE. *Rediscovering Northwest Denver*, 60. Boulder, 1978; Melrose F. "TB victims found haven at Oakes." RMN April 3, 1983.

51. Holmes AM. "Some problems pertaining to tuberculosis." DMT 20:229, 1900.

52. Wood, "Treatment of consumption."

53. The National Jewish Hospital and the later Jewish Consumptive's Relief Society (JCRS) were unusual among Colorado's sanitaria in that they cared for the indigent and did not charge their patients. They are discussed in the next section.

54. *Colorado Souvenir Book for the International Congress on Tuberculosis, 1908*, 157 - 58; Edson CE, Bergtold WH. "The Agnes Memorial Sanitarium"; Trans Amer Climatol Assn 20:164, 1904. It was located on the present site of Lowry Air Force Base. Phipps, although he and his family became prominent Coloradans, had made his fortune in western Pennsylvania and preference was given to applicants from that area.

55. Ibid., Edson and Bergtold.

56. As the number of tuberculosis patients declined, Agnes became prohibitively expensive to maintain, and it was closed in 1931. It was offered to the state, but the offer was rejected.

57. Harper F. *The Story of Tuberculosis and the Evangelical Lutheran Sanitarium*. Denver, 1980. Dr. Harper's book is an excellent source of material, not only on what is now Lutheran Hospital, but also on tuberculosis in early Denver and Colorado.

58. Edmonds WE. "The YMCA Health Farm." J Outdoor Life 5:211, 1908; *The Association Health Farm*, 5th edition. Denver, 1904; *Colorado Souvenir Book*. The Health Farm was located in suburban Edgewater, "1 1/2 miles west of the 29th Avenue car line." There were other tent colonies in the Denver vicinity, including the Rocky Mountain Industrial Sanitarium (1901) and the Craig Colony (1909).

59. *Illustrated Denver*, 1. Denver, 1893.

60. In addition to cited sources, information on many of Colorado Springs' sanitaria is provided by M. D. and E.R. Ormes' *The Book of Colorado Springs*. Colorado Springs, 1933. Douglas R. McKay's *Asylum of the Gilded Pill: The Story of Cragmor Sanitarium* (Denver, 1983) is an excellent study of Cragmor.

61. Solly SE. "Sanatorium treatment of tuberculosis in Colorado." Tran Amer Climatol Assn 18:182, 1902.

62. Sprague M. "Healers in Pike's Peak history." Denver Westerners Roundup 23 (12): 3, 1967.

63. The journal's name was derived from normal body temperature in degrees Fahrenheit—symbolic of recovery.

64. These and the following instances are from the April and May, 1925, issues of *Ninety-Eight-Six*.

65. After years of financial difficulty, in the 1950s Cragmor became a federal government-sponsored sanitarium for tuberculous Navajo Indians. In 1964, the University of Colorado acquired it as its Colorado Springs' campus.

66. The name and the sanitarium's therapeutic regimen were derived from the Nordrach Sanitarium in Germany's Black Forest. One former patient compared the sanitarium to "a prison" and recalled that its medical director was referred to as "the Master Warden." (McKay DR. "A history of the Nordrach Ranch." Colo Mag 56:179, 1979). Other private sanitaria included Sunnyrest, Star Ranch in the Pines, and Idlewild.

67. Hafen LR (editor). *Colorado and Its People*, IV. New York, 1948; Ormes, *Colorado Springs*.

68. In 1939, Spencer Penrose founded the Penrose Tumor Institute at what would become, in 1946, the Glockner-Penrose Hospital.

69. CM 7:164, 1910.

70. *The Modern Woodmen Sanatorium for Tuberculosis*. NP, ND ca. 1910.

71. In 1919 the sanitarium published a follow-up report on its former patients. Of 1,654 patients who had been discharged for at least four years and for as long as nine years, 47% were still alive. Rutledge JA, Crouch JB. "The ultimate results in 1,654 cases of tuberculosis treated at the Modern Woodmen of America Sanatorium." Ann Rev Tuber 1:755, 1919. Woodmen Sanitarium was closed in 1947. Following a rumor that it was to become the "Summer" White House, Woodmen was converted into a convent. Kitch JI, Kitch BB. *Woodmen Valley*. Palmer Lake, Colorado, 1970.

72. Anfaenger ML. *Birth of a Hospital; The Story of the Birth of the National Jewish Hospital in Denver, Colorado*. Denver, 1942; Schaefer S., Parsons E. "A brief history of the National Jewish Hospital at Denver." Colo Mag 5:191, 1928. Much of the impetus for a free sanitarium had come from the earlier work of the late Frances Wisebart Jacobs. National Jewish Hospital has always been located at its present site, Colorado Boulevard and Colfax Avenue.

73. Muller A. "The National Jewish Hospital for Consumptives." CMJ 10:309, 1904.

74. Dr. John Elsner was one of the hospital's founders. Drs. Robert Levy and Saling Simon served on the original Board.

75. Uchill IL. *Pioneers, Peddlers, and Tsadikim*, 241. Denver, 1957.

76. *First Annual Report of The Jewish Consumptives' Relief Society at Denver, Colorado, 1905*. Denver, 1905.

77. Charles Spivak was born in Russia. In trouble because of his anti-czarist activities, he came to the United

States in 1882, worked as a laborer and mill hand, became a teacher, and graduated from Jefferson Medical College. Because of his wife's poor health, they moved to Denver in 1896. In addition to his practice, and, for its first twenty-five years, Spivak was the major medical force at the JCRS. Hornbein M. "Dr. Charles Spivak of Denver." Western States Jewish Historical Quarterly 11:195, 1979; Uchill, *Pioneers*. Other early physicians who contributed to the JCRS included Drs. A. Zederbaum and Phillip Hillkowitz.

78. *First Annual Report*, JCRS.

79. The Outlook, cited in Hornbein, "Spivak."

80. Abrams J. "East European Jews, Tzedakah, and the Jewish Consumptives' Relief Society." Rocky Mountain Jewish Historical Notes. Vol. 6, Nos. 1,2 Fall, 1983.

81. Eventually, as the need for such an institution decreased, JCRS was replaced by the American Medical Center, an institution which specializes in cancer research, and "JCRS" was memorialized as the name of a shopping center now located on the sanitarium's former grounds. NJH recently changed its name to the National Jewish Center for Immunology and Pulmonary Diseases, a leading institution for research in those areas.

82. Boggs AE. "The history and development of the Tuberculosis Assistance Program in Colorado." Master's thesis, University of Denver, 1943.

83. Cooper CE. "Tuberculosis in its relations to public health." CM 1:309, 1904.

84. Galbreath, *Chasing the Cure*.

85. Bird IL. *A Lady's Life in the Rocky Mountains*, 3rd edition, 178. New York, 1881.

86. Hershey EP. "The patient in Colorado." DMT 19:568, 1899.

87. Fisk SA. In discussion of Gardiner CF. "Light and air in the treatment of tuberculosis in Colorado." Trans Amer Climat Assn 15:19, 1899.

88. Wetherill HG. "Health resorts of the West and Southwest". Med News Dec. 16, 1893.

89. Manly CS. "Unfavorable cases of phthisis for altitude treatment." Colo Climatol 1:144, 1895 Dr. Manly died that year—of tuberculosis.

90. Eliot SA. "The migration of invalids." Proc Natl Conf Charities Corrections, 90. Nineteenth Annual Session, 1892.

91. *The Opinions of the Judge and the Colonel*, 11. 1894.

92. Municipal Facts 1:18, 1918.

93. Sewall H. "Suggestions for the administrative control of tuberculosis in . . . Denver." CM 4:52, 1907.

94. Galbreath, *Chasing the Cure*.

95. Bonney SG. Some phases of the tuberculosis problem in Colorado. Philad Med J. Oct 13, 1900.

96. Galbreath, *Chasing the Cure*.

97. CMJ 11:24, 1905.

98. Myers JA. "James Johnston Waring." The Journal—Lancet 84:4, 1962. Waring later became chairman of the Department of Medicine at the University of Colorado and a specialist in pulmonary diseases.

99. JAMA 34:1430, 1900.

100. J Outdoor Life 6:155, 1909.

101. DMT 15:409, 1895 - 96.

102. Beggs WN. "The duty of the consumptive." J Outdoor Life 4:13, 1911.

103. Burrage S. "The migratory consumptive in Colorado." CM 17:26, 1920.

104. Munn W. *Official Report of the Bureau of Health of the City of Denver*, 58. Denver, 1895.

105. DMT 16:405, 1896 - 97.

106. Personal communication—Ida L. Uchill.

107. Beggs, "The duty . . ."

108. Sanitarian 44:342, 1900.

109. Ibid.

110. Munn W. *Annual Report of the Bureau of Health of Denver, 1896 - 97*. Denver, 1897.

111. *Official Report, 1895*.

112. *Annual Report, 1896 - 97*.

113. J Outdoor Life 7:81, 1910.

114. "Tuberculosis—Notification of cases and control of. Chap 125, Mar. 17, 1913." Public Health Reports 29:593, 1914.

115. Pyle GS. "The development of the field of public health in Colorado," 76 - 79. Master's thesis, University of Denver, 1946.

116. "Education a la Eskimo". Municipal Facts 6:12, 1922. Cheltenham Annex School was located at 1580 Julian Street. According to Dr. Spivak, between 1900 and 1920, 46% of the 3,649 deaths among Denver's Jews were due to tuberculosis—an astounding figure. Spivak CD. "The mortality of the Jews in Denver." CM 20:46, 1923.

Chapter 16

1. Gardiner CF. *Doctor at Timberline*. Caldwell, Idaho, 1938.

2. Hopkins DR. *Princes and Peasants. Smallpox in History*. Chicago, 1983.

3. Karzon, DT. "Smallpox vaccination in the United States: The end of an era." Journal of Pediatrics 81:600, 1972.

4. Mumey N. *Vaccination: Bicentenary of the Birth of Edward Jenner*. Denver, 1949.

5. Hopkins, *Princes*, 263.

6. Bloom LB. *Early vaccination in New Mexico*. Santa Fe, 1924.

7. James E. *Account of an Expedition from Pittsburgh to the Rocky Mountains*, 434. Philadelphia, 1823.

8. Grinnell GB. "Bent's old fort and its builders." Collections Kansas State Historical Society 15:43, 1923.

9. Spencer EDR. *Green Russell and Gold*, 165. Austin, 1966.

10. Hill KL. "A history of public health in Denver, 1859-1900," 13. Master's thesis, University of Denver, 1970.

11. RMN, Feb. 15, 1862.

12. *Second Annual Report of the State Board of Health of Colorado, 1877*.

13. Beshoar B. *Hippocrates in a Red Vest*, 186. Palo Alto, 1973.

14. *Second Annual Report*, 130.

15. *Pioneers of the San Juan Country*, II, 57. Colorado Springs, 1946.

16. Byrne BJ. *A Frontier Army Surgeon*, 132. Cranford, 1935.

17. *Pioneers*, IV, 115.

18. Mumey N: *Silver Heels Stories*, 1970.

19. Lake City Times, July 6, 1899. Cited in Houston G. *Lake City Reflections*, 105. 1976.

20. *Laws Passed at the Ninth Session of the General Assembly of the State of Colorado, 1893*, 386 -87.

21. CMJ 6:554, 1900; CMJ 9:183, 1903.

22. *Second Annual Report*, 134.

23. U.S. Public Health Reports 16:137, 1901.

24. *Fifth Report of the State Board of Health of Colorado, 1894-1900*.

25. CMJ 5:79, 1899.

26. Hill, "History of public health," 69.

27. CMJ 5:165, 1899.

28. *Second Annual Report of the Social Welfare Department of the City and County of Denver, 1914*, 92. Denver, 1914. The original pesthouse was located at the site of the Botanical Gardens' parking lot.

29. Fallis EH. *When Denver and I Were Young*, 35. Denver, 1956.

30. Stuver E. DMT 22:71, 1902.

31. Hall JN. *Tales of Pioneer Practice*, 111. Denver, 1937.

32. CMJ 7:179, 1901.

33. CM 8:79, 1911.

34. DMT 31:62, 1911-12.

35. CMJ 6:117, 1900.

36. Critique 8:107, 1901.

37. *Seventh Report of the State Board of Health, 1903 - 04*, 60.

38. *Eighth Biennial Report of the State Board of Health, 1905-06*, 4.

39. CM 8:79, 1911.

40. *Social Welfare Department, Denver*, 16.

41. CM 17:107, 1920.

42. CM 18:259, 1921.

43. CM 20:90, 1923.

44. DMB Feb. 3, 1923.

45. Hopkins, *Princes*, 291.

Chapter 17

1. Bancroft FJ. "On the sanitary condition of Denver." RMN, March, 1878.

2. "Report of the City Physician." RMN, Mar. 21, 1873. At the same time, Dr. Bancroft requested "an ordinance restricting the driving of wild cattle" through the city

streets. Many years later, Denver remains sensitive to the epithet "cow town." The term "miasma" referred to the "bad air" that was thought to be responsible for various diseases such as malaria.

3. RMN, March 22, 1873.

4. Bancroft, "Sanitary condition."

5. Denver Tribune, March 20, 1879.

6. RMN, August 23, 1885.

7. "Laws and Regulations of the Union District, Clear Creek County, Colorado Territory." October 21, 1861.

8. In addition to the references cited below, information on the State Board of Health was obtained from: Pyle GS. "The development of the field of public health in Colorado." Master's thesis, University of Denver, 1946.

9. RMN, April 12, 1876.

10. Rogers EJA. "Address." TCSMS 24:48, 1894.

11. Bancroft FJ: "Annual address of the President." *Annual Reports of the State Board of Health of Colorado for the Years 1879 and 1880*. Denver, 1881.

12. Rogers, "Address."

13. *Laws of Colorado*, 1893, Sec. 2, 398.

14. *Fifth Report of the State Board of Health of Colorado, 1894-1900*.

15. *Eighth Report of the State Board of Health of Colorado, 1905-1906*.

16. *Report of the Secretary, State Board of Health*, 1898, 35.

17. *Sixth Report of the State Board of Health of Colorado, 1901-1902*.

18. *Eighth Report, 1905-1906*.

19. *Eleventh Biennial Report of the State Board of Health, 1911-1912*.

20. In addition to references cited, information on Denver's Board of Health and public health in Denver, was obtained from Hill KL. "A history of public health in Denver, 1859 - 1860." Master's thesis, University of Denver, 1970. An excellent source of information.

21. Dr. Steele had come to Colorado from Ohio in 1870. He soon became one of the state's leading physicians—a founder and early president of the Colorado Medical Society, a founder and the first dean of the state's first medical school, president of the Denver School Board, and, when it was reestablished in 1892, president of the State Board of Health. Sewall H. "Memoir of Dr. Henry King Steele." DMT 22:598, 1903.

22. Munn WP. "The history of the Denver Health Department." CMJ 7:523, 1901.

23. Rogers P. "Address by the Mayor to the Denver and Arapahoe Medical Society," 1892.

24. Munn had come to Denver, at the age of 36 "for his health." He was appointed Assistant Health Commissioner in 1891 and to the State Board of Health in 1893. It was said that "one always knew . . . that Munn would say and do what he thought" and, as a result, he had many admirers and enemies. Sewall H. "Dr. William P. Munn—The man and friend." DMT 22:542, 1903.

25. *Annual Report of the Bureau of Health of the City of Denver for the Year Ending December 31, 1896*. Denver, 1897. The budget included $2,500 for the Commissioner's salary, $75 a month for sanitary inspectors, and a total of $920 for diphtheria antitoxin and smallpox vaccine. In addition, $1,500 was designated for "the removal of dead animals and $4,800 for garbage removal.

26. CMJ 2:131, 1896. Munn had an even more intensive battle with the Denver Water Company. He died in 1903.

27. Kauvar SS, et al. Health—Twenty years late." Amer J Public Health 40:170, 1950.

28. Newspaper clippings from the F.J. Bancroft scrapbook, referring to Dr. Bancroft's presentation to the Denver Medical Association, March 12, 1878.

29. *Annual Report of the Bureau of Health*, 1896.

30. Letter in the collection of Dr. Michael Arnall.

31. JAMA 47:598, 1906.

32. McLauthlin HW. "The prevention and suppression of contagious diseases in rural communities." CMJ 3:407, 1897.

33. CMJ 2:58, 1896.

34. Denver Municipal Facts 1:13, 1919.

35. McGraw HR. "Fumigation of private houses after contagious diseases." TCSMS 36:47, 1906.

36. *Board of Health, 1905 - 06*.

37. *Board of Health, 1901 - 02*.

38. *Board of Health, 1894 - 1900*.

39. TCSMS 28:19, 1898.

40. CM 8:300, 1911.

41. CM 8:268, 1911.

42. Bancroft, "Sanitary condition."

43. Lemen HA. "Typhoid fever—History of an epidemic in Denver." *Board of Health, 1879 and 1880*.

44. Wetherill HG. "Health resorts of the West and Southwest." Med News, Dec. 16, 1893.

45. Bancroft, "Sanitary conditions."

46. City of Denver 1:10, 1913.

47. CM 46:73, 1916.

48. Wetherill, "Health resorts."

49. Problems with the composition, as well as the unwarranted claims, of drugs, patent medicines, nostrums, and the like are discussed in Chapters 12, 18, and 21.

50. *Annual Report of the Health Commissioner, Bureau of Health, Denver, 1895*, 10, 96.

51. DMT 24:253, 1905.

52. Formaldehyde was used as a preservative in milk, meats, wines, broken eggs, and oysters. It was known by a variety of euphemisms, including freezine, icelene, preservaline, and milk sweet. Hill EC: "Food adulterations in relation to health." CM 5:190, 1908.

53. CM 3:203, 1906.

54. Golden Globe, January 2, 1904. Cited in *More Than Gold. History of Arvada*, 187. Boulder, 1976.

55. *Ninth Biennial Report of the Colorado State Board of Health, 1907 - 1908*.

56. "Annual Report of the Secretary of the State Board of Health," DMT 29:313, 1910.

57. Hill, "History of public health."

58. CM 48:227, 1918.

59. *Fourth Annual Report of the Denver Chamber of Commerce, 1886*.

60. McLauthlin DW. "Public health in Colorado." TCSMS 16:61, 1887.

61. Although its infectious basis and means of spreading were suspected in the 1850s, the microorganism was not described until 1880 and not isolated from patients until 1884.

62. Death is usually due to dehydration and electrolyte imbalance or intestinal perforation. Innumerable therapeutic measures—all non-specific and virtually useless—were used in the pre-antibiotic era. Although typhoid continues to be a major problem in areas of the world where water purification and sewage control are inadequate, most of the 500 or so cases which continue to occur annually in the U.S.A. are in international travelers or immigrants.

63. *Fourth Report of the State Board of Health of Colorado, Including Reports for the Years 1892, 1893, and 1894*.

64. Lemen, "Typhoid fever."

65. Various aspects of the history of Denver's water are to be found in Arps LW. *Denver in Slices*. Denver, 1959; King CL. *History of the Government of Denver*. Denver, 1911; Hill, "History of public health"; Mills WFR, "Evolution of the water system." Municipal Facts 3:8, 1920. The Water Company's board included its president, Colonel James B. Archer and its treasurer, banker and railroad magnate David H. Moffat, and directors, financier Walter S. Cheesman, politician James B. Chaffee, and Governor Edward M. McCook.

66. Lemen, "Typhoid fever." An excellent discussion of the argument, and the role of the newspapers, is presented in Claman G. "The typhoid fever epidemic and the power of the press in Denver in 1879." Colo Mag 56:143, 1979. Interestingly, the predominantly conservative and Republican physicians found themselves allied, on this issue, with the liberal and Democratic *Rocky Mountain News* against Republican businessmen and political leaders.

67. RMN, Dec. 12, 1879; Undated newspaper clipping included in the minutes of the Denver Medical Association meeting of Dec. 9, 1879, cited in Hill, "History of public health," 62.

68. "RMN, undated clipping."

69. RMN, December 12, 1879.

70. RMN, December 13, 1879.

71. RMN, February 12, 1881.

72. *Official Report of the Bureau of Health of the City of Denver for the Year, 1895*. Denver, 1896.

73. McIntyre JA. *Report of the City Engineer of Denver, 1891*, 51.

74. *Ninth Annual Report of the Denver Chamber of Commerce . . . , 1892*, 117.

75. DMT 16:189, 1896.

76. McLauthlin HW. "The recent epidemic of typhoid fever at the County Hospital, Denver." TCSMS 26:152, 1896.

77. RMN, January 1, 1897.

78. *Annual Report of the Bureau of Health of Denver, Colorado, for the Year, 1896*. Denver, 1897.

79. CMJ 2:333, 1896.

80. Hughes CA. "Impressions of Denver." DMT 18:59, 1898.

81. McLauthlin HW. "The prevention and suppression of contagious diseases in rural communities." CMJ 3:407, 1897.

82. M'Hugh PJ. "The late epidemic of typhoid fever in Fort Collins, Colorado." TCSMS 31:198, 1901.

83. *Board of Health, 1894 - 1900.*

84. Colorado State Board of Health Sanitary Bulletin. 4:6, 1904.

85. Garwood HG. "Typhoid fever." CM 6:35, 1909.

86. *Board of Health*, 1904.

87. Leadville News Dispatch, Jan. 19, 1904.

88. Hall IC. "Typhoid fever death rates in Denver and Colorado." CM 24:212, 1927.

Chapter 18

1. From a letter written in February 1859. Quoted in Larimer WHH. *Reminiscences of General William Larimer and of His Son*, 168. Lancaster, Pennsylvania, 1918.

2. Reed JW. *Map and Guide to the Kansas Gold Region*, 9. 1859. Reprint. Denver, 1959.

3. Simonin, L. *The Rocky Mountain West in 1867*. 33. Lincoln, 1966.

4. *Denver City and Auraria. The Commercial Emporium of the Pike's Peak Gold Regions*, 30. 1859.

5. Later, in a more sober mood, the city fathers changed its name to Jimtown.

6. Manning JF. *Leadville, Lake County and the Gold Belt*, 13. 1895.

7. Whitmore, EA. "Observations on the effects of great altitudes." DMT 18:537, 1898-99.

8. Gibbons JJ. *In the San Juan, Colorado; Sketches*, 151. Chicago, 1898.

9. Critique 11:355, 1904.

10. Eskridge JT. Trans Amer Climatol Assn 7:171, 1892.

11. Material relating to the Doctors-Ministers controversy was derived from 1) Hill KL. "A history of public health in Denver, 1859 - 1900," 34-36. Master's thesis, University of Denver, 1970; including clippings from the *Denver Daily Tribune, Rocky Mountain News* and *Denver Times* dated Feb. 13, 1878 and 2) Elder CS. "Medicine, public health and hospitals." In *Colorado and Its People*, II, 393 - 94. Edited by LR Hafen. New York, 1948.

12. DMT 6:80, 1886.

13. CM 6:404, 1909.

14. TCSMS 32:93, 1902. Recall that "proof" is double the percentage of alcohol, and that "hard liquor" is generally 80 to 90 proof.

15. DMT 25:258, 1905 - 06.

16. DMT 33:491, 1913 - 14.

17. Twain M. *Roughing It*, 1872.

18. Whiteside HO. "The drug habit in nineteenth century Colorado." Colo Mag 55:47, 1978. An excellent review.

19. Bennett AL. "Report of the State Medical Inspector of Chinese." *Sixth Report of the State Board of Health of Colorado, 1901 - 02.*

20. *Eighth Biennial Report of the Bureau of Labor Statistics of the State of Colorado, 1901-1902*, 299-300.

21. TCSMS 26 :167, 1896.

22. Courtney JE. "Report of cases of morphinism." CM 4:19, 1907.

23. Berlin WCK. "Novel method of administering morphine by a habitual." DMT 34:430, 1914.

24. Knowles EW. "Narcotics addiction." CM 8:286, 1911.

25. Girard F. *Durango. The End of the Trail*, 22. Durango, 1975.

26. Whiteside, "Drug habit," 64.

27. Ibid., 55; Musto DF. *The American Disease*, 7. New Haven, 1973.

28. DMT 22:23, 1902.

29. Stedman A. "Address." TCSMS 9:29, 1879.

30. TCSMS 32:96, 1902.

31. City of Denver, 3:16, 1914.

32. Johnson C. "Suicides." Med News 64:540, 1894.

33. Sears MH. "Morphine poisoning." TCSMS 14:107, 1884.

34. Inglis J. "Morphinism." DMT 22:391, 1903.

35. CMJ 10:539, 1904.

36. Aspen Times, November 5, 1892.

37. *American Disease*, 5.

38. Knowles, "Narcotics addiction."

39. Inglis, "Morphinism," 392.

40. DMT 35:438, 1905 - 06.

41. JAMA 11:885, 1888.

42. CM 12:165, 1915.

43. *Second Annual Report of the Social Welfare Department of the City and County of Denver, Colorado for the Year Ending December, 31, 1914*, 12.

44. CM 26:343, 1929.

45. Stuver E. "Prophylaxis of syphilis." CMJ 6:339, 1900.

46. RMN, Oct. 12, 1872.

47. DMT 22:451, 1903.

48. Stover GH. "What shall we do with syphilis?" DMT 13:367, 1894.

49. Hershey EP. "Modes of infection." CMJ 6:275, 1900.

50. Ewing S. "The medico-legal supervision of prostitution." DMT 19:290, 1899.

51. DMT 22:451, 1903.

52. Corwin RW. "Education vs. legislation." CMJ 2:20, 1905.

53. Stuver, "Prophylaxis."

54. "Fee Bill of the Jefferson Medical Society," June 4, 1860.

55. "Fee Bill of the Denver Medical Association," June 15, 1871.

56. "Constitution, By-laws and Fee Bill of the Denver and Arapahoe Medical Society," 1895.

57. CM 6:109, 1909.

58. Cox GW. "The social evil." TCSMS 12:65, 1882.

59. Bancroft FJ. "Annual Report of the City Physician for 1874." RMN Jan 30, 1875.

60. Letter to the editor of the "Democrat" - unsigned, in F. J. Bancroft scrapbook, 1875.

61. DMT 22:451, 1903.

62. CM 12:35, 1915.

63. Jarvis, M. *Come on in Dearie, or Prostitutes and Institutes of Early Durango*, 17. Durango, Colorado, 1976.

64. Thomas L. *Good Evening Everybody*. New York, 1976.

65. Parkhill F. *The Wildest of the West*, 48. New York, 1951.

66. Hall JN. *Tales of Pioneer Practice*, 82. Denver, 1937.

67. Levine B. *Lowell Thomas' Victor*, 21. Colorado Springs, 1982.

68. Salida Mail, Jan 5, 1897. Quoted in Pasquale CJ, et al. *One Hundred Years in the Heart of the Rockies*, 91. Salida, Colorado, 1980.

69. The Great Divide, July, 1892. Cited in Denver Westerners Roundup, February, 1960.

70. Boulder County Herald, May 15, 1889. Cited in Gladden SC. *Ladies of the Night*, 21. Boulder, 1979.

71. Miller M, Mazzulla F. *Holladay Street*, 48, 58, 63. New York, 1971.

72. Pasquale, *One Hundred Years*, 92.

Chapter 19

1. New Mex Med. J. 9:91, 1912-13.

2. *Biennial Report of the Colorado Bureau of Labor Statistics, 1901 - 1902*, 407 - 11. Denver, 1903.

3. *First Annual Report of the Railroad Commissioner of the State of Colorado for the Year Ending June 30, 1885*. Denver, 1886.

4. Reports of the Coroner of Arapahoe County, 1903.

5. "Railway accidents: Their cause and prevention - an essay by a railroad employee." The Railway Surgeon 8:180, 1901.

6. "Railway accidents for six months of 1901." The Railway Surgeon 9:30, 1902.

7. JAMA 10:207, 1888.

8. *Third Annual Report of the Hospital funds of the Denver and Rio Grande Railroad Company*. March 31, 1887.

9. Trickle EH. "That cinder in your eye." The Railway Surgeon 8:254, 1902.

10. Ibid. Comments by Dr. William C. Bane.

11. JAMA 16:207, 1891.

12. *Third Annual Report, 1887.*

13. Fairbrother HC. "Legal railway surgery." The Railroad Surgeon 9:136, 1902.

14. *Third Annual Report, 1887.*

15. Fairbrother, "Legal railway surgery."

16. Grant WW. "Railway spine and litigation symptoms." JAMA 30:956, 1898.

17. Thompson WG. *The Occupational Diseases*, 550. New York, 1914.

18. *Third Annual Report, 1887.*

19. Davis WB. "Is railroad and other contract practice unethical?" The Railroad Surgeon 8:183, 1901.

20. *Third Annual Report, 1887.*

21. Everett GG, Hutchison WF. *Under the Angel of Shavano.* Denver, 1963; Pasquale CJ, et al. *One Hundred Years in the Heart of the Rockies*, 28, 53, 59. Salida, 1980. In 1899 the hospital burned down. It was replaced in 1901 by a new, more impressive structure costing $45,000. JAMA 37:520, 1901.

22. *Third Annual Report, 1887.*

23. *Bureau of Labor, 1901 - 02.*

24. CMJ 3:135, 1902.

25. CM 13:195, 1916. Dr. Cochems closed his hospital in 1941.

26. *Colorado and Southern Railway Company Medical Department Instructions to Surgeons, 1899.*

27. *A.T. & S.F. Hospital Association Financial and Operating Report for 1927.*

28. Grant WW. "Railway hygiene and emergency equipment." JAMA 34:395, 1900.

29. Harbison AB. "Report of the Committee on General Hygiene." April 9, 1900. *Fifth Report of the State Board of Health of Colorado, 1894 - 1900*, 80.

30. Advertisement in the Critique, 1901.

31. *Fifth Report*, 24.

32. *Fourth Report of the State Board of Health of Colorado, Including Reports for the Years 1892, 1893 and 1894*, 23 - 28.

33. Ibid.

34. The Railway Surgeon 9:318, 1903.

35. Grant, "Railway hygiene."

36. CMJ 6:165, 1900.

37. JAMA 35:956, 1900.

38. *Seventh Report of the Colorado State Board of Health, 1902-04*, 100 - 103.

39. Hall JN. *Tales of Pioneer Practice*, 106. Denver, 1937.

40. CM 13:391, 1916.

Chapter 20

1. Arbogast BA. "Castration the remedy for crime." TCSMS 27:324, 1895.

2. Hall JN. *Tales of Pioneer Practice*, 73. Denver, 1937.

3. Elsner J. "Reminiscences." DMT 28:1, 1908.

4. Stone WF. *History of Colorado*, III, 192. Chicago, 1918.

5. Gardiner CF. *Doctor at Timberline*, 34. Caldwell, Idaho, 1938.

6. Stone, *History*, I, 770.

7. Cathell DW. *Book on the Physician Himself*, . Ninth Edition, Revised and Enlarged, 141 - 42. Philadelphia, 1890.

8. Hall, *Tales*, 73.

9. Carden WD. "Nineteenth century physicians in Clear Creek County, Colorado, 1865 - 1895." Master's thesis, University of Denver, 1968.

10. Hall, *Tales*, 56.

11. Gardiner, *Doctor*, 233 - 35.

12. Cook J. *Hands Up.*, 132. Denver, 1897.

13. Stanley F. *The Private War of Ike Stockton*, 154. Denver, 1959.

14. McClelland WF. "Aseptic qualities of the Colorado atmosphere twenty-five years ago." DMT 17:484, 1897-8; McLoughlin D. *Wild and Woolly. An Encyclopedia of the Old West*, 46, 475. Garden City, NY, 1975.

15. Stanley F. *Clay Allison*, 164. Denver, 1956.

16. Segale B. *At the End of the Santa Fe Trail*, 74 - 76. Milwaukee, 1948.

17. Stone, *History*, III, 191.

18. Bentley MV. *The Upper Side of the Pie Crust*, 178. Evergreen, Colorado, 1978.

19. Baskin OL. *History of the Arkansas Valley, Colorado*, 576. Chicago, 1881.

20. DMT 7:713, 1888.

21. Varnell JM. "A Colorado country doctor." CM 77:89, 1980.

22. Hall JN. "The expert witness." CMJ 2:128, 1896.

23. DMT 12:493, 1893.

24. Hall, "Expert witness."

25. Hall JN. "The medico-legal value of powder stains in gun-shot wounds." TCSMS 20:94, 1890; "Diagnosis in a murder trial." RMMJ 35:230, 1938.

26. Axtell ER. "The medico-legal examination of the red stains found on the clothes of Charles Ford." JAMA 25:139, 1895.

27. Hall JN. "Arsenical poisoning from an unusual source." CM 1:175, 1904.

28. *General Laws of the State of Colorado*, Chapter XXII, 1876.

29. JAMA 46:517, 1906.

30. Hall JN. "A plea for medical examiners." TCSMS 15:191, 1885.

31. DMT 5:249, 1885.

32. Wetherill HG. "Our relations to the public and to public institutions." CMJ 8:1, 1902.

33. Newspaper article in the Dr. Charles Denison scrapbook, Denison Memorial Library, University of Colorado Health Sciences Center. Undated, source not cited, ca. 1875.

34. Coroner's Records of Custer County, 1888 - 1915. Cited in Mazzulla FM. "The county coroner," Denver Westerners Roundup. April, 1955.

35. CMJ 7:190, 1901.

36. *Mortality Statistics.* Seventh Annual Report of the Bureau of the Census—1906. Department of Commerce. Washington, D. C., 1907.

37. *First Annual Report of the Social Welfare Department of the City and County of Denver, Colorado, 1913*, 80. There were 26 inquests and 38 autopsies. The coroner, Dr. Charles Jaeger, was paid $900 for the year, and the entire budget, including the cost of the autopsies, was $2,701.

38. Reports of the Coroner of Arapahoe County, 1901 - 05.

39. Dr. Henry Hewett was Deputy U. S. Marshall in California Gulch's early mining camp days. Baskin, *Arkansas Valley*, 345.

40. Schultz MM. *Tenderfoot Schoolmarm*, 22. Baltimore, 1977.

41. CMJ 3:29, 1897.

42. CMJ 8:518, 1902.

43. Byers WN. *Encyclopedia of Biography of Colorado*, 375. Chicago, 1901.

44. Van Meter SD. "Medical forgeries." CM 22:169, 1925.

45. DMT 12:59, 1882 - 1883.

46. Baskin, *Arkansas Valley*, 554, 563.

47. Parkhill F. "He drove the West wild." Denver Westerners Brand Book, XIV, 75. Edited by N Mumey. Denver, 1959.

48. Dougan DH. "Report of Committee on the State Charitable Institutions." *Annual Reports of the State Board of Health of Colorado for the Years 1879 and 1880.*

49. CM 19:131, 157 1922; CM 20:230, 1923.

50. CMJ 11:82, 1905.

51. CMJ 9:389, 1903.

52. DMT 21:194, 1901.

53. Arbogast, "Castration."

54. Cook, *Hands Up*, 164.

55. Hill AP. *Tales of Colorado Pioneers*, 106. Denver, 1884.

56. DMT 6:200, 1886.

57. DMT 20:307, 1900.

58. Ibid.

59. JAMA 36:38, 1901.

Chapter 21

1. CMJ 4:385, 1898.

2. RMN, April 11, 1885. Cited in Colorado Prospector, November 1985.

3. DMT 19:521, 1899.

4. Critique 10:29, 1903.

5. Critique 10:435, 1903.

6. Smythe SS. "Homeopathy in Denver." Critique 10:202, 1903.

7. Critique 10:468, 1903.

8. CMJ 3:73, 1897.

9. Powell C. "Cults." CM 22:178, 1925.

10. CMJ 3:73, 1897.

11. *Boulder Daily Camera Souvenir Edition*, 9. Boulder, 1902.

12. CMJ 3:111, 1897.

13. *The Morgan County Medical Society, 1908 - 1960*. NP,ND.

14. Aberg A. "Massage vs. osteopathy." CMJ 10:581, 1904.

15. DMT 18:121, 1898 - 99. Originally the Western Institute of Osteopathy, it was founded in 1895 by Drs. Jeanette H. and Newton A. Bolles, both former students of Still's. It was closed in 1904. Whitehead RW, Perkin RL. "Medical education in Colorado, 1881 - 1971." RMMJ 68:135, 1971.

16. Powell, "Cults." Actually, Powell's prediction has only only partially been fulfilled, with osteopathy, its physicians, schools, and degree having achieved equivalence with regular medicine.

17. Ibid.

18. Powell C. "Modern pseudo-medical cults. 2. Chiropractic." CM 12:117, 1915. The college was located on Colfax Avenue in Denver.

19. J.M. "Sweet and Low." DMB September 23, 1922. Despite intense opposition from the medical community, chiropractic survived in Colorado, culminating in the opening of the Spears' Hospital in Denver. A 1930s edition of the Spears' Clinic News consists of 24 pages of articles with titles such as " Whooping Cough Responds to Chiropractic" and "Colon Irrigations Wash Away Many Evils."

20. Palmer EW. "Letter to the editor." Critique 10:380, 1903.

21. Blaine JM. "Fallacies of Christian Science." CMJ 5:116, 1899.

22. Wetherill HG. "The first epistle from George and to George." DMT 30:398, 1911.

23. Critique 11:87, 1904.

24. DMT 21:415, 1900 - 01.

25. CMJ 9:210, 1903.

26. DMB May 19, 1923.

27. Stone WG. *The Colorado Handbook*, 84. Denver, 1892.

28. Golden City Transcript, January 6, 1875.

29. Aspen Times, March 8, 1893.

30. RMN, November 12, 1895.

31. CMJ, September 1901.

32. Advertisement, source unknown, ca. 1910.

33. DMT 30:354, 1910 - 11.

34. Garden of the Gods Magazine, April, 1903.

35. Advertisement, source unknown, ca. 1905 - 10. The ingredients, and their percentages, were listed on the label. The product was manufactured by Denco, Inc., Denver.

36. Material kindly lent by Dr. Michael Arnall. Letter to Dr. W.E Driscoll from Reed and Carnrick Company, Jersey City, N.J. dated October 23, 1905; Letter to Dr. W. E. Driscoll from Katharomon Chemical Company, St. Louis, Missouri, December 14, 1905.

37. CM 4:412, 432, 472, 1907.

38. DMT 12:164, 1892.

39. Pennock VR. "Electricity in general practice." CMJ 4:330, 1898.

40. Stover GH. "Comments." DMT 15:420, 1905 - 06.

41. CM 3:92, 1906.

42. CMJ 5:377, 1899.

43. Advertisement, source unknown, ca. 1890.

44. Grant WW. "The present status of radium." CM 11:172, 1914.

45. CM 11:2, 1914.

46. Grant, "Radium."

47. Bruyn K. *Uranium Country*, 76, 111. Boulder, 1955.

48. Advertisement, source unknown, ca. 1910.

49. Davis WB. "What is sauce for the goose is sauce for the gander." DMT 21:270, 1901. Dr. Davis, had previously won a contest, sponsored by the Colorado Medical Society, for the best essay on quackery. TCSMS 31:22, 97 1901.

50. Hawes J. "Charlatanism in Colorado." TCSMS 13:37, 1883.

51. Denver Tribune, May, 1879.

52. TCSMS 8:22, 1878.

53. CM 3:101, 1906.

54. *Life of Francis Schlatter. The Great Healer . . . or . . .*

New Mexico Messiah. Denver, ca. 1895. This was a promotional pamphlet published by The Knox Company of Denver.

55. Denver Times, November 16, 1895.

56. Hyde AB. Quoted by Bluemel CS. "Faith healers." CM :143, 1921.

57. Schaetzel J. *Memoirs of Denver*, 47. Denver, 1970.

58. DMT 15:294, 1895.

59. CMJ 3:322, 1897.

60. The Great West 2:14, 1891.

61. Butterfield RO. "Methods of the cancer quack." Western Medical Times 38:361, 1919.

62. DMT 30:354, 1910 - 11.

63. RMN November 14, 1875.

64. Stuver E. "The attitude of the newspapers toward regular physicians and scientific medicine." DMT 19:280, 1899; Editorial. "Chinese quackery." DMT 8:159, 1889.

65. Ibid., Stuver.

66. "Chinese quackery."

67. Davis, "Sauce for the goose."

68. Hall JN. "The work of the State Board of Medical Examiners." TCSMS 21:103, 1891. Another account states that Gun Wa was actually an Irishman named W.H. Hale who had begun his medical career selling aphrodisiacs in Denver's Hop Alley. Miller M. *Holladay Street*, 144 - 45. New York, 1962.

69. Mumey N: *History of Tin Cup, Colorado*, 155 - 56. Boulder, 1963.

70. Advertisement. *Illustrated Denver. The Queen City of the Plains*, 111. Denver, 1895.

71. Ormes MD, Ormes ER. *The Book of Colorado Springs*, 228. Colorado Springs, 1933.

72. Daily Herald and Solid Muldoon, Jan. 1, 1893. Cited in *Pioneers of the San Juan*, I, 82. Colorado Springs, 1942.

73. CMJ 3:318, 1897.

74. DMT 12:513, 1893.

75. DMT 30:59, 1910.

76. CM 9:67, 1912.

77. CM 17:171, 1920.

78. CM 20:304, 1923.

Chapter 22

1. CM 15:21, 1918.

2. Morris RB. *Encyclopedia of American History*. New York, 1961.

3. CM 12:161, 213, 1915.

4. RMMJ 39:689, 1942.

5. CM 15:227, 1918.

6. Magruder AC. " 'I'll go when I am needed'." CM 14:260, 1917.

7. Wetherill HG. "The nation's need of doctors and nurses for the Army." CM 15:271, 1918.

8. Fraser MEV. "The Medical Women's War Service League." CM 15:31, 1918.

9. De Mund M. *Women Physicians of Colorado*, 35. Denver, 1976.

10. CM 14:141, 1917.

11. CM 15:227, 1918.

12. CM 15:72, 1918.

13. Municipal Facts, October 1918.

14. JAMA 253:3521, 1985.

15. Katz RS. "Influenza 1918 - 1919: A study in mortality." Bull Hist Med 48 :416, 1974.

16. *Mortality Statistics. Twentieth Annual Report of the Bureau of the Census - 1919*, 28 - 30. Department of Commerce Washington, D.C. 1921. The mortality rate in Colorado was 8.4 per 1,000 population.

17. Municipal Facts, October 1918.

18. Municipal Facts, November 1918.

19. Sewall H. "A brief study of influenza for two months at the Denver County Hospital." CM 49:33, 1919.

20. *Biennial Report of the Board of Regents of the University of Colorado, 1917 - 1918*.

21. Fritz PS. "Tungsten and the road to war." Univ of Colo., Series C, Studies in the Social Sciences, vol 1, No. 2, 1942.

22. Gilliland ME. *Summitt - A Gold Rush History of Summitt County, Colorado*, 186. Silverthorne, Colo. 1980.

23. Coquoz RL. *The History of Medicine in Leadville, and Lake County, Colorado*, 12. NP, 1967.

24. "Dr. (Walter W.) King recalls Cripple Creek epidemic." Univ of Colo Scl of Med Quart, 14. Winter, 1964.

25. Benham J. *Silverton*, 59. Ouray, Colorado, 1977.

26. Wyman L. *Snowflakes and Quartz*, 38. Silverton, Colorado, 1977.

27. Childs SB. "Medicine today and tomorrow." CM: 316. 1928.

28. *Yearbook of the State of Colorado*, 1928 - 1929. Denver, 1929. Much of the information on the state, except where otherwise cited, is derived from this source.

29. *Mortality Statistics. Twenty-ninth Annual Report of the Bureau of the Census - 1928*. Department of Commerce. Washington, D.C., 1930. Much of the data on health and disease in Colorado was obtained from these two sources.

30. CM 20:64, 1923; Sewall H. "Tuberculosis in Colorado." CM 24:104, 1927.

31. Hall IC. "A summary of two year's bacteriological testing of Denver city water." CM 25:391, 1928.

32. CM 27:18, 57 1930. Denver's Dr. F. P. Gengenbach, a pediatrician, published an analysis of this "scandal" in 1932. J Peds 1:719, 1932.

33. CM 27:57, 1930.

34. Spivak CD. "A bio-ethnological study of the organized medical profession of the state of Colorado." CM 23:188, 1926.

35. Denver Post, April 1929.

36. CM 17:109, 1920.

37. The *Colorado Yearbook for 1928-1929* lists 32 "approved" hospitals, and the ratio of hospital beds is an estimate, excluding tuberculosis sanitaria and military hospitals. There were also a number of small, "unapproved" hospitals, mainly in rural communities. Several Denver hospitals, including Presbyterian, Colorado General (University), and Beth Israel, had been recently opened.

38. DMB September 16, 1922.

39. Spivak, "Bio-ethnological study."

40. CM 25:43, 1928.

41. DMB, May 15, 1926.

42. Levens M. *The Incomes of Physicians*. Chicago, 1932.

43. Sewall H. "On the cost of medical care." CM 25:324, 1928.

44. Childs, "Medicine today."

45. C.E. Cooper. Comments in Wetherill HG. "A paramount problem of modern medicine." CM 25:320, 1928.

46. Hillkowitz P. "Medicine and publicity." CM 20:43, 1923.

47. Childs, "Medicine today."

48. Hillkowitz, "Medicine and publicity."

49. CM 19:271, 1922.

50. Hillkowitz, "Medicine and publicity."

Index